AF776785

Fostering Healthcare through Artificial Intelligence

In this book, readers can explore the transformative power of artificial intelligence (AI) in reshaping modern healthcare. The book dives deep into how cutting-edge technologies are revolutionizing diagnostics, patient care, and medical research. From the predictive analytics that anticipate disease outbreaks to intelligent systems that enhance clinical decision-making, this book reveals how AI technologies are playing a transformative role in healthcare domain. Designed for healthcare professionals and AI enthusiasts, this book presents real-world applications, ethical considerations, and visionary insights from researchers and industry. The book provides readers a comprehensive understanding of AI's potential to drive meaningful change.

This book:

- Covers high-performance computing field programmable gate array networks for machine learning-based biomedical applications.
- Presents machine learning algorithms for cancer susceptibility, recurrence, and survival prediction.
- Discusses the use of high-performance computing (HPC) in the execution of low-power processors for healthcare devices.
- Demonstrates detailed performance analysis of wearable healthcare devices.
- Highlights the use of Pix2pix generative adversarial networks for mammographically occult breast cancer detection.

Whether you're navigating the complexities of digital health transformation or simply curious about AI's role in medicine, *Fostering Healthcare through Artificial Intelligence* is your essential guide to understanding how technology can foster a healthier, smarter future for all.

Fostering Healthcare through Artificial Intelligence

A High-Performance Computing Approach

Kavita Khare, Zainab Aizaz, and Nilay Khare

CRC Press
Taylor & Francis Group
Boca Raton London New York

CRC Press is an imprint of the
Taylor & Francis Group, an **informa** business

Designed cover image: shutterstock

MATLAB® and Simulink® are trademarks of The MathWorks, Inc. and are used with permission. The MathWorks does not warrant the accuracy of the text or exercises in this book. This book's use or discussion of MATLAB® or Simulink® software or related products does not constitute endorsement or sponsorship by The MathWorks of a particular pedagogical approach or particular use of the MATLAB® and Simulink® software.

First edition published 2026
by CRC Press
2385 NW Executive Center Drive, Suite 320, Boca Raton FL 33431

and by CRC Press
4 Park Square, Milton Park, Abingdon, Oxon, OX14 4RN

CRC Press is an imprint of Taylor & Francis Group, LLC

© 2026 Kavita Khare, Zainab Aizaz, and Nilay Khare

Reasonable efforts have been made to publish reliable data and information, but the author and publisher cannot assume responsibility for the validity of all materials or the consequences of their use. The authors and publishers have attempted to trace the copyright holders of all material reproduced in this publication and apologize to copyright holders if permission to publish in this form has not been obtained. If any copyright material has not been acknowledged please write and let us know so we may rectify in any future reprint.

Except as permitted under U.S. Copyright Law, no part of this book may be reprinted, reproduced, transmitted, or utilized in any form by any electronic, mechanical, or other means, now known or hereafter invented, including photocopying, microfilming, and recording, or in any information storage or retrieval system, without written permission from the publishers.

For permission to photocopy or use material electronically from this work, access www.copyright.com or contact the Copyright Clearance Center, Inc. (CCC), 222 Rosewood Drive, Danvers, MA 01923, 978-750-8400. For works that are not available on CCC please contact mpkbookspermissions@tandf.co.uk

Trademark notice: Product or corporate names may be trademarks or registered trademarks and are used only for identification and explanation without intent to infringe.

ISBN: 9781032821184 (hbk)
ISBN: 9781032821191 (pbk)
ISBN: 9781003503033 (ebk)

DOI: 10.1201/9781003503033

Typeset in Sabon
by Newgen Publishing UK

Contents

Preface xi
Acknowledgments xiii
About the authors xv

1 Introduction to AI and high-performance computing in the healthcare domain **1**
1.1 *Introduction to artificial intelligence* 1
1.1.1 *History of artificial intelligence* 1
1.1.2 *Components of high-performance computing* 1
1.1.3 *Artificial intelligence: a rapidly evolving technology* 2
1.2 *Subfields of artificial intelligence* 4
1.3 *Applications of artificial intelligence* 5
1.3.1 *Applications of artificial intelligence for healthcare* 6
1.4 *Scope of AI in the field of biomedical analysis, disease prediction, and treatment* 9
1.5 *Conclusion* 10

2 Introduction to ML algorithms for biomedical applications **14**
2.1 *Machine learning* 14
2.1.1 *Understanding machine learning* 14
2.1.2 *Types of machine learning* 14
2.1.3 *Principle of operation of machine learning algorithms* 15
2.2 *Applications of machine learning* 17
2.3 *Scope of machine learning in biomedical analysis, disease prediction, and treatment* 19
2.4 *Deep learning* 20
2.4.1 *Understanding deep learning* 20
2.4.2 *Components of deep learning* 20
2.4.3 *Types of deep learning* 23
2.4.4 *Applications of deep learning* 23

2.5 *Evaluation measures* 25
2.6 *Contribution of DNN in data augmentation, training set expansion, and simulation creation* 27
2.7 *Significant role of deep neural network in advancing the healthcare industry* 31
2.8 *Scope of deep learning in biomedical analysis, disease prediction, and treatment* 32
2.9 *Conclusion* 34

3 Biomedical signal and image processing using machine learning **38**
3.1 *Introduction* 38
3.2 *Image processing using machine learning* 39
3.3 *Biomedical image analysis* 42
3.3.1 *Medical imaging modalities* 43
3.4 *Application of AI algorithm in biomedical signal processing* 45
3.5 *Deep learning in biomedical signal processing and state-of-the-art applications* 51
3.6 *Revolutionizing healthcare: advantages of electronic health records (EHRs) and how AI can be useful in EHR management* 55
3.6.1 *Advantages of EHR over traditional paper systems* 56
3.7 *Conclusion* 59
Questions 61

4 Machine learning algorithms for cancer susceptibility, recurrence, and survival prediction: viability, challenges, and survey on the state-of-the-art **65**
4.1 *Introduction to recent trends in cancer research* 65
4.2 *Some preliminaries of machine learning algorithms* 67
4.3 *Viability of AI in the cancer domain* 69
4.3.1 *Is AI an appropriate tool for cancer research?* 69
4.3.2 *The success of supervised learning in cancer* 72
4.4 *Cancer susceptibility* 73
4.5 *Cancer recurrence* 78
4.6 *Cancer survival* 80
4.7 *Challenges of AI in cancer* 83
4.8 *Conclusion* 88

5 AI technologies for diagnosis, prognosis, and survival of neurological, cardiovascular, and infectious diseases: state-of-the-art analysis **95**
5.1 *Introduction* 95

5.2 *Assessment of AI methods in diagnosis and prediction 97*
5.3 *State-of-the-art AI techniques for diagnosis and treatment of diseases 99*
5.3.1 *Implications of AI algorithms in the diagnosis and treatment of motor neuron diseases (MND) 99*
5.3.2 *Implications of DNN in diagnosis and treatment of epilepsy 101*
5.3.3 *Implications of DNN in diagnosis and treatment of Alzheimer disease 112*
5.3.4 *Application of DNN in diagnosis and treatment of Alzheimer's disease 115*
5.3.5 *Implications of DNNs in diagnosis and treatment of stroke and hypertension 121*
5.3.6 *Implications of DNNs in diagnosis and treatment of chronic heart disease 126*
5.3.7 *Implications of DNNs in diagnosis and treatment of neurophysical disorder 130*
5.4 *Conclusion 139*

6 Case studies 149
Pix2Pix GANs for breast cancer detection 149
6.1 *Introduction 149*
6.1 *Generative adversarial networks (GAN) for cancer: the case study 150*
6.3 *Application of Pix2pix GAN for detection of breast cancer 151*
6.4 *Results 155*
The role of AI in revolutionizing dentistry 156
6.5 *Abstract 156*
6.6 *Vital discoveries and benefits of AI integration 156*
6.7 *Periodontal disease management with AI 157*
6.8 *Operational efficiencies and patient experience 158*
6.9 *Broader impacts and future prospects 160*
6.10 *Conclusion 160*

7 Application of machine learning to gynecological cancers 164
7.1 *Introduction 164*
7.1.1 *Image processing in medical diagnosis 167*
7.2 *Cancer diagnosis using image processing 168*
7.2.1 *Preprocessing 168*
7.2.2 *Image segmentation 170*
7.2.3 *Feature extraction 171*
7.3 *Importance of feature extraction in image processing 173*
7.4 *Gynecological cancers detection approaches 175*
7.4.1 *Cervical cancer 175*

7.4.2 *Ovarian cancer* 177
7.4.3 *Endometrial cancer* 178
7.5 *Publicly available dataset* 178
7.5.1 *SIPaKMeD* 178
7.5.2 *UCI risk factors* 180
7.5.3 *Mendeley data* 181
7.5.4 *Herlev dataset* 182
7.5.5 *Histopathological image dataset for EC diagnosis* 183
7.5.6 *Histopathological whole slide images dataset for ovarian cancer* 184
7.6 *Conclusion* 186

8 Wearable healthcare devices 191
8.1 *Introduction* 191
8.2 *The medical field and wearable technology* 192
8.3 *Types of wearable devices* 194
8.4 *Benefits of wearable technology* 195
8.5 *Barriers to use wearable technology* 196
8.6 *Wearable medical devices using FPGA* 199
8.6.1 *RNS-based FPGA accelerators for high-quality 3D medical image* 199
8.6.2 *Hardware accelerator for medical image processing* 201
8.7 *RNS-based hardware accelerators* 203
8.8 *FPGA design considerations for medical imaging* 205
8.8.1 *Selection of development tools* 205
8.8.2 *FPGA programming languages* 205
8.8.3 *Resource management and optimization* 206
8.8.4 *Safety and reliability concerns* 206
8.8.5 *Compliance with regulatory standards* 207
8.9 *Conclusion* 207

9 High-performance computing systems for healthcare 213
9.1 *Introduction to high-performance computing in healthcare* 213
9.2 *Medical equipment using high-performance computing with low-power processors: cutting-edge commercial design environments* 215
9.3 *Reconfigurable integrated circuits in healthcare* 218
9.4 *Comparative analysis of FPGA with other ICs* 219
9.4.1 *FPGAs and ASICs* 222
9.4.2 *FPGAs and CPLD* 222
9.4.3 *FPGAs and microcontroller* 222
9.5 *Advantages of using FPGAs in healthcare* 223
9.6 *Limitations of using FPGAs in healthcare* 224

9.7 FPGA applications in medical diagnostics 224
9.7.1 Real-time signal processing in diagnostics 225
9.7.2 Diagnostic tools using FPGA 225
9.7.3 Use of FPGA in biomedical imaging 226
9.8 FPGA design considerations for medical imaging 228
9.8.1 Selection of development tools 228
9.8.2 FPGA programming languages 228
9.8.3 Resource management and optimization 229
9.8.4 Safety and reliability concerns 229
9.8.5 Compliance with regulatory standards 230
9.8.6 Challenges and ethical considerations 230
9.9 Conclusion 231

10 Quantum computing in medical informatics: unlocking revolutionary potential 234
10.1 Quantum computing and healthcare 234
10.1.1 Fundamental concepts 234
10.2 Role of quantum computing advancing healthcare 236
10.3 Quantum computing requirements in healthcare 242
10.4 Designing an effective quantum computing architecture for healthcare applications 247
10.5 Quantum computing security considerations in healthcare 247
10.6 Outstanding challenges and future research avenues 248
10.7 Conclusion 251

Index 258

Preface

The healthcare domain has always been at the forefront of innovation in technology and medicine. This is driven by the requirement for accurate diagnoses, really effective treatments, and better patient care. In the last two decades, artificial intelligence (AI) has emerged as a transformative force, that has revolutionized the medical data in analysis, diseases detection, and healthcare solutions. This book, *Fostering Healthcare through Artificial Intelligence: A High-Performance Computing Approach*, provides an in-depth explanation of the latest advancements in AI technology, machine learning (ML) algorithms, and high-performance computing (HPC) applications which are continuously reshaping the modern medicine.

The book begins with Chapter 1 which is an introduction to AI and HPC in healthcare. The chapter lays the groundwork for understanding how computational power and intelligent algorithms are being leveraged to solve critical medical challenges. The chapter also introduces foundational machine learning algorithms specifically designed for biomedical applications.

Chapter 2 explains the concepts of machine learning and deep learning in much detail. This is especially useful as the algorithms are complex, and for understanding their applications in healthcare, readers must have some introductory knowledge of how they work.

Chapter 3 is dedicated to biomedical signal and image processing using AI. These two fields have shown immense promise in early disease detection and patient monitoring. This chapter includes medical image modalities and diverse image processing algorithms useful for disease diagnoses. The chapter also throws light on the application of AI algorithms in very important procedures such as computed tomography and X-rays is discussed in detail.

Chapters 4 and 5 discuss the cutting-edge AI technologies that are explored for the diagnosis, prognosis, and survival prediction of various diseases, including neurological, cardiovascular, and infectious conditions, providing a state-of-the-art analysis of contemporary methodologies.

Chapter 6 shows two case studies. Firstly, a pix2pix generative adversarial networks (GAN) being used for identifying breast cancer in which no abnormality is detected on screening mammography. GANs are applied here to generate modifications from the initial photos in the dataset. This means that new dataset can be artificially generated. The study also combines convolutional neural networks (CNNs) to construct this framework for cancer detection. Compared to the transfer learning method, the suggested methodology exhibits higher accuracy for two VGG-16 and Resnet-50 CNNs.

Another insightful case study is AI applications in dentistry, showcasing how artificial intelligence is transforming yet another critical area of healthcare.

In Chapter 7, the role of machine learning in gynecological cancers is examined, demonstrating how AI is making a difference in women's health. The chapter presents a literature survey on the prediction techniques used in the field of gynecological cancers such as cervical cancer, ovarian cancer, and endometrial cancer.

This book in the next chapters ventures into the hardware domain. In Chapter 8, a comparison between central processing unit (CPU), graphics processing unit (GPU), and field programmable gate arrays (FPGA) is shown that relates to the next-generation computing devices tailored for healthcare applications. The discussion extends to high-performance computing (HPC) systems, which are crucial for handling massive datasets and performing complex computations in real time. In Chapter 9, the contribution of wearable healthcare devices to the health care is discussed. We have discussed about different types of wearables and how sensors are used for collecting information. Benefits and challenges related to wearables are also discussed.

Furthermore, Chapter 10 is a dedicated chapter on quantum computing which explores its revolutionary potential in healthcare and medicines, offering a glimpse into the future of computational medicine.

Written for researchers and healthcare professionals, this book serves as a comprehensive guide to the current landscape of AI in healthcare. By bridging theoretical concepts with practical implementations, our aim is to provide valuable insights on how AI is reshaping the medical world, improving patient outcomes, and driving the next generation of healthcare innovations.

We hope this book inspires further exploration, research, and innovation in AI-driven healthcare, ultimately leading to a healthier and more technologically advanced future.

Acknowledgments

Writing *Fostering Healthcare through Artificial Intelligence: A High-Performance Computing Approach* has been an incredible journey, and we are deeply grateful to those who supported and inspired us along the way.

First and foremost, we extend our heartfelt thanks to the healthcare professionals, researchers, and AI pioneers whose groundbreaking work continues to transform the landscape of modern medicine. Your dedication and innovation are the foundation of this book's purpose.

We are profoundly grateful to our families and friends for their unwavering encouragement and patience throughout this endeavor. Your belief in us has been our greatest motivation.

A special thanks goes to our colleagues and mentors, whose valuable insights and thoughtful discussions helped shape the ideas presented in this work. Your expertise and support have been invaluable.

Finally, to the readers—thank you for your curiosity and commitment to exploring the intersection of technology and healthcare. We hope this book inspires meaningful conversations and drives positive change in the future of medicine.

About the authors

Kavita Khare received her B. Tech in Electronics and Communication Engineering in 1989, M. Tech. in Digital Communication Systems in 1993, and PhD degree in the field of VLSI Design in 2004. She has nearly 27 years of teaching experience and 200 publications in various international conferences and journals. She has supervised nearly 20 PhD thesis and nearly 42 M. Tech thesis. She also received the Best Paper Award at an international conference in France and is a reviewer of several journals and conference proceedings. Dr Khare cocoordinates short-term courses on VLSI Design organized at MANIT Bhopal. Currently, she is working as a professor at the Department of Electronics and Communication Engineering in MANIT, Bhopal, India. Her areas of interest are VLSI design and Communication Systems, and her research mainly includes design of arithmetic circuits and various communication algorithms related to synchronization, estimation and routing. She is also a Fellow IETE (India) and member of IEEE, Life Member ISTE.

Zainab Aizaz is a VLSI front-end designer and research fellow in the School of Engineering and Informatics at the University of Sussex. She completed her PhD from Maulana Azad National Institute of Technology, Bhopal, India. She has worked as an assistant professor for 6 years in Electronics and Communication Engineering department in Oriental Institute of Science and Technology, Bhopal, Madhya Pradesh, India, and as a research fellow for 3 years in Barkatullah University, Bhopal, Madhya Pradesh, India. She has 17 international journal and conference publications along with three book chapters. She also won the state's annual young scientist award in India in the year 2020 in India. Zainab designs hardware for artificial intelligence systems on Field Programmable Gate Arrays (FPGA). Her recent focus is to design energy efficient Vector Processor as an extension to the RISCV processor. Her research interests include FPGAs, hardware description language, computer architecture, artificial intelligence.

Nilay Khare received his B. Tech degree in 1988, M. Tech. degree in Computer Science Engineering from IIT Delhi in 1995, and PhD degree in the field of VLSI Design in 2009. He has nearly 34 years of teaching experience. His major research work is on hardware implementation of neural network, FPGA implementation of CORDIC processor, machine learning, and data privacy. His PhD thesis is on efficient design of CORDIC processor on FPGA. He has supervised three PhDs in the area of VLSI design namely FPGA implementation of neural networks, hardware implementation of string-matching algorithms, and design and implementation of hardware firewall. He has expertise in AI, machine learning, and deep learning fields, and has supervised many UG and PG projects in these areas. He has published nearly 1000 papers in top journals and conferences. He also has three patents to his name. The primary areas of his expertise are AI, ML, VLSI, theoretical computer science, and IoT.

Chapter 1

Introduction to AI and high-performance computing in the healthcare domain

1.1 INTRODUCTION TO ARTIFICIAL INTELLIGENCE

1.1.1 History of artificial intelligence

The history of artificial intelligence (AI) can be traced back to the 1950s, but it gained significant traction in the 1990s with the invention and development of neural networks, which laid the foundation for modern AI [1–3]. However, despite their potential, the progress of neural networks was limited at the time due to the lack of sufficient computing power to process complex algorithms and large datasets [4]. This computational bottleneck hindered the practical application of AI for several years. Today, advancements in high-performance computing (HPC) have dramatically changed the landscape. With the availability of powerful processors, graphics processing units (GPUs), and parallel computing architectures, we can now efficiently train and deploy AI models at scale. HPC has not only revived the promise of neural networks but has also enabled the rapid evolution of AI across various domains, from healthcare to finance, making AI a transformative force in modern technology.

1.1.2 Components of high-performance computing

HPC plays a critical role in the functioning of AI, primarily through several key components that enhance processing power and efficiency. At the heart of HPC are parallel processing architectures, which allow multiple computations to be carried out simultaneously, significantly reducing the time required to train AI models [5]. GPUs are another vital component, offering massive computational power specifically suited for the matrix and vector operations common in AI and deep learning. Tensor processing units (TPUs), designed specifically for AI workloads, further accelerate the training of neural networks by optimizing operations like matrix multiplication. Cluster computing, where a group of interconnected computers works together as a single system, enables the handling of vast amounts of data and

DOI: 10.1201/9781003503033-1

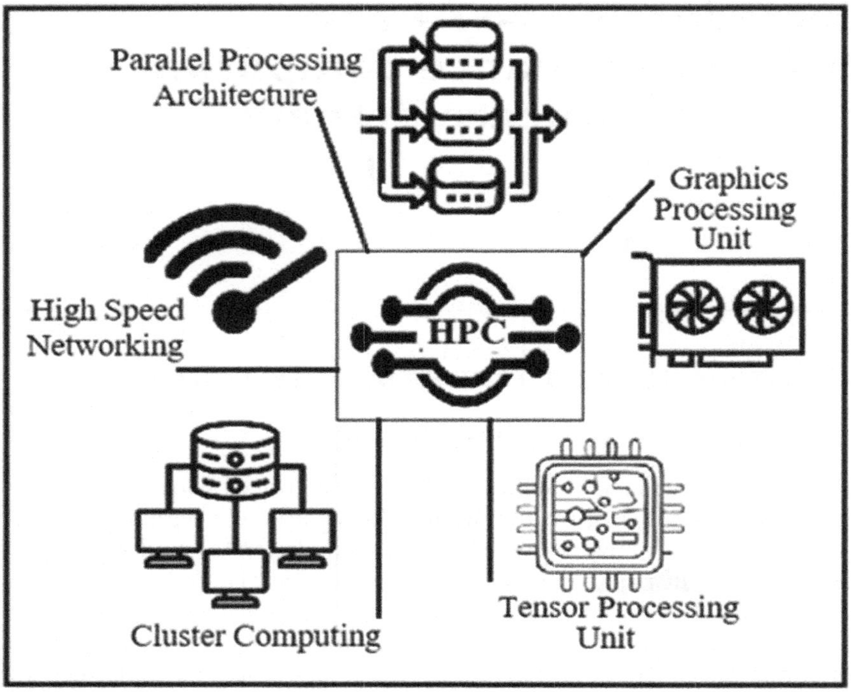

Figure 1.1 Core components of HPC.

complex models. Additionally, high-speed storage systems and networking infrastructure ensure rapid data transfer and accessibility, which are essential for real-time AI applications, as shown in Figure 1.1. Together, these components of HPC provide the computational backbone necessary to support the demanding workloads of modern AI, enabling the development of sophisticated algorithms and real-time data processing capabilities.

1.1.3 Artificial intelligence: a rapidly evolving technology

AI imitates human intelligence in machines that are automated to contemplate and learn in a similar manner like humans do. AI systems can execute tasks that classically necessitate human intelligence, like problem-solving, decision-making, language understanding, and visual perception [6]. AI is an influential and disruptive area of computer science, with the potential to essentially transmute the practice of medicine and delivery of healthcare. It discusses the science and engineering of making intelligent machines, through algorithms or a set of rules, which machine follows to mimic human cognitive functions, like learning and problem solving, which is depicted in Figure 1.2. They have the potential to forestall glitches or deal with issues as they come up and, as such, operate in an intentional, intelligent, and adaptive manner. It's a rapidly advancing field of computer science that seeks to generate systems and technologies proficient at performing tasks that typically necessitate human intelligence. These tasks comprise problem-solving, learning, reasoning, perception, language understanding, and decision-making (clinical decision making). AI systems object to simulate human-like cognitive functions and can be found in a wide range of applications, from voice assistants in our smartphones to self-driving cars and medical diagnostic tools, etc.

AI's development and deployment are ongoing, with continued research and innovation shaping the future of AI. It is built on the premise that machines can be programmed to mimic human thought processes and adapt to new situations. AI incorporates innumerable subfields, such as machine learning (ML), deep learning, natural language processing (NLP), computer vision, and robotics, each with its own set of algorithms and techniques. Its potential is vast and continues to grow as researchers, and engineers develop more sophisticated algorithms and hardware. AI is transforming industries like healthcare, finance, manufacturing, and transportation, offering the promise of improved efficiency, greater convenience, and improved decision-making.

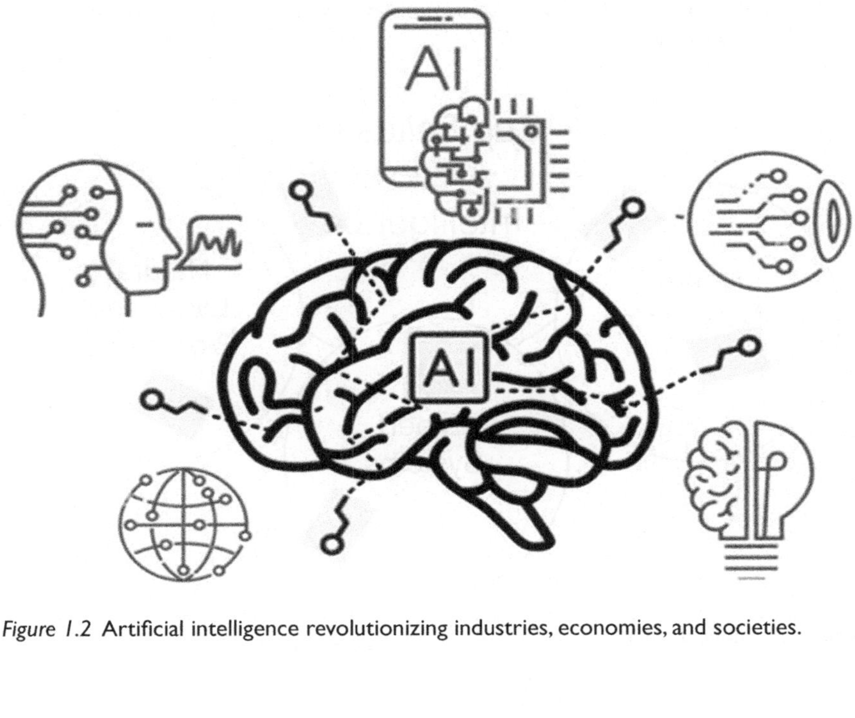

Figure 1.2 Artificial intelligence revolutionizing industries, economies, and societies.

1.2 SUBFIELDS OF ARTIFICIAL INTELLIGENCE

Subfields often overlap, and advancements in one area can contribute to progress in others. AI researchers and practitioners draw upon a combination of these subfields to develop intelligent systems that can perform diverse tasks and solve complex problems. AI is a broad and interdisciplinary field that encompasses various subfields [7].

AI subfields include ML for algorithmic learning, NLP for language interaction, computer vision for visual interpretation, robotics for intelligent automation, expert systems for domain-specific decision-making, and neural networks/deep learning for complex pattern recognition.

AI incorporates several subfields, as shown in Figure 1.3, like ML, deep learning, NLP, computer vision, and robotics. ML, in particular, is

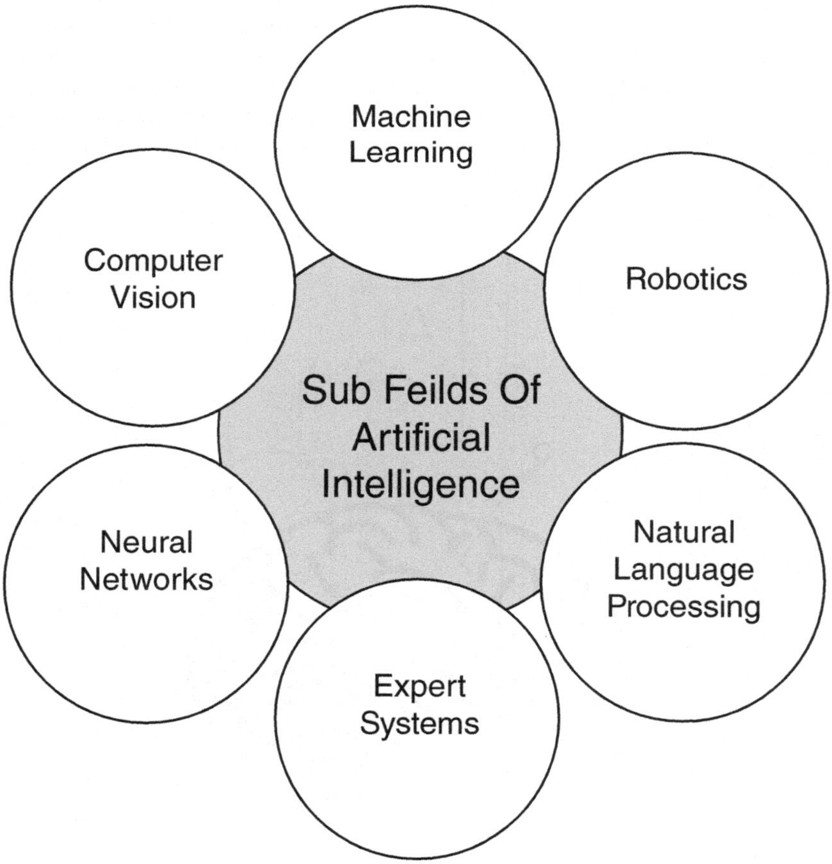

Figure 1.3 Subfields of AI.

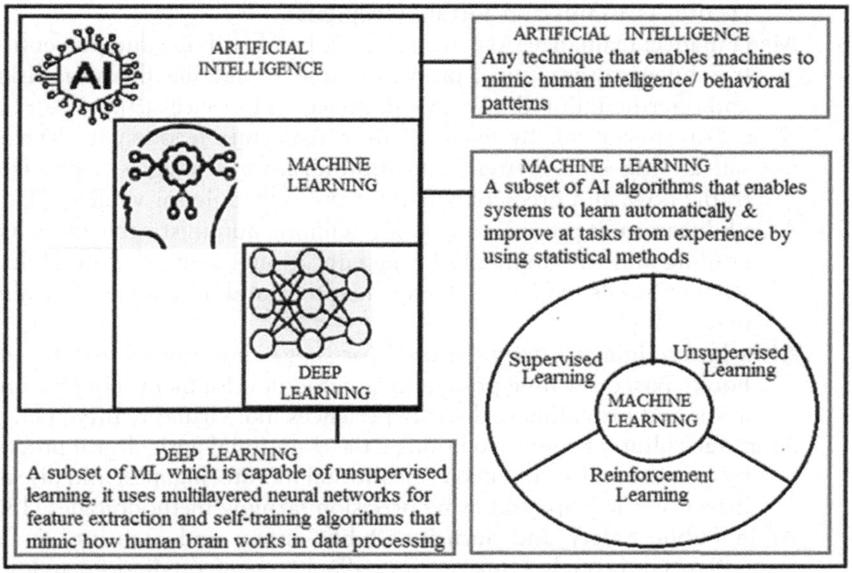

Figure 1.4 Relationship between AI, ML, and deep learning.

a subdivision of AI that emphasizes on developing algorithms that allow computers to learn and advance from experience, often by using large datasets. It has a varied assortment of practical applications in innumerable industries, from healthcare and finance to transportation and entertainment. Some common instances of AI in everyday life comprise virtual assistants like Siri and Alexa, recommendation systems used by platforms like Netflix and Amazon, self-driving cars, and medical diagnostic tools.

The field of AI is continually evolving, and advancements in hardware and software technologies have led to more powerful and capable AI systems. Relationship between AI, ML, and deep learning systems is shown in Figure 1.4.

1.3 APPLICATIONS OF ARTIFICIAL INTELLIGENCE

AI is revolutionizing multiple sectors by enhancing efficiency, accuracy, and decision-making processes. AI in healthcare sector, finance, agriculture, education, and entertainment is reshaping the global scenario and making AI inevitable for the near future.

AI in Healthcare: It can be used for enhancing and analyzing images for accurate diagnosis, forecasting disease outbreaks and patient outcomes, accelerating the identification and development of new drugs [8], providing personalized treatment and medicines, providing 24/7 support and guidance to patients (by using Virtual Health Assistants and Virtual Hospitals).

AI in Finance: In finance, AI can contribute by identifying and preventing fraudulent transactions, predicting and mitigating financial risks, and offering tailored investment advice and services [9].

AI in Transportation: By using AI in transportation, one can develop self-driving cars, better route optimization strategies, optimized traffic flow, and predictive maintenance schedule for vehicles [10].

AI in Education: It provides aid in streamlining administrative tasks like grading and scheduling, tailoring educational content to individual student needs and developing adaptive and interactive learning materials [11].

AI in Entertainment: It can be used for suggesting movies, music, and books based on user preferences, game development, content creation and providing realistic experiences like virtual reality [12].

AI in Agriculture: It can revolutionize the traditional agricultural process by efficient and automated crop and soil monitoring, pest and disease detection for crops and using precision farming methodologies [13].

AI in Public Safety and Security: Public safety and security can be enhanced through AI-driven surveillance, crime prediction, and disaster response [14].

1.3.1 Applications of artificial intelligence for healthcare

Fostering healthcare through AI is a swiftly growing and promising area that has the potential to transform various aspects of healthcare industry. AI is implemented in healthcare for tasks like medical image analysis, drug discovery, predictive analytics, and patient management [15]. It can improve diagnosis and treatment, enhance research, and reduce healthcare costs. AI can be applied in numerous ways to improve patient care, diagnosis, treatment, and the overall efficiency of healthcare systems. Table 1.1 demonstrates key Applications of AI in healthcare domain.

The integration of AI into healthcare is a dynamic and evolving field, with continuous advancements that have the potential to significantly improve patient outcomes, reduce costs, and transform the delivery of healthcare services.

AI has the potential to transform healthcare by reducing costs and enhancing the overall healthcare experience. As technology and research continue to advance, integration of AI into healthcare is likely to become more widespread, leading to better and more efficient healthcare services. Healthcare organizations have started the optimization of AI to improve the efficiency of all kinds of processes and procedures, beginning with tasks from backoffice to patient care [16].

Table 1.1 Key Applications of AI in healthcare domain

AI application in healthcare	*Explanation*
Medical imaging and diagnostics	AI is used for analyzing medical images such as X-rays, MRIs, and CT scans to detect abnormalities, tumors, and other conditions. Deep learning algorithms can help improve diagnostic accuracy and speed up the interpretation of images
Predictive analytics and risk stratification	AI algorithms analyze patient data to identify individuals at high risk for certain conditions. This helps healthcare providers intervene early, customize treatment plans, and improve patient outcomes. Predictive analytics are applied to conditions like diabetes, heart disease, and sepsis
Drug discovery and development	AI accelerates drug discovery by analyzing vast datasets to identify potential drug candidates, predict their efficacy, and optimize treatment regimens. This can significantly reduce the time and cost associated with bringing new drugs to market
Personalized medicine	AI analyzes genetic, clinical, and lifestyle data to tailor treatment plans to individual patients. This approach considers genetic variations, allowing for more precise and effective interventions, especially in cancer treatment
Virtual health assistants and chatbots	Virtual assistants and chatbots powered by AI provide information, answer queries, and offer basic healthcare advice. They can help patients schedule appointments, manage medications, and provide support for mental health
Natural language processing (NLP)	NLP enables the extraction of valuable information from unstructured clinical notes, medical records, and research literature. This helps in better understanding patient histories, improving documentation, and supporting clinical decision-making
Remote patient monitoring	AI facilitates continuous monitoring of patients' health using wearable devices and other remote sensors. This allows for real-time tracking of vital signs, early detection of anomalies, and proactive intervention, particularly for chronic disease management
Fraud detection and security	AI is employed to detect fraudulent activities in healthcare billing and insurance claims. It enhances the security of patient data through advanced encryption, authentication, and monitoring systems
Robot-assisted surgery	AI-powered robotic systems assist surgeons in performing minimally invasive surgeries with precision. These systems enhance the surgeon's capabilities, reduce recovery times, and improve overall surgical outcomes
Clinical decision support systems (CDSS)	AI-driven CDSS assists healthcare professionals in making informed decisions by providing evidence-based recommendations. It considers patient data, medical literature, and best practices to support diagnosis and treatment planning

(*continued*)

Table 1.1 (*Cont.*)

AI application in healthcare	*Explanation*
Epidemiological modeling and outbreak prediction	AI is used to model and predict disease outbreaks by analyzing various factors such as travel patterns, climate data, and demographic information. This aids in early detection and proactive measures to control the spread of infectious diseases
Healthcare operations and workflow optimization	AI optimizes hospital operations by streamlining workflows, managing resources more efficiently, and predicting patient admission rates. This leads to improved resource allocation, reduced waiting times, and enhanced overall healthcare delivery

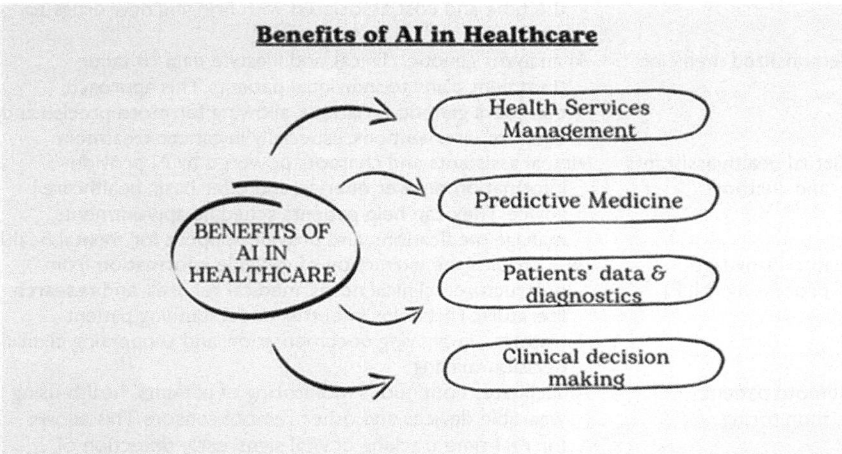

Figure 1.5 Benefits of AI in healthcare.

Utilization of AI can encompass the benefits in the area where its utilization can be beneficial for the automation and help the hospital staff to keep the process and management up to date and other time-consuming mundane tasks.

Healthcare amenities that scrutinize data properly reach inferences that save patient's lives [17]. AI in healthcare companies build ML algorithms, NLP-based solutions, and deep learning proficiencies to scrutinize enormous expanses of data.

For instance, scrutinizing a patient's medical history and test reports can assist companies deliver better care by considering patterns in health. They can classify whether a person is further susceptible to certain diseases, has any sort of glitches that might lead to forthcoming illnesses, or shows symptoms of something fatal. Figure 1.5 summarizes the benefits of AI in healthcare.

1.4 SCOPE OF AI IN THE FIELD OF BIOMEDICAL ANALYSIS, DISEASE PREDICTION, AND TREATMENT

The scope of AI in the fields of biomedical analysis, disease prediction, and treatment is vast and promising [18]. AI technologies offer several applications and tools that can transform healthcare in significant ways.

As AI technologies advance [19, 20], they offer the potential to transform healthcare by refining patient consequences, enhancing the efficiency of healthcare systems, reducing costs, and accelerating medical discoveries. Table 1.2 shows the scope of AI in healthcare domain.

Table 1.2 Scope of AI in healthcare domain

Scope of AI	*Basic operations*	*Scope*
Medical imaging analysis	AI can scrutinize medical images like X-rays, CT scans, MRIs, and pathology slides. Basic operations include image segmentation, feature extraction, and pattern recognition	AI can support radiologists in the initial recognition of diseases, like cancer, and improve the accuracy of diagnoses by identifying anomalies and abnormalities in medical images
Disease prediction and risk assessment	AI utilizes machine learning and predictive modeling to analyze patient data, which involves data preprocessing, feature selection, and model training	AI can predict disease risk and patient consequences by investigating electronic health records, genomic data, and lifestyle factors. It helps in identifying at-risk individuals and tailoring preventive interventions
Drug discovery and development	AI-driven drug discovery involves scrutinizing large datasets, virtual screening, molecular modeling, and predicting the efficacy of drug compounds	AI accelerates drug development by identifying potential drug candidates, discovering new therapeutic uses for existing drugs, and optimizing treatment protocols
Clinical decision support	AI analyzes patient data and provides evidence-based recommendations to clinicians, including risk assessment and treatment suggestions	AI supports healthcare professionals in making additional conversant and accurate decisions, leading to improved patient care and reduced medical errors
Remote patient monitoring	AI enables real-time monitoring of patients using wearable devices and IoT sensors. It involves data collection, data analysis, and alert generation	AI continuously tracks patients' vital signs and health metrics, allowing for early intervention, remote patient management and reduced hospital readmissions
Natural language processing (NLP)	NLP involves text analysis, language understanding, and information extraction from clinical notes and research papers	AI-driven NLP can help in clinical documentation, extracting insights from unstructured data and improving communication between healthcare providers

(*continued*)

Table 1.2 (Cont.)

Scope of AI	*Basic operations*	*Scope*
Treatment personalization	AI scrutinizes patient data and clinical guidelines to customize treatment plans based on discrete characteristics	AI optimizes treatments by tailoring them to a patient's genetic profile, medical history, and responses to therapy, leading to additional operative and personalized care
Disease monitoring and progression prediction	AI analyzes patient data over time to predict disease progression and therapeutic response	AI aids in monitoring chronic diseases and provides insights for treatment adjustments to improve patient outcomes
Vaccine development and epidemic prediction	AI models analyze viral genomes, epidemiological data, and vaccine candidate properties	AI supports the development of vaccines and helps predict disease outbreaks, as seen in the context of COVID-19 pandemic

1.5 CONCLUSION

As AI continues to progress, it holds the promise of solving complex problems, increasing automation and efficiency, and improving our eminence of life. However, it likewise elevates imperative ethical and societal enquiries, like those related to privacy, bias, accountability, and impact on the job market. Components of AI work together to create intelligent systems capable of understanding, learning from, and responding to complex information in a manner that simulates human intelligence.

On one hand, it promises increased productivity, efficiency, and innovation. On the other, it raises concerns about job displacement, data security, and ethical dilemmas. As AI continues to evolve, the need for responsible AI development, regulation, and international collaboration becomes paramount. Addressing ethical concerns and fostering transparency will be essential to ensure that AI benefits humanity as a whole.

The conclusion is that AI's trajectory holds the potential for extraordinary advancements, and as stewards of this technology, it is our responsibility to navigate its development with care and foresight.

REFERENCES

[1] M. Ida, *A narrative history of artificial intelligence: The perpetual frontier of information technology*. Springer Nature, 2024.

[2] S. Russell and P. Norvig, *Artificial intelligence: A modern approach*, 4th ed. Pearson, 2021.

[3] J. Schmidhuber, "AI history, where are we headed?" *AI Magazine*, vol. 42, no. 1, pp. 10–20, 2021.

[4] I. Goodfellow, Y. Bengio, and A. Courville, *Deep learning*. MIT Press, 2016.

[5] Y. LeCun, Y. Bengio, and G. Hinton, " Deep learning." *Nature*, vol. 521, no. 7553, pp. 436–444, 2015.

[6] N. Bostrom and E. Yudkowsky, "The ethics of artificial intelligence." in *The Cambridge handbook of artificial intelligence*, K. Frankish and W. M. Ramsey, Eds., Cambridge University Press, 2014, pp. 316–334.
[7] N. Thompson, K. Greenewald, K. Lee, and G. Manso, "The computational limits of deep learning." *Proc. Natl. Acad. Sci.*, vol. 118, no. 46, 2021.
[8] S. Esteva, A. Kuprel, and R. A. Novoa, "Dermatologist-level classification of skin cancer with deep neural networks." *Nature*, vol. 542, pp. 115–118, 2017.
[9] A. B. Miller and G. Turner, "AI and fraud detection in financial services." *AI J.*, vol. 34, no. 7, pp. 12–18, 2020.
[10] C. L. Wang, "Autonomous vehicles and the future of transportation." *Transp. Res. J.*, vol. 11, no. 2, pp. 75–80, 2019.
[11] J. Zhang and R. K. Wong, "AI in education: Opportunities and challenges." *Educ. Tech. J.*, vol. 25, pp. 45–60, 2021.
[12] D. Silver et al., "Mastering the game of Go with deep neural networks and tree search." *Nature*, vol. 529, pp. 484–489, 2016.
[13] S. B. Kang et al., "Precision agriculture using AI-based crop monitoring." *Agric. Res. J.*, vol. 22, no. 3, pp. 58–65, 2020.
[14] S. Omori and N. T. Hayashi, "AI-driven disaster response: Innovations and challenges." *Sec. Technol. J.*, vol. 15, pp. 23–33, 2021.
[15] R. Ching et al., "AI and machine learning for healthcare: Challenges and opportunities." *Med. Sci. J.*, vol. 49, no. 3, pp. 201–210, 2022.
[16] A. Jha et al., "Artificial intelligence and the healthcare revolution." *Health J.*, vol. 62, pp. 125–140, 2021.
[17] K. P. Murphy, *Machine learning: A probabilistic perspective.* MIT Press, 2012.
[18] T. Dean et al., "AI in hospitals: Applications and future prospects." *Hosp. Mgmt. Rev.*, vol. 18, no. 5, pp. 31–44, 2020.
[19] G. E. Hinton, S. Osindero, and Y. Teh, "A fast learning algorithm for deep belief nets." *Neural Comput.*, vol. 18, pp. 1527–1554, 2006.
[20] R. Smith et al., "Deep learning in healthcare: Impacts on patient care." *J. Med. Inform.*, vol. 34, pp. 15–28, 2022.

Subjective Questions (Short Answers)

Q1. How does AI contribute to personalized medicine in healthcare?
Q2. Explain how AI and HPC can be used together to improve drug discovery?
Q3. What are some challenges of integrating AI and HPC in healthcare?
Q4. Discuss the importance of data quality in leveraging AI and HPC for healthcare.
Q5. What is the significance of real-time predictive analytics in managing patient care?

Subjective Questions (Long Answers)

Q1. Discuss the role of Artificial Intelligence (AI) in transforming healthcare. How have AI technologies contributed to improving diagnostics, treatment plans, and patient outcomes? Provide examples to illustrate your answer.

Q2. Explain the importance of HPC in accelerating AI applications in healthcare. How does HPC enable the processing of large-scale healthcare data, and what are its benefits in medical research and real-time healthcare applications?

Q3. Discuss the ethical considerations and potential risks involved in applying AI and HPC to healthcare. How do issues like patient privacy, data security, and algorithmic bias impact the adoption of these technologies? Propose solutions to address these challenges.

Q4. How has the integration of AI and HPC impacted medical imaging, such as MRI or CT scans, in healthcare? Provide examples of AI techniques (like deep learning) used in medical imaging and explain how HPC enhances the efficiency and accuracy of these methods.

Q5. Explore the future potential of AI and HPC in healthcare. What emerging technologies, such as quantum computing or advanced AI algorithms, could further revolutionize healthcare delivery and medical research? What challenges must be overcome to realize this future?

Objective Questions

Q1. Which technology is essential for running complex simulations in healthcare data analysis?
A) Cloud computing
B) High-performance computing (HPC)
C) Quantum computing
D) Edge computing
Answer: B) High-performance computing (HPC)

Q2. How does AI assist in drug discovery?
A) By synthesizing new drugs
B) By identifying potential drug candidates and predicting their effectiveness
C) By manufacturing drugs
D) By conducting clinical trials
Answer: B) By identifying potential drug candidates and predicting their effectiveness

Q3. What is a major challenge when integrating AI into clinical practice?
A) Lack of data
B) High computational costs
C) Over-reliance on human intuition
D) Lack of AI algorithms
Answer: B) High computational costs

Q4. In what way does HPC enhance real-time data analysis in healthcare?
A) By reducing data accuracy

B) By increasing data storage capacity
C) By accelerating data processing and analysis
D) By simplifying data collection methods
Answer: C) By accelerating data processing and analysis

Q5. What role does AI play in medical imaging?
A) Replacing radiologists
B) Analyzing and interpreting images to identify abnormalities
C) Printing medical images
D) Conducting physical examinations
Answer: B) Analyzing and interpreting images to identify abnormalities

Q6. Which of the following is an advantage of combining AI with HPC in healthcare research?
A) Increased research time
B) Slower data processing
C) Enhanced ability to analyze large datasets quickly
D) Decreased accuracy of research findings
Answer: C) Enhanced ability to analyze large datasets quickly

Q7. Which type of AI application is commonly used for predicting disease outbreaks?
A) Natural language processing
B) Predictive analytics
C) Computer vision
D) Reinforcement learning
Answer: B) Predictive analytics

Q8. In what way does AI impact the management of electronic health records (EHRs)?
A) By replacing human doctors
B) By automating data entry and improving data accuracy
C) By eliminating the need for EHRs
D) By slowing down data retrieval
Answer: B) By automating data entry and improving data accuracy

Q9. Which of the following is NOT a typical use case of AI in healthcare?
A) Disease diagnosis
B) Patient scheduling
C) Image analysis
D) Automated drug manufacturing
Answer: D) Automated drug manufacturing

Q10. What is a critical factor for ensuring the effectiveness of AI models in healthcare?
A) High data complexity
B) Randomized data inputs
C) Availability of diverse and representative datasets
D) Minimal data collection
Answer: C) Availability of diverse and representative datasets

Chapter 2

Introduction to ML algorithms for biomedical applications

2.1 MACHINE LEARNING

2.1.1 Understanding machine learning

Machine learning (ML) enables computers to generalize patterns and similarities within data in order to make predictions on new and unnoticed data. Choice of model, data quality, and effective feature engineering play crucial roles in the success of a ML system [1]. Furthermore, the iterative nature of training, evaluation, and refinement contributes to the continuous improvement of ML models. Its fundamental principle revolves around the idea for enabling computers to interpret existing data and progressively make their performance better on a given task.

ML can be regarded as a subset of artificial intelligence (AI) which has emphasized the development of techniques and models that make computers to understand data and then make predictions or decisions based on that data. Its primary goal is to build systems that can inevitably advance their performance over time without being explicitly programmed to do so. It achieves this by identifying patterns, relationships, and insights within datasets [2].

The essence of ML is to improve systems in terms of their performance to learn a specific task through experience when data is given as input to that system. This iterative learning process allows machines to adapt and evolve without human intervention.

2.1.2 Types of machine learning

ML has three major categories of learning approaches, and each of them is suited to a variety of problems and data. The three main broad categories of ML are supervised learning, unsupervised learning, and reinforcement learning [3, 4]. These categories are based on the type of learning process and the nature of the input data.

DOI: 10.1201/9781003503033-2

Supervised Learning: In this type of learning, the algorithm demands a labeled dataset. A labeled dataset means that correct answers are provided, which are called labels. The algorithm then learns to make predictions based on features of input data and their corresponding labels.

Unsupervised Learning: In this type of learning, the answers are not provided in advance and algorithms work with unlabeled data. The goal is to discover relationships or patterns or groups within data, for example, clustering similar data points.

Reinforcement Learning: In this type of learning, an agent interrelates with an environment and learns to make a sequence of decisions to maximize a reward. It's commonly used in applications like games and robotics.

2.1.3 Principle of operation of machine learning algorithms

ML principles are depicted in Figure 2.1. The key components of ML vital to developing effective ML systems, including data, which serves as the essential input for any model, and Features, which are the specific attributes extracted from this data that are crucial for accurate predictions. Then comes the algorithms that learn from the data, forming the core of the ML process [5, 6]. The process also involves model training, where these algorithms are trained on the data, and model evaluation phase, where the model's

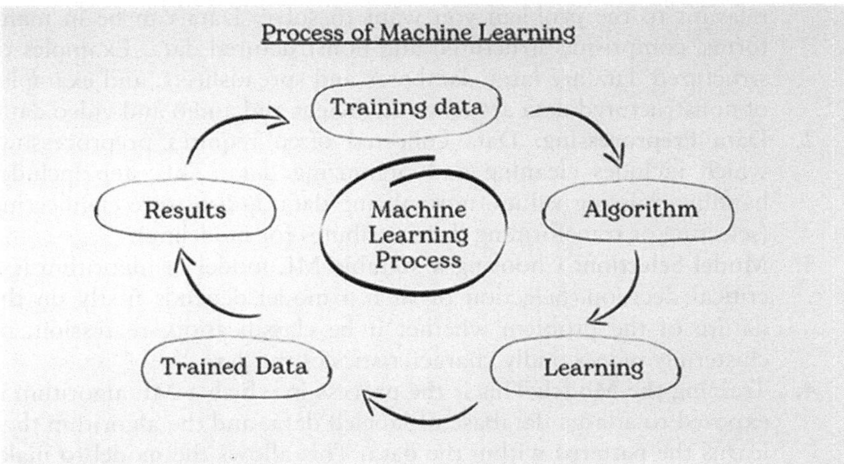

Figure 2.1 Principle of operation of machine learning.

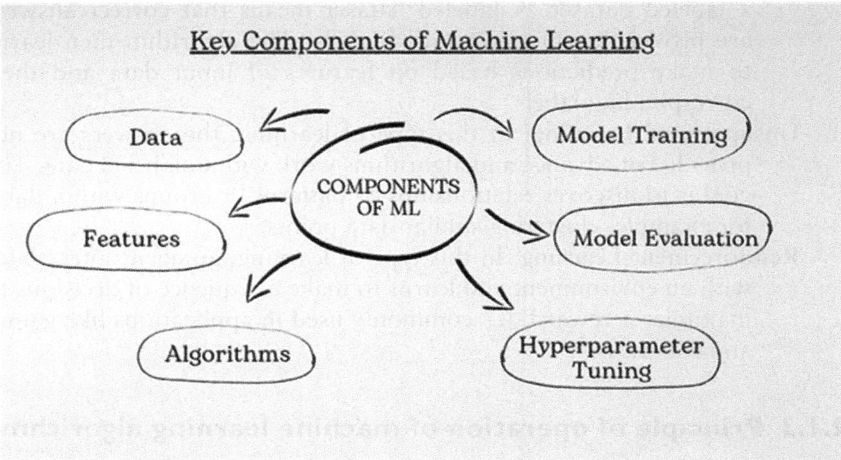

Figure 2.2 Key components of machine learning.

performance is assessed to ensure accuracy. Finally, using hyperparameter tuning, the model finetunes itself to optimize its performance. Figure 2.2 shows the key components of ML systems.

The following points summarize how ML algorithms work:

1. **Data Collection:** The ML process begins with the collection of data relevant to the problem you want to solve. Data can be in many forms, comprising structured and nonstructured data. Examples of structured data are large databases and spreadsheets, and examples of nonstructured data are text and images and audio and video data.
2. **Data Preprocessing:** Data collected often requires preprocessing, which includes cleaning and organizing data. This step includes handling missing values, normalizing data, and feature engineering (selecting or transforming data attributes for modeling).
3. **Model Selection:** Choosing a suitable ML model or algorithm is a critical decision. Selection of such a model depends firstly on the nature of the problem whether it be classification, regression, or clustering and secondly characteristics of the data.
4. **Training the Model:** This is the process in which a ML algorithm is exposed to a large database of labeled data, and the algorithm then learns the patterns within the data. This allows the model to make estimations or classifications on unseen and novel data.
5. **Model Learning:** During the training process, a model modifies its internal parameters to curtail the difference between its predictions

Table 2.1 Components of machine learning

Component	*Principle*
Input data	The fundamental idea is to learn from available data. The two major factors that determine the effectiveness of the learning process are the quality and quantity of data
Model generalization	Aim of machine learning is to create models that can generalize well to new, unseen data. Generalization is crucial for the model to make accurate predictions on data it has not encountered during training
Feature representation	Features are the attributes of the data used by the model to make predictions. Effective feature representation is essential for learning meaningful patterns from data. Features that capture relevant information and relationships in the data
Supervised and unsupervised learning	Machine learning encompasses both supervised and unsupervised learning paradigms
Evaluation and feedback	Continuous evaluation and feedback are crucial for model improvement
Bias and fairness	Addressing bias and ensuring fairness are important considerations in machine learning
Model interpretability	Interpretability is important for understanding and trusting machine learning models. Interpretable models are easier to understand, validate, and trust
Model complexity and overfitting	Balancing model complexity is essential to avoid overfitting. Overfitting takes place when a model learns from the training data too much because of capturing noise. The balance between a model complexity and generalization of data is the most important challenge in machine learning

and correct outputs in training data. The process is frequently guided by an optimization algorithm that updates the model parameters iteratively.

Table 2.1 explains several components of machine learning in detail.

2.2 APPLICATIONS OF MACHINE LEARNING

The sphere of ML applications is vast, comprising image and speech recognition, recommendation systems, natural language processing (NLP), healthcare [7], finance, manufacturing, etc. It allows businesses and organizations to leverage data for automation, decision-making, and insights, making it an influential tool for solving complex glitches and enhancing efficiency.

Image and Speech Recognition: Recognizing objects, faces, and speech in various applications like facial recognition, voice assistants, and autonomous vehicles. It has the ability to perform tasks without explicit instructions and relying on patterns [8]. Its emphasis is on enabling computers to perform tasks without explicit programming. ML is applied in an extensive assortment of applications, comprising:

NLP: It refers to understanding human language and then processing it for identification, manipulation, and learning. This is used in chatbots, language translation, sentiment analysis, and text summarization [9].

Recommendation Systems: Recommendation of movies, music, and other content purely on users' past preferences. This can be easily experienced on platforms like Amazon and Netflix.

Healthcare: Medical image analysis, disease prediction, personalized treatment, and drug discovery.

Finance: Credit scoring, fraud detection, algorithmic trading, and risk assessment.

Manufacturing: Control over quality and inputs, maintenance, and supply chain optimization.

ML is a compute-intensive tool with an extensive assortment of practical applications, and its importance continues to grow as more data becomes accessible and computing power upsurges [10, 11]. Figure 2.3 shows applications of ML.

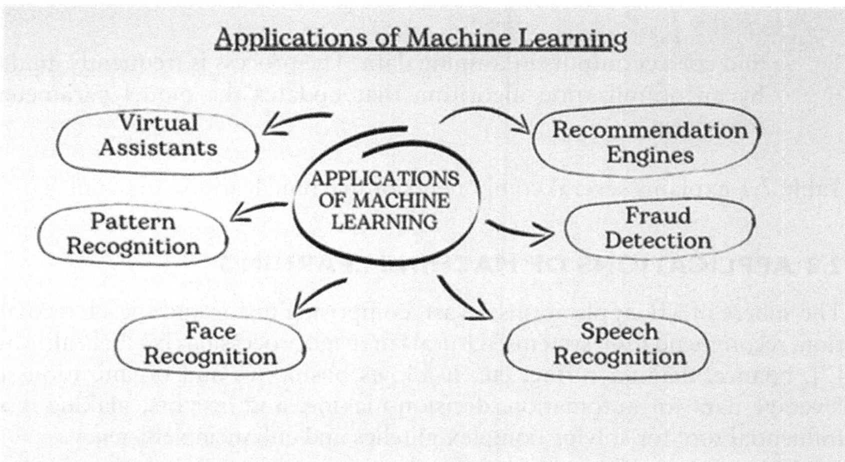

Figure 2.3 Applications of machine learning.

2.3 SCOPE OF MACHINE LEARNING IN BIOMEDICAL ANALYSIS, DISEASE PREDICTION, AND TREATMENT

The scope of ML in biomedical analysis, disease prediction, and treatment is incessantly escalating, driven by the availability of vast healthcare data, advancements in machine learning techniques, and the prerequisite for more precise and efficient healthcare solutions. This is demonstrated in Table 2.2. As ML endures to evolve, it is latent to enhance early disease detection, treatment efficacy, patient care, and the overall understanding of complex medical conditions. However, ethical and regulatory considerations, data

Table 2.2 Scope of machine learning in healthcare domain

Scope of ML	*Scope*
Medical imaging analysis	Used to investigate medical images for X-ray, CT scans, MRIs, and pathology slides. Detection and diagnosis of diseases, automated tumor detection, image segmentation, disease staging, and quantifying disease progression
Disease diagnoses and risk assessment	Used to analyze large datasets containing patient information, genetic data, and lifestyle factors for predicting risk and assess a patient's vulnerability to specific conditions. Predicting the risk of diseases like diabetes, heart disease, Alzheimer's, and cancer, and identifying high-risk individuals for preventive measures
Drug discovery and development	Drug discovery by identifying potential drug candidates, understanding molecular interactions, and predicting efficacy. Virtual screening, drug repurposing, target identification, and optimizing clinical trial designs
clinical decision support	Evidence-based recommendations, predicting patient outcomes, and optimizing treatment strategies
Personalized Treatment	Precision medicine for cancer patients, individualized drug dosages, and targeted therapy recommendations
Remote patient monitoring	Machine learning powers wearable devices and IoT sensors that track vital signs, monitor patients' health conditions, and provide early intervention when needed. Remote monitoring for chronic disease management, telehealth, and timely alerts for deteriorating health
Natural language processing (NLP)	Automatic medical report generation, clinical note extraction, and information retrieval from vast medical databases
Disease monitoring and progression prediction	Machine learning models analyze longitudinal patient data to envisage disease progression and therapeutic response. Monitoring chronic diseases, adjusting treatment plans, and improving patient outcomes
Vaccine development and epidemic prediction	Machine learning aids in identifying vaccine candidates, analyzing viral genomes, and predicting disease outbreaks. Accelerating vaccine development, understanding viral evolution, and early detection of epidemics

privacy, and responsible use of AI in healthcare remain important factors in this field.

2.4 DEEP LEARNING

2.4.1 Understanding deep learning

Deep learning is a subfield of ML that is based on particularly deep neural networks to model and unravel complex glitches. Deep learning algorithms are inspired by the structure and function of the human brain and consist of interconnected layers of artificial neurons, referred to as artificial neural networks [12]. These networks have multiple hidden layers (hence "deep") that enable them to mechanically learn and represent hierarchical features from data.

2.4.2 Components of deep learning

A hierarchical diagram of the relationship between AI, ML and deep learning is shown in Figure 2.4. The layers are defined as an input layer, one or more hidden layers, and output layer. In deep learning, many hidden layers are present between the input and the output layer. These multiple layers enable the network to learn increasingly abstract and complex features from the data. Deep learning excels at automatically learning and extracting features from raw data. This process permits the model to identify

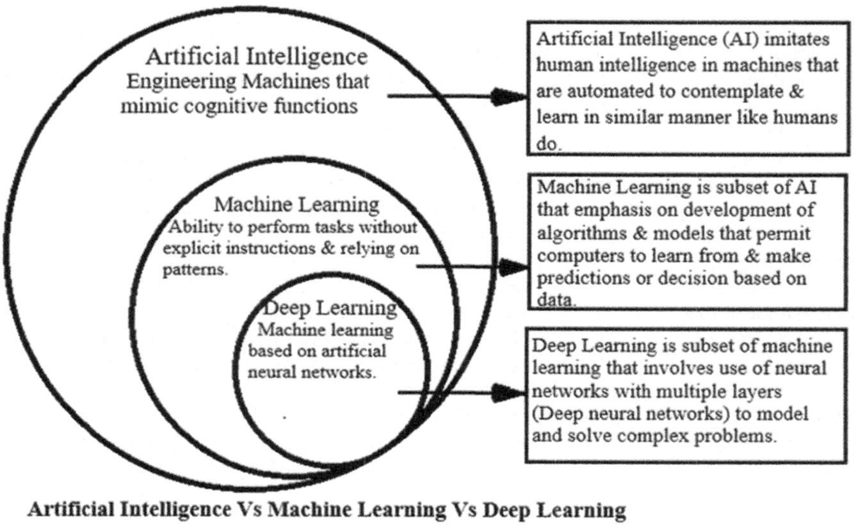

Figure 2.4 Artificial intelligence versus machine learning versus deep learning.

patterns, representations, and abstractions that are essential for solving complex problems. Deep learning models use backpropagation, a technique that regulates model's internal parameters during training by manipulating gradients of the loss function thus allowing the model to minimize errors. Activation functions are fundamental mathematical operations that introduce nonlinearity in neural networks and enable them to model complex connections in data. Some commonly used activation functions comprise Rectified Linear Unit, also called RELU, sigmoid, and tanh. Understanding these fundamental principles provides a foundation for effectively designing,

Table 2.3 Components of deep learning

Component	*Principle*	*Explanation*
Representation learning	Deep learning focuses on learning hierarchical representations of data	Every layer must learn different levels of abstraction. The lower layers are designed to capture basic features and higher layers are designed to combine the lower layers to form more complex representations. This hierarchy allows the model to understand and differentiate between intricate patterns in the data
End-to-end learning		Traditional machine learning often involves multiple stages, including data preprocessing and feature engineering. In deep learning, the model understands important features from raw data and enables end-to-end learning, which reduces the reliance on human-crafted features
Nonlinearity and activation functions	Nonlinear activation functions are used between layers	These functions introduce nonlinearity to the model to capture intricate relationships in the data. Linearity would limit the expressive power of the model, hindering its ability to learn intricate patterns
Backpropagation and training		During training, predictions are made by model, and the error between predicted and actual outcomes is used to adjust the model's parameters iteratively. Backpropagation involves calculating gradients with respect to the error and updating the model's weights to minimize this error. This iterative optimization process refines the model's ability to make accurate predictions
Adaptability and generalization	These models demonstrate adaptability	They aim to learn underlying patterns and relationships in the data. The adaptability of these models is crucial for handling diverse datasets and real-world applications
Scalability	These models can be scaled for handling large and complex data	The depth and complexity of neural networks allow them to handle high-dimensional input spaces and learn intricate patterns. This scalability is especially important for applications where large amounts of data are available

training, and deploying deep learning models in various domains. These principles guide the development of architectures and techniques that contribute to the success of deep learning in solving complex problems. Table 2.3 summarizes the components of deep learning.

Deep neural networks (DNNs) typically have an input layer, more than two hidden layers, and an output layer. Figure 2.5 shows the concept of DNNs. Each layer comprises multiple neurons connected to neurons in adjacent layers through weighted connections. Deep networks have many hidden layers, enabling them to learn intricate patterns and relationships within data. DNNs are trained using algorithms such as backpropagation and stochastic gradient descent, in order to adjust the weights and biases for minimizing the difference between predicted and real outputs. Figure 2.6 shows feedforward and backpropagation in neural networks. Training requires large labeled datasets to learn meaningful representations of input data. DNNs excel at automatically learning hierarchical representations of data, extracting increasingly abstract features at deeper layers. In this way, hierarchical learning enables DNNs to grasp complex patterns and variations within the data, thus making them suitable for image recognition, speech recognition, and NLP. Apart from revolutionizing the world, DNNs have certain challenges to overcome. Training and optimizing DNNs can be computationally intensive and require substantial computational resources. DNNs are also prone to overfitting,

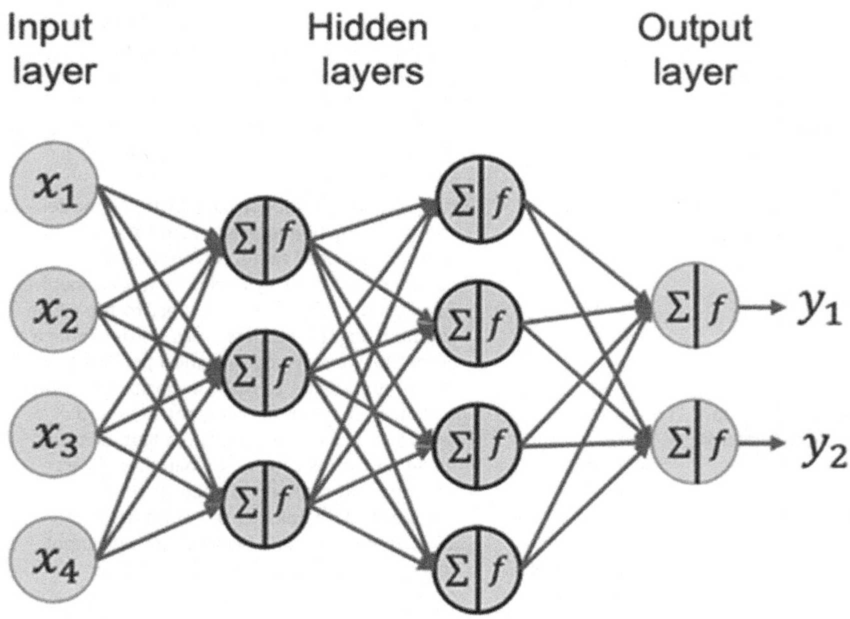

Figure 2.5 Deep neural network with layers.

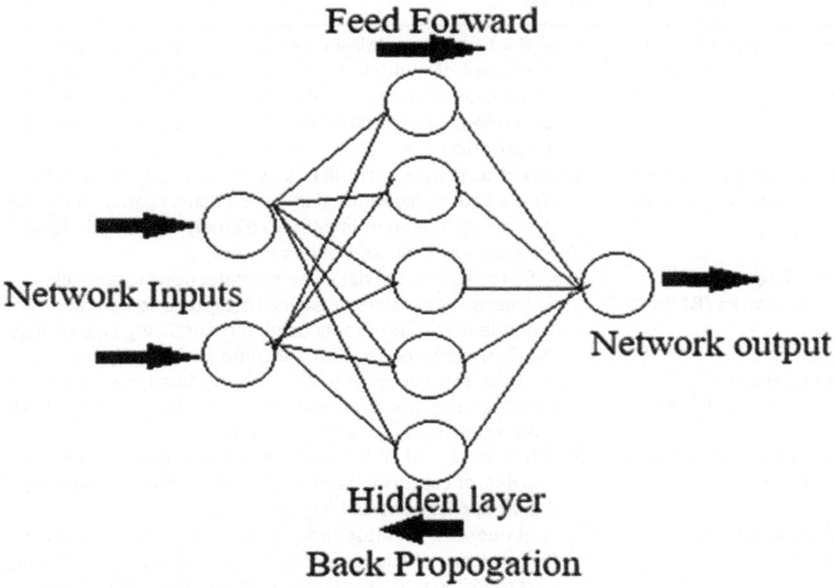

Figure 2.6 Feedforward and backpropagation in DNNs.

in which it fails to generalize to unseen data. Addressing these challenges requires careful design, regularization techniques, and hyperparameter tuning. There is a lot of research going on improving model architectures, training algorithms, and regularization methods for DNNs. Future directions include advancing interpretability and explainability of DNNs, enhancing their robustness to adversarial attacks, and enabling efficient deployment on resource-constrained devices for edge computing applications.

2.4.3 Types of deep learning

Deep learning encompasses various types of neural network architectures and techniques, each designed to address specific types of problems and data. These are explained in Table 2.4.

2.4.4 Applications of deep learning

Deep learning has found extensive applications in a variety of fields [13], including:

Computer Vision: Deep learning powers image and video analysis, object detection, facial recognition, and image classification.

Table 2.4 Types of deep learning

Feedforward neural networks (FNNs)	Also identified as multilayer perceptrons (MLPs). FNNs are composed of multiple layers of interconnected neurons. Foundation of deep learning is used for an extensive assortment of applications, comprising image and text classification
Convolutional neural networks (CNNs)	Intended to process grid-like data, for example, images and videos. Use convolutional layers to learn spatial hierarchies of features hidden in images. Extremely effective in tasks like image recognition and object detection
Recurrent neural networks (RNNs)	Specific for sequential data. Their connections loop back on themselves making it easier to capture temporal dependencies. Commonly used in natural language processing (NLP), speech recognition, and time series analysis
Long short-term memory (LSTM)	One of the categories of RNN with modified mechanisms for handling long-range dependencies. Extensively used in NLP tasks, speech, and music generation
Gated recurrent units (GRUs)	Another variant of RNNs that are simpler than LSTMs. Capable of capturing long-range dependencies, often used in similar applications as LSTMs
Autoencoders	Neural network architectures used for unsupervised learning., Aim to learn efficient representations of data by reducing its dimensionality. Variational autoencoders (VAEs) and denoising autoencoders are common types
Generative adversarial networks (GANs)	GANs are made up of two neural networks, a generator and adiscriminator, that compete in game. Used to generate artificial data, such as images, and have applications in image generation, style transfer, and data augmentation
Transformer networks	Attention-based models designed for sequential and parallel data processing. Revolutionized NLP and are used in large-scale language models like BERT, GPT, and T5
Capsule networks (CapsNets)	More recent developments in deep learning are intended to handle hierarchical data. Used in computer vision tasks like object recognition
Radial basis function networks (RBFNs)	Use radial basis functions as activation functions and are well-suited for problems involving function approximation, pattern recognition, and interpolation
Deep reinforcement learning (DRL)	Combines deep learning with reinforcement learning and is used in applications like game playing, robotics, and autonomous agents
Siamese networks	Designed for similarity and distance metric learning. Used in applications like face recognition, signature verification, and recommendation systems

Convolutional neural networks (CNNs) are commonly used for these tasks.

NLP: In NLP, deep learning models, including recurrent neural networks (RNNs) and transformer architectures like BERT and GPT, have significantly improved tasks like text classification, sentiment analysis, language translation, and chatbots.

Speech Recognition: Deep learning is widely employed in speech recognition systems, such as virtual assistants and transcription services.

Recommendation Systems: Deep learning models are used to make personalized product recommendations, content recommendations, and more.

Healthcare: Deep learning has been applied to medical image analysis, disease diagnosis, drug discovery, and treatment optimization.

Autonomous Vehicles: Deep learning is a vital technology in self-driving cars, helping them perceive their environment, make decisions, and navigate safely.

Deep learning has demonstrated remarkable capabilities in handling complex and large-scale data, making it a critical technology in solving a wide range of problems, but it often requires substantial computational resources and extensive training data. As a result, it continues to drive innovations and breakthroughs in various fields. Figure 2.7 shows applications of deep learning.

2.5 EVALUATION MEASURES

The evaluation measures of classification quality can be computed using the confusion matrix, where each element represents:

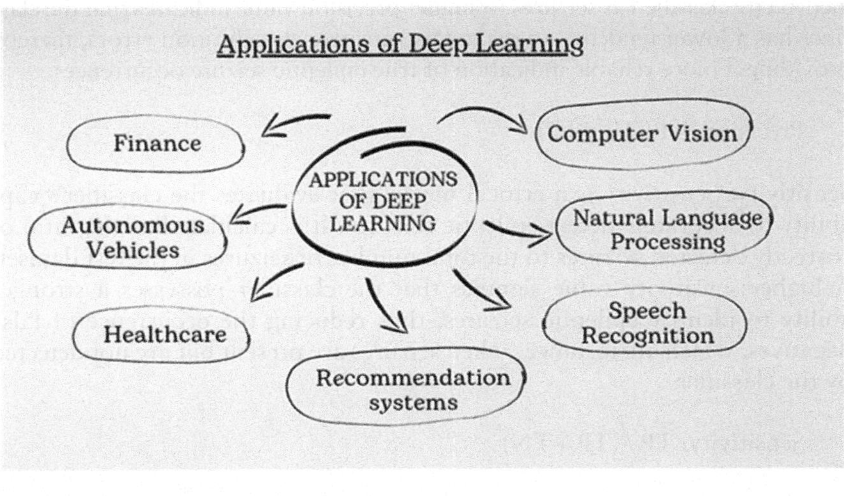

Figure 2.7 Applications of deep learning.

- True Negative (TN): The number of cases correctly classified as nonseizure periods.
- False Positive (FP): The number of cases incorrectly classified as epileptic seizures when they are nonseizure periods (Type I error).
- False Negative (FN): The number of cases incorrectly classified as nonseizure periods when they are epileptic seizures (Type II error).
- True Positive (TP): The number of cases correctly classified as epileptic seizures.

Based on a comparison between predicted and actual classes, various measures of classification quality can be calculated, such as accuracy, sensitivity, specificity, precision, etc. These measures help assess the effectiveness of the classifier and understand how well it performs on new, unknown data. **Accuracy:** Accuracy is a fundamental metric in evaluating classifier performance, as it represents the ratio of correctly classified instances (both positive and negative) to the total number of instances. A higher accuracy value signifies that the classifier effectively categorizes instances into their respective classes. It provides a comprehensive measure of overall classifier effectiveness in classification tasks.

Accuracy: (TP + TN) / (TP + TN + FP + FN)

Precision: Precision is a crucial metric that assesses the classifier's ability to accurately identify epileptic seizures among all signals classified as seizures. Mathematically, it is calculated as the ratio of correctly classified epileptic seizures to the sum of correctly classified epileptic seizures and other signals incorrectly classified as seizures. A higher precision value indicates that the classifier has a lower tendency to make false positive classification errors, thereby providing a more reliable indication of true epileptic seizure occurrences.

Precision: TP/(TP + FP)

Sensitivity: Sensitivity is a critical metric that evaluates the classifier's capability to accurately detect epileptic seizures. It is calculated as the ratio of correctly detected seizures to the total number of seizures in the test dataset. A higher sensitivity value signifies that the classifier possesses a stronger ability to identify epileptic seizures, thus reducing the occurrence of false negatives, which are instances when seizures are present but are not detected by the classifier.

Sensitivity: TP / (TP + FN)

Specificity: Specificity is a crucial metric that evaluates the classifier's ability to accurately classify nonseizure signals. It is calculated as the ratio of correctly classified nonseizure signals to the sum of correctly classified nonseizure signals and signals incorrectly classified as seizures. A higher specificity value indicates that the classifier exhibits a lower tendency to make false positive classification errors, thereby enhancing its reliability in distinguishing nonseizure signals from seizure signals.

Specificity: TN / (TN + FP)

DNNs represent a powerful class of ML models capable of learning complex representations from data. Their ability to automatically extract hierarchical features has led to significant advancements across a wide range of applications, with promising opportunities for further innovation and impact in the future. They comprise of layers of nonlinear computational units, or neurons, structured to progressively extract intricate, robust, and distinctive features from input data. In contemporary era, DNNs have revolutionized the field of AI, with numerous research breakthroughs enhancing the efficacy of projects in this domain. These advancements empower developers to attain superior and more durable outcomes, leading to the gradual displacement of traditional ML approaches. They are type of artificial neural network characterized by multiple layers of interconnected nodes, or neurons, organized in a hierarchical fashion. Each layer processes input data received from previous layer, with each subsequent layer extracting increasingly abstract and complex features from input. DNNs leverage nonlinear activation functions and learn through the process of training on large datasets using techniques like backpropagation. They excel at tasks like pattern recognition, classification, regression, and feature extraction across various domains, including computer vision, NLP, speech recognition, etc. They have significantly advanced the field of AI and ML, enabling the development of sophisticated models capable of handling complex real-world problems. DNNs have demonstrated remarkable capabilities in generating synthetic medical images, offering numerous benefits for various applications in healthcare. By leveraging techniques such as generative adversarial networks (GANs) and variational autoencoders (VAEs), DNNs can generate high-fidelity images that closely resemble real medical data.

2.6 CONTRIBUTION OF DNN IN DATA AUGMENTATION, TRAINING SET EXPANSION, AND SIMULATION CREATION

DNNs have emerged as effective tools for enhancing pattern recognition efficiency across diverse anatomical regions in medical imaging. These models exhibit promising outcomes in organs like the kidney, liver, brain, bone, breast, chest, eyes, and beyond. Their capacity for precise and automated analysis of medical images holds promise for improving diagnostic accuracy, facilitating treatment planning, and monitoring disease progression. Synthetic medical images generated by DNNs serve multiple purposes, including augmenting data, expanding training sets, and developing realistic simulations for training and testing in healthcare.

Data Augmentation: Synthetic medical image generation enables the augmentation of existing datasets by creating additional samples with diverse variations. This process helps address the challenge of limited annotated data, which is common in medical imaging tasks. By generating synthetic images with different anatomical variations, pathologies, imaging modalities, and imaging artifacts, DNNs enhance the robustness and generalization of ML models trained on these augmented datasets.

Training Set Expansion: Deep learning models require large and diverse training datasets to learn complex patterns and generalize well to unseen data. However, collecting annotated medical images can be time-consuming, costly, and limited by factors such as patient privacy regulations and rare clinical conditions. Synthetic image generation enables the expansion of training sets by synthesizing realistic images that supplement the available data. This approach enhances the model's ability to capture the variability and complexity of real-world medical scenarios, leading to improved performance and reliability.

Creating Realistic Simulations: Synthetic medical images serve as valuable resources for developing realistic simulations for training and testing purposes. By generating images that mimic various clinical scenarios, DNNs enable researchers and clinicians to simulate diagnostic procedures, surgical interventions, and medical treatments in a controlled and safe environment. These simulations facilitate training and skill development for healthcare professionals, enhance medical education and training programs, and enable the evaluation of new imaging techniques and diagnostic algorithms in virtual settings. Moreover, synthetic medical images offer advantages in scenarios where obtaining real patient data is impractical or ethically challenging, such as rare diseases, experimental treatments, or invasive procedures. Additionally, by controlling the generation process, researchers can manipulate specific parameters to study the impact of different factors on imaging outcomes, such as noise levels, imaging protocols, or disease progression. However, it is essential to validate the realism and clinical relevance of synthetic medical images to ensure their utility and reliability in practical applications. Incorporating expert knowledge, domain-specific constraints, and quality assurance measures into the generation process helps produce synthetic images that faithfully represent real clinical data and support meaningful insights and decision-making in healthcare. DNNs have indeed transformed various aspects of medical image processing, leading to significant advancements in diagnosis, treatment planning, and patient care.

Their ability to leverage large-scale datasets and extract meaningful features from medical images has revolutionized the field in several ways:

Improved Diagnostic Accuracy: DNNs excel at detecting subtle patterns and abnormalities in medical images, leading to enhanced diagnostic accuracy across a wide range of conditions. From identifying tumors and lesions in radiological images to detecting early signs of diseases such as Alzheimer's or cancer, DNNs empower healthcare professionals with more precise and reliable diagnostic tools.

Enhanced Treatment Planning: By providing detailed insights into the morphology, structure, and function of anatomical and physiological systems, DNNs enable more informed treatment planning and decision-making. Clinicians can utilize DNN-derived information to tailor treatment strategies, optimize surgical interventions, and personalize therapies based on individual patient characteristics and disease profiles.

Facilitated Image Analysis: DNNs automate and streamline the process of medical image analysis, saving time and reducing the burden on healthcare professionals. Tasks such as segmentation, registration, and feature extraction, which were previously labor-intensive and subjective, can now be performed rapidly and consistently with the help of DNN-based algorithms. This enables clinicians to focus on interpreting results and formulating clinical judgments rather than on manual image processing tasks.

Early Disease Detection and Prevention: DNNs contribute to early disease detection and prevention by identifying subtle indicators and biomarkers in medical images that may precede clinical symptoms. By detecting diseases at an earlier stage, healthcare providers can initiate timely interventions, monitor disease progression, and implement preventive measures to improve patient outcomes and mitigate long-term complications.

Support for Clinical Decision-Making: DNNs serve as valuable decision support tools for healthcare professionals, providing additional insights and recommendations based on quantitative analysis of medical images. Integrating DNN-based algorithms into clinical workflows enhances decision-making processes, reduces diagnostic errors, and increases confidence in treatment planning and patient management.

Adoption of DNNs in medical image processing has transformed the practice of medicine, offering unparalleled opportunities to advance diagnostic capabilities, optimize treatment strategies, and improve patient outcomes. As DNN technologies continue to evolve and mature, their impact on healthcare is expected to grow, paving the way for more personalized, precise, and effective patient care across various medical specialties and settings. They have become instrumental in optimizing medical imaging workflows and enhancing clinical care delivery. DNNs have become essential tools in

Table 2.5 Types of deep learning for specific healthcare technology

Types of deep learning	*Healthcare technology*
Image segmentation	Computer-aided diagnosis (CAD) and prognosis
Image registration	Lesion/landmark detection
Image fusion	Microscopic image analysis
Image annotation	Computer-aided diagnosis (CAD)

the field of medical imaging for several reasons, mentioned below are the reasons:

Efficiency in Image Analysis: DNNs excel at automating and streamlining image analysis tasks, such as segmentation, classification, and detection of abnormalities. By leveraging large datasets, DNNs can learn complex patterns and features from medical images, enabling them to perform these tasks with high accuracy and efficiency. Table 2.5 gives types of deep learning for images in healthcare technology.

Speed and Consistency: DNN-based algorithms can analyze medical images much faster than manual methods, allowing for rapid interpretation of results. Moreover, DNNs ensure consistency in analysis across different cases and healthcare providers, reducing variability and improving reliability in diagnostic assessments.

Enhanced Diagnostic Accuracy: DNNs have demonstrated the ability to identify subtle patterns and abnormalities in medical images that may not be apparent to the human eye. This can lead to improved diagnostic accuracy, earlier detection of diseases, and more timely interventions, ultimately enhancing patient outcomes.

Personalized Medicine: DNNs enable the extraction of detailed quantitative information from medical images, facilitating personalized treatment planning and monitoring. By analyzing imaging data at the individual patient level, DNNs help healthcare providers tailor interventions to the specific needs and characteristics of each patient, leading to more effective and targeted care.

Workflow Optimization: By automating repetitive tasks and reducing manual intervention, DNNs optimize medical imaging workflows, allowing healthcare providers to focus their time and expertise on more complex and critical aspects of patient care. This increases operational efficiency, reduces turnaround times, and enhances overall productivity in healthcare settings.

Research and Development: DNNs serve as powerful tools for research and development in medical imaging, enabling the exploration of novel imaging techniques, biomarkers, and diagnostic algorithms. By facilitating the analysis of large-scale imaging datasets, DNNs contribute to the advancement of medical knowledge and the development of innovative diagnostic and therapeutic approaches.

DNNs have become indispensable assets in optimizing medical imaging workflows and enhancing clinical care delivery. Their ability to automate tasks, improve diagnostic accuracy, and facilitate personalized medicine makes them valuable tools for healthcare providers in their pursuit of better patient outcomes.

2.7 SIGNIFICANT ROLE OF DEEP NEURAL NETWORK IN ADVANCING THE HEALTHCARE INDUSTRY

In modern times, the prevalence of cardiovascular disease (CD) is on the rise, leading to an increasing fatality rate. However, wearable devices, although capable of real-time patient monitoring, are not universally embraced due to discomfort, especially among children and the elderly. In response, deep learning emerges as a solution for data collection, leveraging wearable devices' capabilities while minimizing patient discomfort. This integration of deep learning with wearable technology enables the real-time assessment of patient conditions. Moreover, modern healthcare systems are leveraging smart technologies such as computational learning systems, structural health monitoring (SHM), Internet of Things (IoT), and expert medical professionals to address acute diseases like diabetes, Alzheimer's disease, genetic disorders, cancer, and respiratory ailments. By incorporating these technologies and expertise, healthcare providers can detect patient conditions in real time and predict future health trajectories. The prevalence of CDs is alarming, affecting approximately 30% of the population. To address this challenge, computational and robotic learning techniques are deployed for smart health monitoring. This approach combines health monitoring devices, IoT infrastructure, and AI to provide comprehensive healthcare solutions. AI, particularly ML algorithms, is instrumental in analyzing healthcare data and deriving actionable insights. Deep learning models, such as CNNs, are specifically adept at processing medical imaging data, including ultrasound, MRI, CT scans, and X-rays.

Integration of deep learning, wearable technology, and smart healthcare systems holds immense promise for revolutionizing patient monitoring, disease detection, and treatment planning in the modern era. By harnessing the power of AI and advanced technologies, healthcare providers can deliver more effective, personalized, and efficient care to patients, thereby mitigating the burden of CDs and other acute health conditions. Healthcare industry is entering a new era abundance of biomedical data is assuming increasing significance. Precision medicine, as an example, strives to

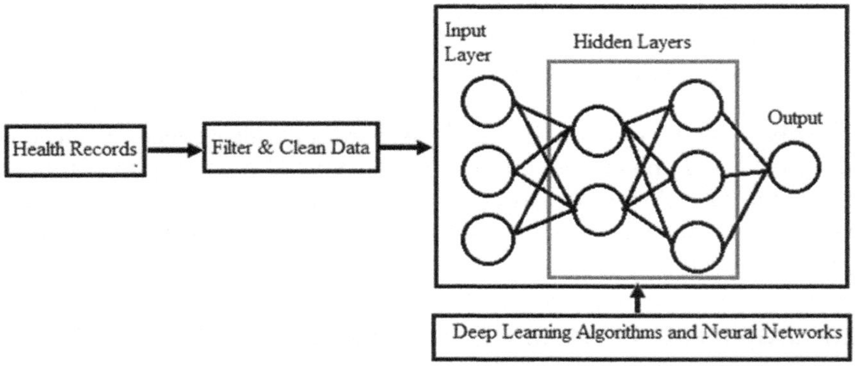

Figure 2.8 Healthcare informatics utilizes DL techniques.

optimize treatment delivery by considering multiple facets of patient data, such as variability in molecular traits, environmental factors, electronic health records, and lifestyle choices [14–16]. The vast availability of biomedical data presents both significant opportunities and challenges in healthcare research. A fundamental challenge lies in exploring the associations among the myriad pieces of information within these datasets. This exploration is essential for developing reliable medical tools using data-driven approaches and ML techniques. Figure 2.8 shows the application of DNN in healthcare.

2.8 SCOPE OF DEEP LEARNING IN BIOMEDICAL ANALYSIS, DISEASE PREDICTION, AND TREATMENT

The scope of deep learning in the field of biomedical analysis, disease prediction, and treatment is incredibly promising. Deep learning techniques have the potential to revolutionize healthcare and have already made significant advancements in various aspects of medical research and practice. This is demonstrated in Table 2.6.

As volume of healthcare data continues to grow, deep learning models have the potential to unlock valuable insights, enhance early disease detection, improve treatment outcomes, and drive innovation in medical research. Though, it is essential to address challenges like data privacy, regulatory compliance, and validation of deep learning models in real clinical settings to ensure their accountability and effective implementation in healthcare.

Table 2.6 Scope of deep learning in healthcare domain

Healthcare technology	*Machine learning model*	*Advantages*
Medical imaging analysis	Deep learning models, predominantly convolutional neural networks (CNNs), have shown remarkable success in analyzing medical images, like X-rays, CT scans, MRIs, and pathology slides. They can assist in early disease detection, image segmentation, and feature extraction	Improving accuracy and efficiency in the diagnosis of conditions like cancer, cardiovascular diseases, and neurological disorders
Disease prediction and risk assessment	Deep learning algorithms can scrutinize vast healthcare datasets, comprising patient records, genomic data, and environmental factors to predict disease risk and assess individual susceptibility	Identifying high-risk individuals, personalizing preventive measures, and enabling early intervention for conditions like diabetes, heart disease, and cancer
Drug discovery and development	Deep learning accelerates drug discovery process by predicting the binding affinity of molecules, simulating drug-protein interactions, and optimizing lead compounds	Faster and more cost-effective drug development, repurposing existing drugs, and exploring new therapeutic targets
Clinical decision support	Deep learning models analyze patient data to provide evidence-based recommendations, diagnose diseases, and predict treatment outcomes	Enhancing clinical decision-making, reducing diagnostic errors, and optimizing treatment strategies
Personalized treatment	Deep learning assists in tailoring treatment plans constructed on individual patient features, like genetic profiles, medical history, and real-time health data	Precision medicine, improving treatment efficacy, and minimizing adverse effects
Natural language processing (NLP)	Deep learning-driven NLP can extract valuable information from unstructured clinical notes, research papers, and electronic health records	Automating medical report generation, extracting insights from vast medical datasets, and improving information retrieval
Disease monitoring progression prediction	Deep learning models analyze patient data over time to predict disease progression, therapeutic responses, and potential complications	Improved management of chronic diseases, early detection of deteriorations, and personalized treatment adjustments
Vaccine development and epidemic prediction	Deep learning techniques support the development of vaccines by identifying potential vaccine candidates and analyzing viral genomes. They can also predict disease outbreaks	Accelerating vaccine development, understanding viral evolution, and early detection of epidemics

2.9 CONCLUSION

AI has revolutionized the world and has impacted our daily life. ML algorithms and deep learning are advanced computing techniques that are very useful for image and video analysis process. In healthcare domain, ML methods are used in several stages of medical image analysis thereby reducing human intervention and also improving quality of outcomes. By using ML algorithms, it is convenient to discover a variety of hidden patterns between the pixels.

REFERENCES

[1] K. P. Murphy, *Machine learning: A probabilistic perspective*. MIT Press, 2012.
[2] T. Mitchell, *Machine learning*. McGraw Hill, 1997.
[3] I. Goodfellow, Y. Bengio, and A. Courville, *Deep learning*. MIT Press, 2016.
[4] Y. LeCun, Y. Bengio, and G. Hinton, "Deep learning." *Nature*, vol. 521, no. 7553, pp. 436–444, 2015.
[5] J. Schmidhuber, "Deep learning in neural networks: An overview." *Neural Networks*, vol. 61, pp. 85–117, 2015.
[6] D. Silver et al., "Mastering the game of Go with deep neural networks and tree search." *Nature*, vol. 529, pp. 484–489, 2016.
[7] M. Esteva, A. Kuprel, R. A. Novoa, et al., "Dermatologist-level classification of skin cancer with deep neural networks." *Nature*, vol. 542, pp. 115–118, 2017.
[8] A. Krizhevsky, I. Sutskever, and G. E. Hinton, "ImageNet classification with deep convolutional neural networks." in *Proc. NIPS*, 2012, pp. 1097–1105.
[9] J. Devlin, M. Chang, K. Lee, and K. Toutanova, "BERT: Pre-training of deep bidirectional transformers for language understanding." in *Proc. NAACL-HLT*, 2019, pp. 4171–4186.
[10] G. E. Hinton, S. Osindero, and Y.-W. Teh, "A fast learning algorithm for deep belief nets." *Neural Comput.*, vol. 18, no. 7, pp. 1527–1554, 2006.
[11] S. Russell and P. Norvig, *Artificial intelligence: A modern approach*, 4th ed. Pearson, 2021.
[12] F. Chollet, *Deep learning with Python*, 2nd ed. Manning, 2021.
[13] T. Dean et al., "AI in hospitals: Applications and future prospects." *Hosp. Mgmt. Rev.*, vol. 18, no. 5, pp. 31–44, 2020.
[14] Precision Medicine Initiative (NIH). www.nih.gov/precision-medicine-initiative-cohort-program Accessed 12 November 2016.
[15] G. H. Lyman and H. L. Moses. "Biomarker tests for molecularly targeted therapies--the key to unlocking precision medicine." *N. Engl. J. Med.*, vol. 375, no. 1, pp. 4–6, 2016. doi:10.1056/NEJMp1604033
[16] F. S. Collins and H. Varmus. "A new initiative on precision medicine." *N. Engl. J. Med.*, vol. 372, no. 9, pp. 793–795, 2015. doi:10.1056/NEJMp1500523

Subjective Questions (Long Answers)

Q1. What are the core principles of machine learning, and how do they differ from traditional programming approaches? Explain the different types of machine learning (supervised, unsupervised, and reinforcement learning) with relevant examples from the healthcare sector.
Q2. Discuss the challenges and limitations of applying machine learning techniques in healthcare and how they can be addressed.
Answer: Some challenges include:
Q3. How does machine learning contribute to personalized medicine in healthcare? Provide examples of its real-world applications.
Q4. What are the primary components of deep learning, and how do they enable more advanced processing of complex data compared to traditional machine learning?
Q5. What are the ethical considerations and potential biases when implementing machine learning and deep learning models in healthcare, and how can they be mitigated?

Subjective Questions (Short Answers)

Q1. Explain the significance of neural networks in deep learning. How do neural networks differ from other machine learning algorithms?
Q2. Describe how hyperparameter tuning and model evaluation impact the performance of machine learning models.
Q3. What are features in machine learning?
Q4. How does high bias in a machine learning model affect patient outcomes in healthcare?
Q5. What is the bias-variance tradeoff in healthcare-focused machine learning models?

Objective Questions:

1. Which type of machine learning is most commonly used for predicting patient outcomes based on historical medical data?
   A) Unsupervised learning
   B) Reinforcement learning
   C) Supervised learning
   D) Semi-supervised learning
   Answer: C) Supervised learning
2. What is the main challenge associated with using machine learning models in healthcare?
   A) Lack of medical data
   B) Ensuring patient privacy and data security

C) The model's inability to process numerical data
D) Lack of clinical applicability
Answer: B) Ensuring patient privacy and data security

3. In healthcare, what is the impact of high variance in a machine learning model?
   A) The model underfits the training data
   B) The model fails to identify key medical features
   C) The model overfits the training data and performs poorly on new patients
   D) The model generalizes well to new patient data
   Answer: C) The model overfits the training data and performs poorly on new patients
4. How can machine learning be applied to healthcare for early disease detection?
   A) By analyzing patient reviews of medical treatments
   B) By using unsupervised learning to cluster patient data and identify early signs of disease
   C) By optimizing hospital resource allocation
   D) By replacing doctors in patient diagnosis
   Answer: B) By using unsupervised learning to cluster patient data and identify early signs of disease
5. In healthcare, what is one of the key benefits of deep learning over traditional machine learning?
   A) It requires less medical data
   B) It can automatically extract features from complex medical images such as MRIs and X-rays
   C) It is easier to train than traditional machine learning models
   D) It reduces the need for medical professionals
   Answer: B) It can automatically extract features from complex medical images such as MRIs and X-rays
6. Which machine learning technique is commonly used in medical image analysis, such as interpreting MRI or CT scans?
   A) Linear regression
   B) Decision trees
   C) Convolutional neural networks (CNNs)
   D) K-means clustering
   Answer: C) Convolutional neural networks (CNNs)
7. In healthcare, which of the following is an example of using unsupervised learning?
   A) Predicting a patient's risk of heart disease
   B) Grouping patients based on symptoms for further analysis
   C) Diagnosing cancer based on historical medical records
   D) Prescribing a treatment plan based on patient data
   Answer: B) Grouping patients based on symptoms for further analysis

8. Which healthcare problem can be addressed using natural language processing (NLP)?
   A) Predicting patient diagnosis from images
   B) Grouping similar patients based on lab results
   C) Analyzing clinical notes to extract useful patient information
   D) Forecasting disease outbreaks based on geographical data
   Answer: C) Analyzing clinical notes to extract useful patient information
9. Which of the following is a key challenge when training machine learning models in healthcare?
   A) The abundance of labeled data
   B) Interpreting patient data that may be noisy or incomplete
   C) The simplicity of healthcare problems
   D) Using outdated data formats
   Answer: B) Interpreting patient data that may be noisy or incomplete
10. What is the role of reinforcement learning in healthcare?
   A) To train models to diagnose diseases using static data
   B) To optimize treatment plans by learning from patient feedback and outcomes
   C) To cluster patients based on medical conditions
   D) To identify patient groups based on symptoms
   Answer: B) To optimize treatment plans by learning from patient feedback and outcomes

Chapter 3

Biomedical signal and image processing using machine learning

3.1 INTRODUCTION

Ongoing research and collaboration between engineers, clinicians, and data scientists continue to drive advancements in this interdisciplinary field. Biomedical engineering involves integrating engineering concepts, methods, and principles into the domains of medicine and biology. The integration of various physiological signals with artificial intelligence (AI) algorithms has opened up new avenues for research and application in healthcare. Algorithms for AI have brought about new methods for virtual and predictive healthcare. The signal-to-noise ratio of biomedical signals obtained by non-invasive sensors can often be low. Advanced signal processing techniques are used to process them. Neural prosthetics and brain–computer interfaces (BCIs) additionally employ these techniques. By establishing automated and computer-aided diagnosis (CAD) systems, smart sensors and modern signal processing techniques play a significant role in the healthcare industry. Advanced signal processing methods are crucial for cleaning and enhancing these signals, ensuring accurate and reliable data for further analysis. Processed biomedical signals are utilized in the classification and analysis of health conditions. AI algorithms aid in prognosis and diagnosis, providing valuable insights into the current state of health and predicting potential future developments. Incorporation of AI with biomedical signals is instrumental in the development and improvement of brain–BCIs. Neural prostheses benefit from AI algorithms for interpreting signals from the nervous system, enhancing communication between the brain and external devices. Smart sensors play a substantial role in collecting high-quality biomedical data. These sensors, when integrated with AI algorithms, enable real-time monitoring and analysis, contributing to early detection and intervention. Automated and CAD systems leverage advanced signal processing techniques. These systems assist healthcare professionals by automating the analysis of biomedical signals, leading to more efficient and accurate diagnoses.

DOI: 10.1201/9781003503033-3

3.2 IMAGE PROCESSING USING MACHINE LEARNING

The process of converting an image into digital form and carrying out specific operations to extract some valuable information from it is known as image processing. Image processing is the use of algorithms and techniques to analyze, enhance, or optimize digital images. Image processing is the process of modifying and examining images in order to improve their quality, identify patterns, or extract information. It can involve analyzing, enhancing, manipulating, and compressing. A detailed description of several image processing techniques is given in Table 3.1. Conventional image processing methods use predetermined rules and algorithms to carry out particular tasks, such as object recognition, image segmentation, and edge detection. Machine learning (ML)-based image processing uses a variety of models and algorithms to evaluate and modify images. Figure 3.1 illustrates integration of image processing with ML.

ML provides an adaptable and versatile method for processing images. ML models can automatically identify patterns and extract pertinent characteristics by training algorithms on big datasets of labeled pictures. ML is a potent tool for image processing and analysis because of its capacity to learn from data and adjust to novel circumstances. Object detection and recognition is one of the main applications of ML in image processing. Some of the goals of image processing are shown in Figure 3.2. ML algorithms can learn to recognize and locate things of interest in new images by training

Table 3.1 Image processing techniques

	Techniques	*Description*
1	Image enhancement	Techniques to improve image quality, such as contrast stretching, histogram equalization, and filtering
2	Image segmentation	Dividing an image into meaningful regions for analysis, often used for tumor detection, organ delineation, or anatomical measurements
3	Image registration	Aligning images from diverse modalities or time points to enable comparative analysis, critical in treatment planning and follow-up
4	Feature extraction	Identifying and extracting relevant features from images for quantitative analysis, aiding in automated diagnosis
5	3D reconstruction	Generating three-dimensional representations of anatomical structures, valuable for surgical planning and educational purposes
6	Machine learning in image analysis	Utilizing algorithms to automatically learn and identify patterns in medical images, assisting in diagnosis and prognosis
7	Image fusion	Combining information from different imaging modalities to provide a more comprehensive view of the patient's condition

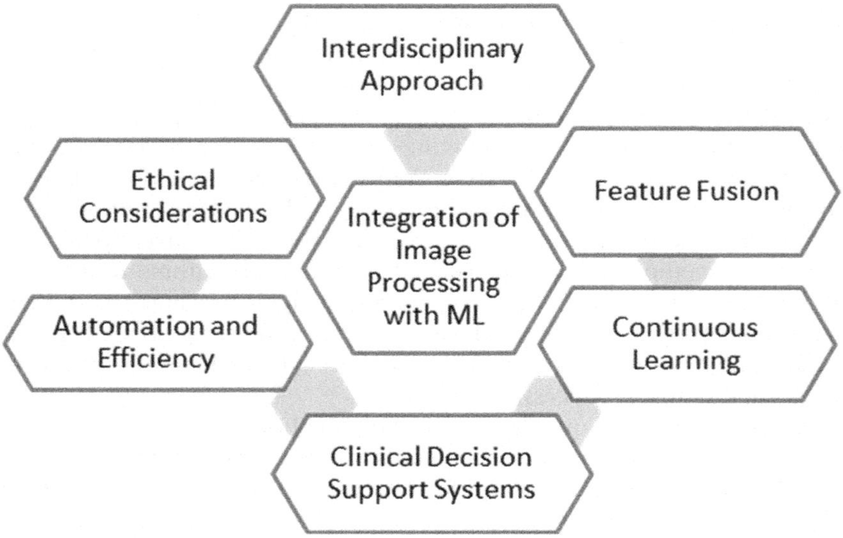

Figure 3.1 Integration of image processing with machine learning.

models that are trained by using labeled images that contain such objects as vehicles, buildings, or people. This feature has important applications in various domains, such as surveillance, where automated object detection can help spot irregularities or possible hazards.

ML algorithms are designed to process data rapidly and efficiently, even when working with smaller datasets. This capability allows them to focus on the most relevant elements of the data without being hindered by extraneous factors. However, it is important to note that accuracy can be compromised when the number of variables in the dataset is reduced. Image classification is one of the applications of ML in image processing. ML algorithms can learn to categorize new images into the right categories by training models using labeled image datasets from various categories, such as landscapes, animals, or medical images. In fields like healthcare, where precise and automated image classification can support medical imaging analysis, disease diagnosis, and treatment planning, such expertise is highly beneficial. In the context of ML intended for data analysis, significant feature extraction or feature representation lies at the midpoint of its success in achieving target assignments.

Considering the accuracy of the model depends on the quality and quantity of data. Having a complex model does not mean a better model. Preparation of a model requires its accuracy and scalability. Depending on the objective, ML methods such as random forest, decision trees, linear regression, logistic regression, support vector machines (SVM), principal

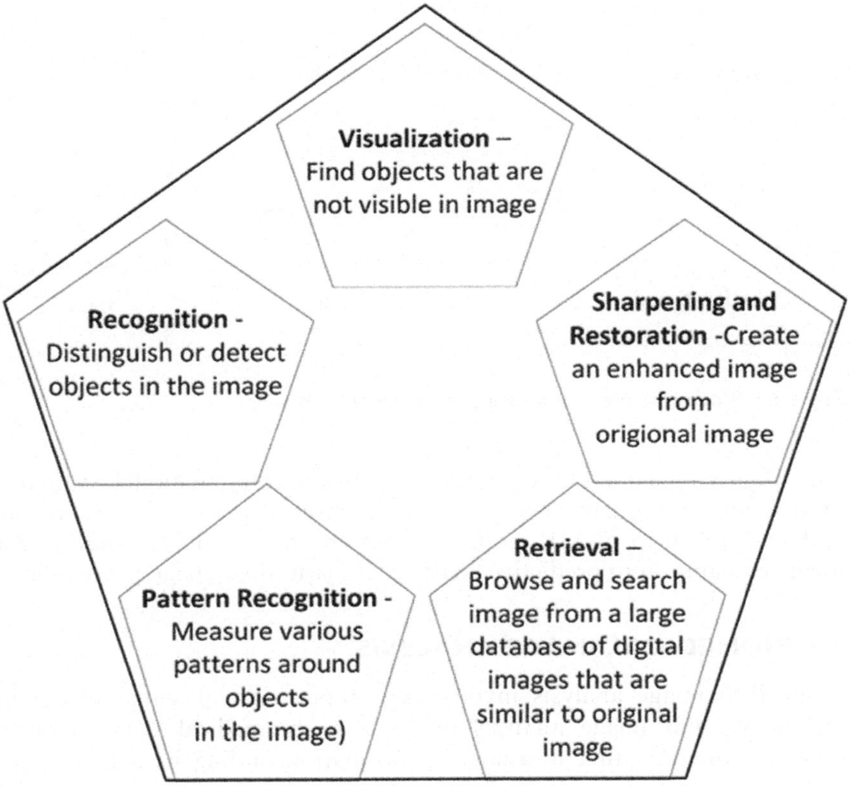

Figure 3.2 Goals of Image processing.

component analysis (PCA), K-means, Naïve Bayes, and neural networks can be used. Coming on to the next step where irrelevant features are removed from the data. It reduces the number of input features or variables in the dataset while retaining essential information. It abridges the dataset by eliminating redundant or irrelevant features, making it computationally more efficient and less prone to overfitting. It captures the most important patterns and relationships in data, preserving its inherent structure and reducing the risk of noise or irrelevant details. For instance, dimensionality reduction includes various methods such as generalized discriminant analysis, linear discriminant analysis (LDA), and PCA. It is performed during the preprocessing stage before building the model to enhance performance. Training a model forms the basis of ML by training data, and predictions of model can be improved. Every cycle in the training model involves updating weights and biases in each training step. Figure 3.3 illustrates processes involved in image processing through ML. After processes of collecting

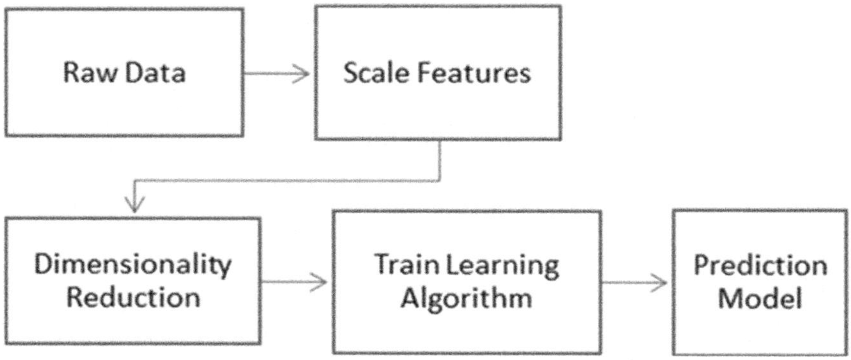

Figure 3.3 Process of image processing using machine learning.

data, preparing data, selecting an ML algorithm, training model, evaluating model, and tuning parameters, next step involved is to make predictions, and with the help of ML model, predictions can be made ranging from image recognition to predictive analytics to natural language processing.

3.3 BIOMEDICAL IMAGE ANALYSIS

Biomedical image analysis involves the application of signal processing techniques and image analysis methods to biomedical data, with the objective of extracting meaningful information, aiding in diagnosis and monitoring physiological parameters related to a disease. A significant field of research is the quantitative multiparametric analysis of biological imaging. Figure 3.4 demonstrates the collaboration of image processing algorithms and data science within a single biomedical image analysis workflow. This collaboration between different disciplines enables advanced image analysis workflows. Biomedical image analysis is one of the most imperative jobs in determining uptime, and misdiagnosis can be costly and dangerous. In the dynamic landscape of modern healthcare, the role of medical imaging is paramount in enabling precise diagnosis, treatment planning, and therapeutic monitoring. Medical image modalities have evolved significantly, presenting a diverse array of technologies that provide invaluable insights into the intricacies of the human body. Medical imaging plays a decisive role in modern healthcare, providing valuable insights for diagnosis, treatment planning, and monitoring of various medical conditions [1]. The mounting intricacy of medical data necessitates advanced analytical tools, and ML algorithms have emerged as powerful tools [2, 3]. Diverse imaging modalities utilize numerous physical principles to capture internal structures of

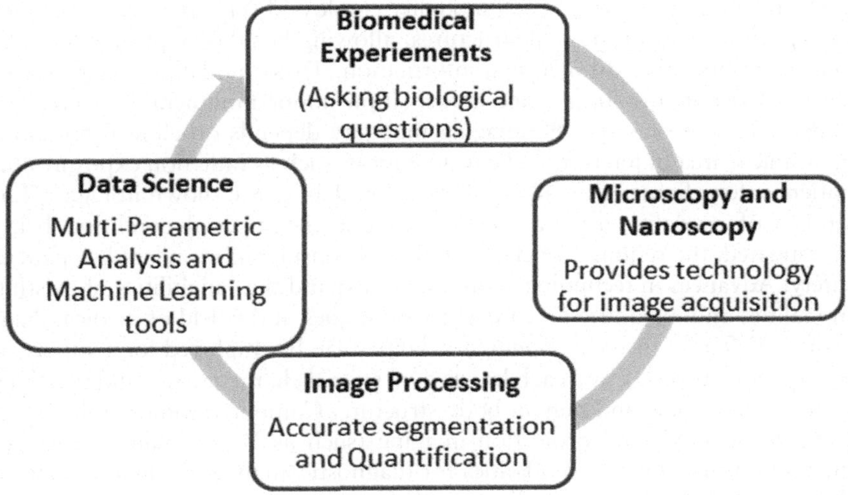

Figure 3.4 Collaboration of image processing algorithms and data science with in single biomedical image analysis workflow.

body. Image processing techniques are then employed to enhance, analyze, and interpret these images. Advancements in medical imaging have transformed landscape of diagnostics and patient care. The demand for medical imaging services such as radiography, endoscopy, computed tomography (CT), ultrasound images, mammography images (MG), magnetic resonance imaging (MRI), nuclear medicine imaging, magnetic resonance angiography, pathological testing and positron emission tomography (PET) has dramatically increased in health care systems. Besides, medical images can often be challenging and time-consuming to analyze due to a shortage of radiologists. Biomedical signal and image processing constitutes a dynamic and critical area of specialization within the broader field of biomedical engineering.

Biomedical signals acquired through noninvasive sensors often have low signal to noise ratio. They are processed using advanced signal processing methods. The classification and analysis of signals are used in prognosis and diagnosis. They are also used in BCIs and neural prostheses. Smart sensors and advanced signal processing techniques play a substantial role in healthcare sector by employing automated and CAD systems.

3.3.1 Medical imaging modalities

Medical imaging modalities refer to a diverse set of techniques and technologies used in healthcare to visualize the internal structures and functions of human body. These modalities play a critical role in medical diagnosis, treatment planning, and monitoring. Each modality employs diverse physical principles to capture images of internal structures, allowing healthcare professionals to assess anatomical and functional information. These modalities offer diverse levels of detail, resolution, and information about innumerable aspects of body. Selection of a specific imaging modality depends on clinical question, anatomical area of interest, and considerations such as radiation exposure and patient safety. Some of the medical image modalities are shown in Figure 3.5. Choice of modality depends on factors like the medical condition being investigated, the required level of detail, and considerations related to patient safety. Advances in technology continue to expand the capabilities of existing modalities and introduce new imaging techniques in the field of medical diagnostics. Different medical imaging modalities can be employed for a variety of therapeutic purposes, and each has its own special characteristics and reactions to the organ tissue and human body structure. Computed tomography (CT), MRI, ultrasound, and projection imaging (such as X-ray imaging) are frequently utilized imaging modalities for diagnostic analysis in clinics. Some of the important modalities are discussed below in brief.

X-ray imaging: They are a cornerstone in medical diagnostics, utilizing ionizing radiation to visualize bones and select soft tissues, facilitating the detection of fractures and pulmonary conditions. CT scans employ advanced X-ray technology to generate detailed cross-sectional images, offering unparalleled visualization of soft tissues and organs.

Magnetic Resonance Imaging (MRI): They are based on magnetic fields and radio waves and excel in capturing high-resolution images of soft tissues with superior contrast.

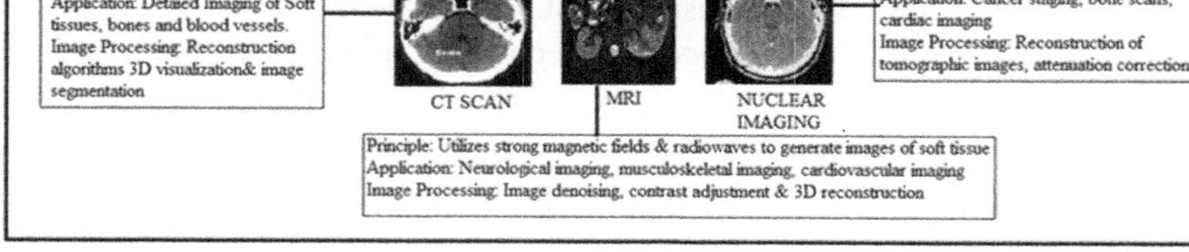

Figure 3.5 Medical image modalities.

Ultrasound imaging: This is a noninvasive modality that uses sound waves and provides real-time imaging of internal structures, commonly used for abdominal and obstetric examinations. Nuclear medicine techniques, such as single photon emission computed tomography (SPECT) and PET, employ radio pharmaceuticals to visualize both anatomical structures and physiological functions.

Fluoroscopy: This technique offers dynamic, real-time X-ray imaging. It finds applications in guiding medical procedures.

Mammography: This technique serves as a specialized X-ray modality for early detection of breast cancer.

Dental imaging: This technique encompasses intraoral and panoramic X-rays, along with cone-beam computed tomography for comprehensive dental examinations.

Endoscopy: This is a versatile modality that involves the insertion of a flexible endoscope into various body cavities to visualize and diagnose conditions, particularly in gastrointestinal and respiratory systems.

3.4 APPLICATION OF AI ALGORITHM IN BIOMEDICAL SIGNAL PROCESSING

In biomedical signal processing, physiological signals are obtained and preprocessed, and relevant information is extracted in order to classify patterns and trends within the signals. Neural activity, cardiac rhythm, muscle contraction, and other physiological processes are examples of biomedical signal sources. Electrocardiograms (ECGs), electroencephalograms (EEGs), and electromyography (EMGs) are examples of noninvasive signals that can be obtained and used as indicators of general health and for diagnosis. Figure 3.6 illustrates the biomedical signal processing workflow. ML techniques are used at various stages of image analysis to reduce human intervention and improve outcomes. Many hidden models and relationships between pixels can be discovered many times using ML. People cannot find many hidden information from images; this is important in many computer vision and imaging applications, such as automatic object detection, biomedical image analysis, analytics, space exploration, bioinformatics, and natural language processing. It has many applications in many disciplines. ML and other image analysis methods based on advanced computational techniques are very useful for applying image analysis techniques. Figure 3.7 shows the components of ML in biomedical signal processing, which are explained as follows.

Data storage: The ability to store and retrieve an enormous amount of data is a crucial part of the learning process.

Abstraction: Procedure for learning about data that has been stored. It entails developing broad notions about data in general. Applying

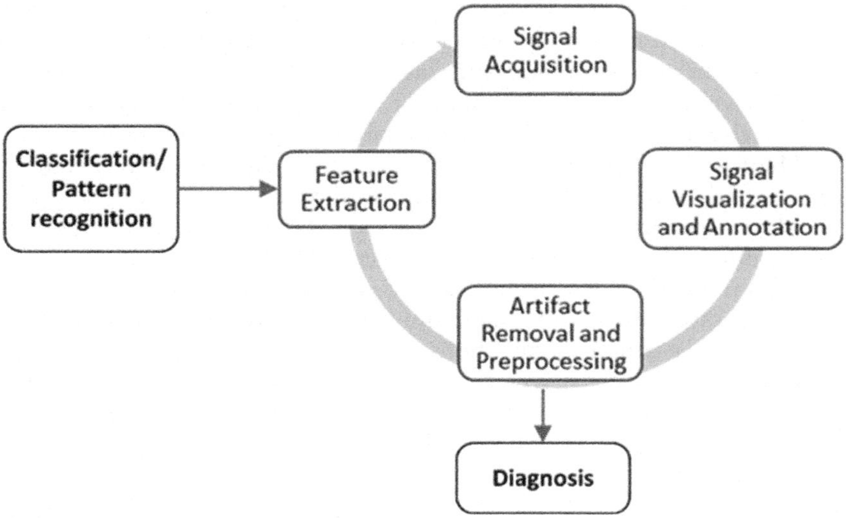

Figure 3.6 Biomedical signal processing workflow.

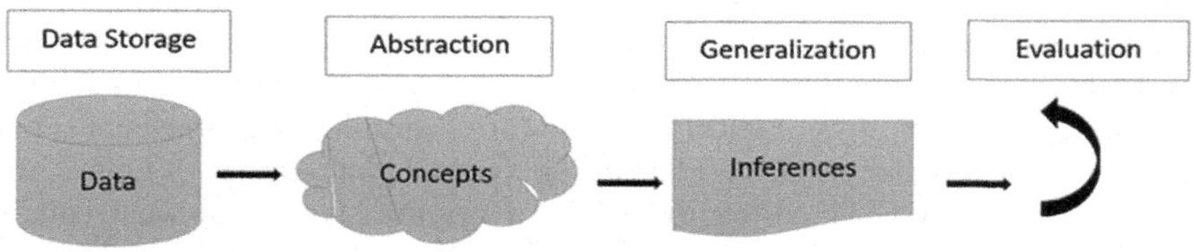

Figure 3.7 Components of machine learning in Biomedical signal processing.

established models and developing new ones are both components of knowledge development. Training is the process of fitting a model to a dataset. After training the model, the data are transformed into an abstract form that condenses the original information.

Generalization: This stage explains how information about stored data is transformed into a format that may be used for further action. These activities are to be performed on tasks that are comparable to those that have been observed previously, but they are not the same. Finding the characteristics of data that will be most important for the next tasks is the aim of generalization.

Evaluation: It is the procedures of providing users with feedback in order to evaluate how useful the knowledge they have learnt is. The entire learning process is then improved by using this feedback.

Integration of ML with biomedical signals is transforming healthcare by providing more accurate, efficient, and personalized approaches to diagnosis, treatment, and monitoring. A cross-section of biomedical signal processing cases, their applications, and the corresponding techniques is shown in Table 3.2.

Figure 3.8 illustrates elements of ML in biomedical signal processing. ML methods are causing significant progress in the field of CAD and helping to develop this field. ML methods combined with image processing techniques make CAD more powerful and reliable.

ML algorithms can assist in signal processing to enhance the quality of biomedical signals. They can automatically extract relevant features, such as peaks, amplitudes, or frequency components. ML models are used for pattern recognition and classification of biomedical signal patterns [4]. They can distinguish normal patterns from abnormal ones. Benefits include automated disease detection, accurate classification of conditions, and early identification of anomalies. ML algorithms use statistical methods to analyze large amounts of data, and thereby, we can identify patterns that can be used to make predictions and prevention. ML models are also able to generate personalized treatment plans based on individual patient characteristics

Table 3.2 Integration of machine learning techniques in context of biomedical signal and image processing [7, 10, 11]

Biomedical signal processing	*Application*	*Machine learning techniques*
Electrocardiogram (ECG) signal processing	Detection of arrhythmias, heart rate variability analysis	Deep learning models for abnormality detection, classification algorithms for arrhythmia recognition
Electroencephalogram (EEG) signal processing	Brain–computer interfaces, epilepsy detection	Convolutional neural networks (CNNs) for feature extraction, classification algorithms for seizure prediction
Electromyogram (EMG) signal processing	Prosthetic control, muscle disorder diagnosis	Pattern recognition algorithms for gesture recognition, neural networks for muscle activity analysis
Magnetic resonance imaging (MRI)	Tumor detection, image segmentation	Convolutional neural networks (CNNs) for image segmentation, generative models for image synthesis
Computed tomography (CT)	Lesion detection, organ segmentation	Deep learning models for image analysis, object detection algorithms
Ultrasound Imaging	Tissue characterization, fetal monitoring	CNNs for image enhancement, classification models for tissue classification

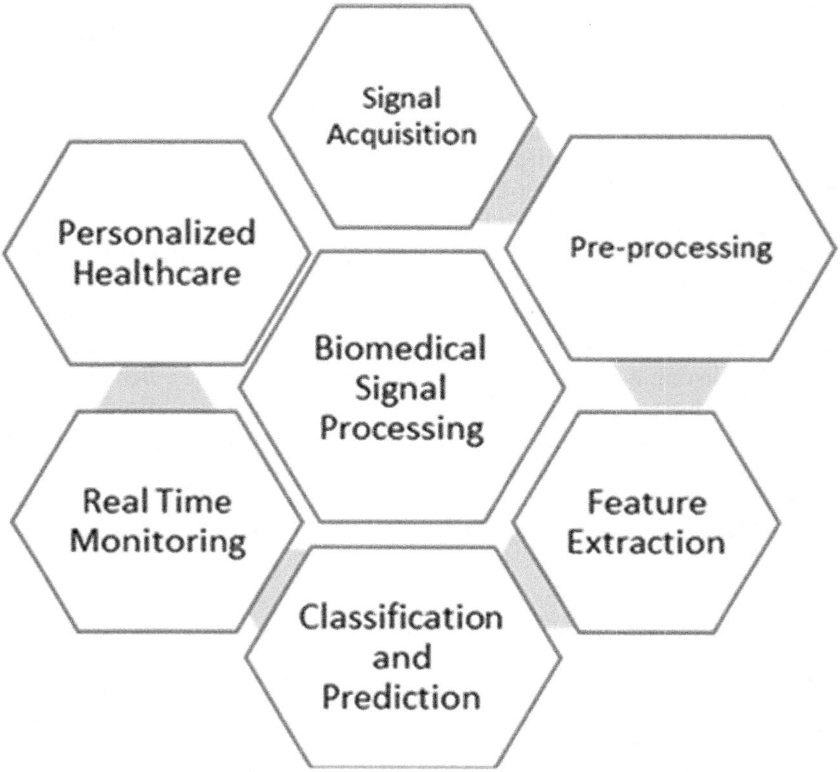

Figure 3.8 Elements of machine learning in biomedical signal processing.

and responses, and therefore, they are used in conjunction with medical imaging modalities to provide comprehensive view of a patient's health. ML is employed in the development of rehabilitation systems and assistive technologies that respond to adapt based on biomedical signals. Moreover, these algorithms can effectively denoise biomedical signals, improving signal clarity and aiding in more accurate analysis. ML models can also analyze longitudinal biomedical signal data to create predictive models for disease progression. At the same time, there are various factors that are challenging the efficient deployment of the ML algorithms to the signal processing. Table 3.3 describes the challenges and considerations at the intersection of ML and biomedical signal and image processing.

ML has found numerous applications in biomedical signal processing, contributing to advancements in diagnostics, patient monitoring, and personalized medicine [5]. Some key applications of ML in biomedical signal processing are discussed as follows:

Table 3.3 Challenges and considerations at the intersection of machine learning and biomedical signal and image processing

Challenges and considerations	*Description*
Data quality and quantity	Limited availability of annotated and diverse biomedical datasets Data augmentation techniques and transfer learning to address data scarcity
Interoperability	The "black-box" nature of some machine learning models Efforts towards developing interpretable models for clinical adoption
Real-time processing	Some applications, especially in clinical settings, require real-time processing Optimization of algorithms and use of hardware acceleration for faster computations
Ethical and regulatory considerations	Privacy concerns regarding patient data Adherence to regulatory standards (e.g., HIPAA) and ethical guidelines in research and deployment

Disease Diagnosis: ML models analyze biomedical signals such as ECG, EEG, or biomarker data, to assist in the diagnosis of diseases. These models can identify patterns associated with specific conditions, enabling early detection and accurate diagnosis.

Cardiovascular Disease Risk Assessment: ML algorithms analyze signals related to cardiovascular health, including blood pressure, heart rate variability, and ECG signals, to assess the risk of cardiovascular diseases. Predictive models help in identifying individuals at higher risk and guiding preventive measures.

Neurological Disorders Diagnosis: ML techniques process EEG signals to aid in the diagnosis of neurological disorders such as epilepsy, Alzheimer's disease, and Parkinson's disease. These models can identify abnormal patterns indicative of specific neurological conditions.

Sleep Monitoring and Disorders Detection: ML is applied to signals such as electroencephalography (EEG) and actigraphy data for sleep monitoring. Algorithms can detect sleep stages, assess sleep quality, and identify sleep disorders based on patterns in signals.

Remote Patient Monitoring: ML models analyze signals from wearable devices, such as smart watches and fitness trackers, to monitor patients remotely. This is particularly valuable for chronic disease management, providing continuous insights into patient's health status.

Detection of Abnormalities in Medical Imaging: ML algorithms are employed for the analysis of medical imaging signals, including MRI, CT, and ultrasound. These models can automatically detect and classify abnormalities such as tumors, lesions, or anomalies in medical images.

Personalized Treatment Planning: ML models analyze biomedical signals and other patient data to create personalized treatment plans. This approach tailors medical interventions based on individual patient's characteristics, improving treatment efficacy.

Drug Response Prediction: ML algorithms analyze genomic and proteomic data to predict how individual patients may respond to specific drugs. This helps in optimizing treatment regimens and minimizing adverse effects.

Biological Signal Processing for Genomics: ML techniques process genomic data to identify patterns associated with genetic variations, mutations, and disease susceptibility. This is crucial for understanding genetic basis of diseases and developing targeted therapies.

Voice and Speech Analysis for Health Monitoring: ML is applied to analyze voice and speech patterns for health monitoring. Changes in speech characteristics can be indicative of conditions such as neurodegenerative diseases or respiratory disorders.

Gait Analysis for Movement Disorders: ML models process signals related to gait and movement to assess and diagnose movement disorders. This is particularly relevant in conditions like Parkinson's disease.

Electromyography (EMG) for Muscular Disorders: ML is used in the analysis of EMG signals to detect and diagnose muscular disorders. This includes conditions such as muscular dystrophy and myasthenia gravis.

Bioinformatics and Computational Biology: ML techniques play a crucial role in processing and analyzing large-scale biological data, including DNA sequences and protein structures, contributing to advancements in bioinformatics and computational biology.

Early Detection of Sepsis: ML models process physiological signals and clinical data to predict and detect sepsis at an early stage. Early identification allows for timely intervention and improved patient outcomes.

Mental Health Monitoring: ML models analyze signals related to mental health, like EEG or heart rate variability, to monitor stress levels, anxiety, and other mental health conditions.

These applications highlight diverse ways in which ML enhances analysis of biomedical signals, providing valuable insights for healthcare professionals and contributing to more personalized and effective medical interventions.

3.5 DEEP LEARNING IN BIOMEDICAL SIGNAL PROCESSING AND STATE-OF-THE-ART APPLICATIONS

Biomedical image analysis methods are gradually changing from manual research to computer-aided solutions to save time and improve diagnostic quality. Biomedical image analysis with the help of deep learning (DL) is one of the main and active areas of research. Several researchers are working in this field, as computer-aided diagnostic solutions with the help of DL are well known for their effectiveness. The application of DL in biomedical signal processing enables more accurate and efficient analysis of complex physiological data, leading to improved diagnostics, patient monitoring, and personalized healthcare. As technology advances, integration of DL models with biomedical signals continues to evolve, offering new possibilities for healthcare innovation. Typically, biomedical images such as X-ray, computed tomography (CT-scan), MRI, PET, microscopy, and ultrasound are reviewed and interpreted by a doctor or radiologist. Human are prone to error and have trouble identifying images accurately, mostly due to the unusual nature of disease. Furthermore, human limitations prevent experts from discovering hidden patterns in biomedical images. To some extent, manual diagnosis can be replaced by computerized diagnosis to diminish labor and error. Integration of DL and biomedical signals offers new possibilities for diagnostics, monitoring, and personalized medicine. DL techniques are well-suited for processing complex and high-dimensional biomedical signal data, providing accurate and automated analyses. Table 3.4 illustrates ways in which DL is integrated with biomedical signals.

Integration of DL with biomedical signals has the potential to revolutionize healthcare by providing more accurate diagnostics, real-time monitoring, and personalized treatment strategies. It allows for more sophisticated analysis, enhanced accuracy, and discovery of intricate patterns that may not be easily discernible through traditional methods. As technology continues to advance, the role of DL in biomedical signal processing is expected to grow, leading to enhanced healthcare outcomes and a deeper understanding of physiological processes. The use of ML techniques in healthcare is expected to contribute significantly to the fight against uncommon diseases. Amyotrophic lateral sclerosis (ALS) is a disease with many unanswered questions. Biomedical signals in ALS show potential as indicators that, when combined with intelligent algorithms, may be helpful for applications within the disease's context. Based on the findings, scientists have distinguished three categories of ML applications in conjunction with biological data inputs in the context of ALS: survival prediction (5.56%), communication (22.22%), and diagnosis (72.22%). Various biomedical signals and algorithmic models have been documented, and there are currently promising methods, irrespective of their classifications [6].

Table 3.4 Integration of deep learning and biomedical signals

Deep Learning	*Application*
Signal denoising and enhancement	Autoencoders and denoising autoencoders can be employed to denoise biomedical signals, enlightening signal quality for more accurate analysis
Feature extraction	DL models, especially convolutional neural networks (CNNs), can automatically extract relevant features from biomedical signals without the need for manual feature engineering
Pattern recognition and classification	DL models, including CNNs and recurrent neural networks (RNNs), excel in recognizing complex patterns and classifying biomedical signals into diverse categories, aiding in disease diagnosis
Diagnostics and disease prediction	Long short-term memory networks (LSTMs) and other recurrent architectures are employed for time-series data, allowing for prediction of disease progression or onset of medical conditions based on continuous monitoring of biomedical signals
Electrocardiogram (ECG) analysis	DL models are used for automated detection of cardiac abnormalities, like arrhythmias or anomalies, in ECG signals
Electroencephalogram (EEG) interpretation	CNNs and recurrent neural networks are applied for analysis of EEG signals, aiding in identification of neurological disorders and brain activity patterns
Biomedical image fusion	Integration of DL with biomedical imaging modalities, like combining MRI and PET images, for more comprehensive understanding of anatomical and functional information
Personalized treatment plans	DL models analyze biomedical signals to predict individual patient responses to specific treatments, allowing for the development of personalized treatment plans
Remote patient monitoring	DL facilitates continuous monitoring of biomedical signals remotely, enabling early detection of health issues and timely interventions
Sleep monitoring and disorders	DL is used for the analysis of signals like respiratory patterns and heart rate variability in sleep studies, aiding in the diagnosis of sleep disorders
Human activity recognition	DL models process signals from accelerometers or gyroscopes to recognize and classify human activities, assisting in health and fitness monitoring
Physiological signal fusion	Integrating information from multiple biomedical signals, like combining ECG and respiration data, to provide a more holistic view of physiological conditions
Drug development and pharmacogenomics	DL contributes to the analysis of genomic and molecular data to predict drug responses and identify potential drug candidates
Rehabilitation technologies	DL is used in the development of assistive technologies and rehabilitation devices that respond to signals related to muscle activity or neural patterns

AI can enhance analysis and interpretation of biomedical signals, contributing to more accurate and efficient diagnostic processes. In their research, AlHinai et al. [7] give an overview of biomedical signal processing using AI, concentrating on different body organs. Later in their chapter, they apply mitigation techniques such as Butterworth filters and finite impulse response filters to reduce noise in the ECG signal. By helping doctors get a second opinion, CAD aims to reduce the rate of incorrect diagnoses. The primary goal of processing biomedical signals, which are data from physiological systems under study, is to extract pertinent information [8]. A signal is a phenomenon that transmits data. Signals utilized primarily to extract information about a biological system for examination are known as biomedical signals. The entire information extraction procedure can be as easy as a doctor using their fingertips to feel a patient's blood pressure pulse and estimate their mean heart rate, or it can be as complicated as using a sophisticated CT machine to analyze the soft tissue structure inside the body.

The DWT technique was used by Doulah et al. [9] to decompose, filter, and extract pertinent features from preprocessed EMG data. Two techniques for classifying subjects in HC and ALS and/or myopathy were included in preprocessing. Features are extracted following frame-by-frame sequential analysis in the direct EMG approach using DWT. In the second method, a collection of features was chosen using the dominating motor unit action potential (MUAP) process, and critical features for classification were retrieved using DWT decomposition. Both suggested approaches were validated in a KNN classifier by Doulah et al. The algorithm's performance was assessed by the authors using different parameters on three different data sets that represented HC, ALS, and OD individuals (10, 8, and 7 subjects, respectively). Both processes presented substantial results for classification of two and three sets (HC, ALS, and OD).

With three sets, the Dominant-MUAP technique achieved 98.8% Acc, demonstrating its constant performance. Promising and statistically significant results were obtained in the process of classifying individuals between HC and ALS (86.6% Acc, 86.6% Spe, 86.6% Sen), HC, ALS, or myopathy (82.2% Acc, 81.89% Sen, 91.31% Spe), and ALS or myopathy (96.6% Acc, 93.7% Sen, 100% Spe) using the ANN-based diagnostic aid strategy proposed by Ambikapathy et al. [10].

Three markers/features for supporting diagnostics—the clustering index, the kurtosis of the EMG signal amplitude histogram, and the kurtosis of the EMG zero crossing-rate expansion—were used by Zhang et al. [11] to define patterns in surface EMG signals. Additionally, a feature vector originating from the concatenation of vectors of the aforementioned attributes was used as input data when the LDA ML algorithm was used in the approach of distinguishing people as HC and ALS. Data from 11 HC volunteers and 10 ALS subjects were analyzed for the experiments in this study. All three features showed distinct and positive outcomes. When used in a synergistic manner with the LDA algorithm, they produced a more robust technique that yielded much more significant results, with a 100% Spe and 90% Sen. This feature suggests positive viewpoints that could potentially be applied to diagnosis support systems.

In order to preprocess and extract characteristics from EMG signals, Hazarika et al. [12] introduced a unique process assessment and inference system with a resilient structure. This structure is made up of steps that first assess the properties of the EMG signal using a method that involves decomposition by DWT and input data partitioning schemes (known as multiview direct). Multidomain multiview discriminant correlation analysis (mmDCA) is then applied. mmDCA synchronizes features from partitions in a single vector, checks for redundancy, evaluates feature correlation, and removes features that are not relevant. The mmDCA-generated vector is used in a variety of ML models, such as KNN, and fed into SVM, the traditional density-based linear classifier, quadratic classifier (QDC), and feedforward back-propagation neural network (FFBP-ANN), which has two hidden layers of eight neurons each. In two real-time EMG signal datasets, the classification of participants into HC, ALS, and myopathy classes was an effective evaluation of each algorithm's performance. The QDC model demonstrated the most robust results in the first dataset, which included 10 healthy participants, 8 with ALS, and 7 with OD, and in the second dataset, which included 4 healthy subjects, 4 with ALS, and 4 with OD: 99.03% Acc and 100% Acc, respectively.

A reliable technique that uses Riemannian geometry to increase the precision of EEG-based emotion classification is covered by Al-Mashhadani et al. [13]. To capture pertinent signal properties and improve classification performance, the suggested method uses PCA in Euclidean space for adaptive feature extraction. The retrieved characteristics are converted into covariance matrices, which are then projected onto the Riemannian manifold. The minimum distance to Riemannian means (MDRM) classifier is used to classify emotions. The technique's generalizability and steady accuracy increase across a range of scenarios were demonstrated by studies conducted on four datasets: DEAP, DREAMER, MAHNOB, and SEED. The validity and effectiveness of applying Riemannian geometry to improve the accuracy of EEG-based emotion categorization were supported by comparisons of classification accuracy and resilience with a number of cutting-edge classification techniques.

Using SVM classifiers with both higher-order crossing and power spectral density features, Pereira et al. [14] demonstrated emotion categorization on the DEAP dataset. The average accuracy of the leave-one-subject-out categorization method was 52.03% for arousal and 53.42% for valence. The link between electrophysiological signals—such as ECG, electromyograms (EMG), and EEG—and functional picture processing, as well as the interactions that result from them, was covered by Jagannath

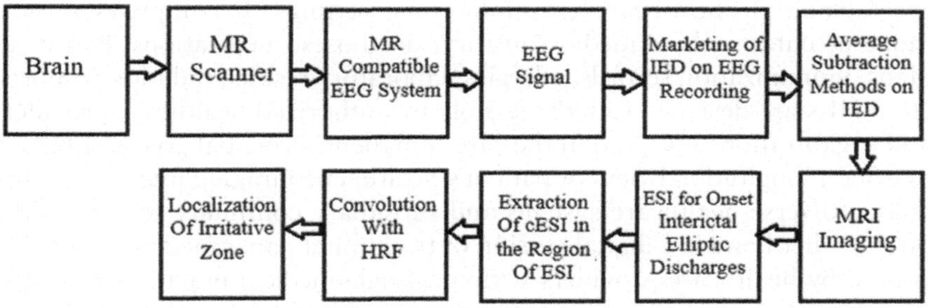

Figure 3.9 Fusion process of EEG signal and MRI imaging for localization of irritative zone in presurgical epilepsy cases (IED, interictal epileptic discharges; ESI, electrical source imaging; Cesi, continuous electrical source imaging; HRF, hemodynamic response function [15]).

et al. [15]. The way information derived from many sources and modalities interacts appears to be highly promising. In the field of information retrieval, sophisticated algorithms and techniques based on time-frequency representation have been studied. Several case studies, including those in the fields of neurology, functional imaging, and the cardiovascular system, have examined examples using a variety of algorithms and techniques. Examples of algorithms that effectively extract electrophysiological signals and functional pictures and have a significant impact on a range of biomedical applications have been reviewed. Figure 3.9 illustrates process of EEG signal and MRI imaging for localization of irritative zone in presurgical epilepsy cases.

3.6 REVOLUTIONIZING HEALTHCARE: ADVANTAGES OF ELECTRONIC HEALTH RECORDS (EHRS) AND HOW AI CAN BE USEFUL IN EHR MANAGEMENT

The electronic version of a patient's paper document, known as an EHR, contains information about the patient's medical history, diagnosis, prescriptions, treatment plans, dates of vaccinations, allergies, radiological pictures, and test results. EHRs are designed to be longitudinal, comprehensive records that offer detailed and up-to-date picture of patient's health. Implementation of EHRs is part of broader efforts to digitize and modernize healthcare systems, pointing to advance patient care, improve coordination among healthcare providers, diminish errors, and upsurge efficiency in healthcare delivery. EHRs play a critical role in ongoing evolution of healthcare information technology.

EHR and electronic medical record (EMR) are terms often used in the context of digital health information systems, but they have distinct meanings.

EHR is inclusive digital record of patient's health information, spanning across multiple healthcare encounters and settings. It comprises a wide range of data, such as medical history, diagnoses, medications, treatment plans, immunization records, allergies, laboratory results, radiology reports, etc. EHRs are designed to be accessible by authorized healthcare providers and organizations involved in the care of patient. Principal goal of EHRs is to offer a longitudinal view of patient's health, encouraging interoperability among diverse healthcare systems and subsidiary continuity of care. EMR on the other hand is a digital version of traditional paper medical chart that is used by healthcare providers within a single medical practice or facility. It comprises patient health information specific to that practice, such as medical and treatment histories, diagnoses, medications, and test results. EMRs are typically created, stored, and managed within a single healthcare organization and are meant to be used by healthcare professionals directly involved in patient's care. While EMRs are more localized and may not be easily shared outside of a specific healthcare facility, they serve the purpose of improving internal documentation, organization, and efficiency. Significant variance between EHR and EMR lies in their scope and interoperability. EHRs are designed to be comprehensive, spanning multiple healthcare organizations and settings, and are meant to support the exchange of information among diverse providers. EMRs, on the other hand, are more localized to a single practice or facility and emphasis on internal management of patient records within that specific context. Terms are sometimes used interchangeably, but understanding their distinctions is important in discussions about healthcare information technology.

3.6.1 Advantages of EHR over traditional paper systems

Adoption of EHR systems offers numerous advantages over traditional paper-based record-keeping systems in healthcare. By taking into account clinical, organizational, and societal results, researchers have carefully examined the advantages of EHRs. Clinical outcomes include reductions in medical errors, enhancements in patient-level metrics that characterize the appropriateness of care, and increases in the quality of care. Conversely, organizational outcomes have incorporated things like financial and operational performance, as well as patient and clinician satisfaction with EHRs. Finally, improving population health and conducting research more effectively are examples of social outcomes.

Accessibility and Availability: EHRs offer instant access to patient information from anywhere with appropriate authorization. Healthcare professionals can access records in real time, improving response times and decision-making.

Interoperability: EHRs promote interoperability, allowing for the exchange of information between diverse healthcare providers and organizations. This augments coordination of care, diminishes duplicate testing, and advances overall healthcare delivery.

Comprehensive Patient Information: EHRs store a wide range of patient data, including medical history, medications, allergies, test results, and treatment plans, providing a more comprehensive view of patient's health.

Reduced Errors and Upgraded Patient Safety: EHRs help diminish errors associated with handwritten records, illegible handwriting, or lost paperwork. Decision support tools within EHRs can alert healthcare providers to potential drug interactions, allergies, and other safety concerns.

Efficiency and Time Savings: EHRs systematize numerous administrative tasks, like appointment scheduling and billing, leading to augmented efficiency and time savings for healthcare professionals. Quick access to digital records streamlines workflow and diminishes time spent searching for and managing paper files.

Cost Savings in Long Run: While initial implementation of EHRs may involve substantial upfront costs, they can lead to cost savings over time by improving overall efficiency and diminishing dependence on paper.

Data Security and Privacy: EHR systems typically have robust security measures, comprising encryption and access controls, to protect patient information. Strict authentication protocols help ensure that only authorized individuals have access to sensitive data.

Patient Engagement: EHRs empower patients by providing them with access to their own health information, fostering more active role in their healthcare. Patients can view test results, medication lists, and other pertinent information through secure patient portals.

Data Analytics and Population Health Management: EHRs support the use of aggregated, deidentified data for analytics, enabling healthcare organizations to identify trends, manage populations, and improve public health outcomes.

Regulatory Compliance: EHR systems help healthcare providers comply with regulatory requirements and standards, which are increasingly emphasizing the use of digital health records.

Scalability and Adaptability: EHR systems are designed to be scalable, accommodating the growth of healthcare facilities and adapting to changing technological landscapes.

While there are clear advantages to adopting EHR systems, it is imperative to note that efficacious implementation requires addressing challenges such as interoperability, data standardization, and user training. Furthermore, the transition from paper to electronic records may involve learning curve for healthcare professionals and organizations.

AI can improve EHRs in many ways; for example, AI can analyze patient data from multiple sources, such as medical files, imaging reports, and laboratories [16]. AI can improve patient care by enhancing treatment planning and creating more accurate medical records. Also, it makes data easier to handle by classifying and organizing. AI can also help in reading and processing human language.

Healthcare professionals can access patient information in real time, leading to more informed and timely decision-making. EHRs facilitate better communication and collaboration among healthcare providers across diverse departments and settings. Multiple healthcare professionals can access and contribute to the same patient record, improving overall coordination of care. EHRs store a wide range of patient data, including medical history, medications, allergies, test results, and treatment plans, offering a more complete view of patient's health. EHRs help minimize errors associated with handwritten records, illegible handwriting, or lost paperwork. Decision support tools in EHRs can alert healthcare providers to potential drug interactions, allergies, and other safety concerns. EHRs automate administrative tasks, such as appointment scheduling, billing, and prescription ordering, leading to augmented efficiency and time savings. Digital records streamline workflows and eliminate the need for manual searching through paper files. While initial implementation costs may be substantial, EHRs can result in long-term cost savings by improving overall efficiency and diminishing dependence on paper.

EHR systems incorporate robust security measures, comprising encryption and access controls, to safeguard patient information. Strict authentication protocols ensure that only authorized individuals have access to sensitive data. EHRs empower patients by providing them with access to their own health information through secure portals. Patients can view test results, medication lists, and other relevant information, fostering more active role in their healthcare. EHRs support the use of aggregated, deidentified data for analytics, enabling healthcare organizations to identify trends, manage populations, and advance public health outcomes. EHR systems help healthcare providers comply with regulatory requirements and standards, comprising those related to privacy and security. EHR systems are designed to be scalable, accommodating growth of healthcare facilities and adapting to evolving technological landscapes. EHRs can integrate with telemedicine platforms, allowing for remote consultations and enhancing access to healthcare services. Overall, EHRs contribute to a more efficient, secure, and patient-centric healthcare system. They play a vital role in improving quality of care, enhancing patient outcomes, and supporting healthcare providers in delivering more effective and coordinated services. EHRs make it easier for physicians to share patient data through HIE once health data is electronically accessible. HIE is the process by which many organizations exchange patient-level electronic health information [17] and can greatly improve the efficiency of health care delivery [18]. Menachemi and Collum [19] presented review and summarized literature on advantages and disadvantages of EHR systems. They have focused on key EHR functionalities, comprising clinical decision support systems, computerized order entry systems, and health information exchange. Their paper describes potential benefits of EHRs that comprise clinical outcomes, organizational outcomes (e.g. financial and operational benefits), and societal outcomes (e.g. enhanced ability to conduct research, improved population health, reduced costs).

3.7 CONCLUSION

AI systems depict a critical role in biomedical signal processing applications and their potential to address challenges faced by physicians during diagnostic process [20]. ML approaches involve feature extraction, and domain experts are needed to choose the best features for a given problem [21, 22]. Biomedical signal analysis has recently benefited greatly from ML technology, particularly DL [23, 24]. Training ML and DL techniques has also considerably improved medical image analysis (MIA). The issue of feature selection is resolved by DL approaches. Clinical impact of precise biomedical signal and image processing cannot be overstated. From early disease detection to treatment monitoring, these techniques play a pivotal role in healthcare decision-making. In this context, ML presents a transformative potential [25]. Recent applications of deep gradient in MIA include various tasks related to computer vision, such as classification, detection, segmentation, and registration. Among the basic and most used tasks are classification, detection, and segmentation. For instance, to diagnose various conditions from medical images, ML has been shown to perform on par with medical experts.

REFERENCES

[1] M. Puttagunta and S. Ravi. "Medical image analysis based on deep learning approach." *Multimed. Tools Appl.*, vol. 80, pp. 24365–24398, 2021. https://doi.org/10.1007/s11042-021-10707-4

[2] G. Litjens et al. "A survey on deep learning in medical image analysis." *Med. Image Anal.*, vol. 42, pp. 60–88, 2017.

[3] V. Cheplygina, M. de Bruijne, and J. P. W. Pluim. "Not-so-supervised: a survey of semi-supervised, multi-instance, and transfer learning in medical image analysis." *Med. Image Anal.*, vol. 54, pp. 280–296, 2019.

[4] S. K. Zhou et al. A review of deep learning in medical imaging: Image traits, technology trends, case studies with progress highlights, and future promises. Proceedings of the IEEE1-19, 2020.

[5] X. Liu et al. "A comparison of deep learning performance against healthcare professionals in detecting diseases from medical imaging: a systematic review and meta-analysis." *Lancet Dig. Health*, vol. 1, no. 6, pp. E271–E297, 2019.

[6] F. Fernandes, I. Barbalho, D. Barros, et al. "Biomedical signals and machine learning in amyotrophic lateral sclerosis: a systematic review." *Biomed. Eng. Online*, vol. **20**, p. 61, 2021. https://doi.org/10.1186/s12938-021-00896-2

[7] N. AlHinai. "Chapter—introduction to biomedical signal processing and artificial intelligence." In W. Zgallai, editor. Biomedical signal processing and artificial intelligence in healthcare. Developments in biomedical engineering and bioelectronics. Amsterdam: Academic Press; 2020. p. 1–28. https://doi.org/10.1016/B978-0-12-818946-7.00001-9

[8] A. Cohen. "Chapter 1–biomedical signals: Origin and dynamic characteristics; frequency-domain analysis." In J. D. Bronzino, editor. Medical devices and systems. The Biomedical Engineering Handbook. Boca Raton: CRC Press, pp. 1–22, 2006.

[9] A. B. M. S. U. Doulah, S. A. Fattah, W. P. Zhu, and M. O. Ahmad. "Wavelet domain feature extraction scheme based on dominant motor unit action potential of EMG signal for neuromuscular disease classification." *IEEE Trans. Biomed. Circuits Syst.*,vol. 8, no. 2, pp. 155–164, 2014. https://doi.org/10.1109/TBCAS.2014.2309252

[10] B. Ambikapathy, K. Kirshnamurthy, and R. Venkatesan. "Assessment of electromyograms using genetic algorithm and artificial neural networks." *EvolutIntell*, vol. 14, pp. 1–11, 2018.

[11] X. Zhang, P. E. Barkhaus, W. Z. Rymer, and P. Zhou. "Machine learning for supporting diagnosis of amyotrophic lateral sclerosis using surface electromyogram." *IEEE Trans. Neural Syst. Rehab. Eng.*,vol. 22, no. 1, pp. 96–103, 2014. https://doi.org/10.1109/TNSRE.2013.2274658

[12] A. Hazarika, L. Dutta, M. Barthakur, and M. Bhuyan. "A multiview discriminant feature fusion-based nonlinear process assessment and diagnosis: application to medical diagnosis." *IEEE Trans. Instrum. Meas.*, vol. 68, no. 7, pp. 2498–506, 2019. https://doi.org/10.1109/TIM.2018.2866744

[13] Z. Al-Mashhadani, N. Bayat, I. F. Kadhim, R. Choudhury, and J.-H, Park. "The efficacy and utility of lower-dimensional Riemannian geometry for EEG-based emotion classification." *Appl. Sci.*, vol. 13, no. 14, p. 8274, 2023. https://doi.org/10.3390/app13148274

[14] E. T. Pereira and H. Martins Gomes. The role of data balancing for emotion classification using EEG signals. In Proceedings of the 2016 IEEE International Conference on Digital Signal Processing (DSP), Beijing, China, 16–18 October 2016; pp. 555–559.

[15] J. Rajeswari and M. Jagannath. "Advances in biomedical signal and image processing – A systematic review." *Inform. Med.*, vol. 8, pp. 2352–9148, 2017. https://doi.org/10.1016/j.imu.2017.04.002.

[16] U. Kumar and S. Yadav. Application of machine learning to analyse biomedical signals for medical diagnosis. Chapter 11, from the book *Handbook of Research on Disease Prediction Through Data Analytics and Machine Learning*, 2021. doi:10.4018/978-1-7998-2742-9.ch011

[17] K. B. Eden, A. M. Totten, S. Z. Kassakian, P. N. Gorman, M. S. McDonagh, B. Devine, M. Pappas, M. Daeges, S. Woods, and W. R. Hersh. Barriers and facilitators to exchanging health information: a systematic review. *Int. J. Med. Inform.*, vol. 88, pp. 44–51, 2016. https://doi.org/10.1016/j.ijmedinf.2016.01.004
[18] J. Walker, E. Pan, D. Johnston, et al. "The value of health care information exchange and interoperability." *Health Aff (Millwood)* W5-10–W5-18, Jan–Jun, 2005.
[19] N. Menachemi and T. H. Collum. "Benefits and drawbacks of electronic health record systems." *Risk Manag. Healthc. Policy*, vol. 4, pp. 47–55, 2011. doi:10.2147/RMHP.S12985
[20] I. Noushad and G. V. Smitha. "Parkinson's disease prediction and prevention using machine learning." *Int. J. Eng. Res. Technol.*, vol. 11, no. 6, 2023.
[21] I. Galić, M. Habijan, H. Leventić, and K. Romić. "Machine learning empowering personalized medicine: A comprehensive review of medical image analysis methods." *Electronics*, vol. 12, no. 21, p. 4411, 2023. https://doi.org/10.3390/electronics12214411
[22] M. Rana and M. Bhushan. "Machine learning and deep learning approach for medical image analysis: Diagnosis to detection." *Multimed. Tools Appl.*, vol. 24, pp. 1–39, 2022. doi:10.1007/s110402-022-14305-w
[23] B. Feng, T. Yu, H. Wang, K. Liu, W. Wu, and W. Long. "Editorial: Machine learning and deep learning in biomedical signal analysis." *Front. Hum. Neurosci.*, vol. 17, p. 1183840, 2023. doi:10.3389/fnhum.2023.1183840
[24] C. Cao, F. Liu, H. Tan, D. Song, W. Shu, W. Li, Y. Zhou, X. Bo, and Z. Xie. "Deep learning and its applications in biomedicine." *Genom. Proteom. Bioinform.*, vol. 16, no. 1, pp. 17–32, 2018. doi:10.1016/j.gpb.2017.07.003
[25] G. Zhu, B. Jiang, L. Tong, Y. Xie, G. Zaharchuk, and M. Wintermark. "Applications of deep learning to neuro-imaging techniques." *Front. Neurol.*, vol. 10, p. 869, 2019. doi:10.3389/fneur.2019.00869

Questions

1. What are present techniques of ML and DL used for medical imaging?
2. What are considered parameters while selecting classifiers?
3. What are evaluation metrics used to evaluate classification models?
4. What are several medical image modalities for classifying diseases?
5. What are the tools and techniques used for medical imaging?
6. What are several datasets used by several researchers in the domain of healthcare?
7. What are the outcomes of comparative analysis of ML classifiers and DL models based on experiments using the MRI dataset?
8. What are prominent AI methods used in medical image analysis?
9. In what medical imaging tasks have AI methods shown the most promising results?
10. What are commonly observed anatomical structures and available datasets for the development of AI algorithms?

11. How can AI-driven medical image analysis be effectively translated into clinical practice?
12. What are techniques used in biomedical signal processing?
13. What are neural networks in biomedical signal processing?
14. What are the applications of signals in the biomedical field?
15. What generates biomedical signals?
16. What is the use of machine learning in signal processing?
17. How can machine learning algorithms be categorized in the context of biomedical engineering?
18. Explain the importance of data in training machine learning models for biomedical applications.
19. Discuss the role of machine learning in predicting and diagnosing diseases based on patient data.
20. Explain how machine learning can be applied in drug discovery and development.
21. What are the ethical considerations in using machine learning for medical decision-making?
22. Discuss the challenges of interpreting machine learning models in the context of healthcare.
23. How can biases in training data impact the performance of machine learning algorithms in biomedical applications?
24. Discuss the potential impact of machine learning on the design and optimization of medical implants.
25. Discuss strategies to ensure the security and privacy of sensitive patient data used in machine learning models.
26. What are the potential risks and regulatory considerations related to the use of machine learning in healthcare?
27. What is machine learning, and how does it differ from traditional programming in the context of biomedical engineering?
28. Provide examples of how machine learning assists in the early detection of diseases through medical imaging.
29. What is the role of machine learning in developing clinical decision support systems (CDSS) in biomedical settings?
30. How can machine learning algorithms be utilized in processing and analyzing biomedical signals, such as ECGs or EEGs?
31. Discuss the potential of machine learning in enabling remote patient monitoring and management of chronic conditions.
32. Discuss the challenges and benefits of interdisciplinary teams working on projects at intersection of machine learning and biomedical engineering.
33. Discuss the potential impact of explainable AI in gaining trust from healthcare professionals in machine learning models.
34. Explain the importance of validation in ensuring the reliability of machine learning models in healthcare.

35. Discuss methods to enhance the interpretability of machine learning models for clinical practitioners.
36. Identify the major challenges faced in integrating machine learning into biomedical engineering applications. Discuss potential solutions and opportunities for overcoming these challenges.
37. In ECG signal processing, which machine learning technique is commonly used for heartbeat classification?
38. What is a common application of machine learning in medical image analysis?
39. In biomedical signal processing, what is the purpose of feature extraction using machine learning?
40. How is machine learning applied to analyze functional MRI data?

Multiple Choice Questions

1. What is the primary goal of biomedical signal processing using machine learning?
   a) Identifying genetic mutations
   b) Extracting meaningful information from physiological signals
   c) Analyzing chemical compositions
   d) Enhancing medical imaging quality
2. In ECG signal processing, which machine learning technique is commonly used for heartbeat classification?
   a) Linear regression
   b) Decision trees
   c) Support vector machines
   d) Convolutional neural networks (CNNs)
3. What is a common application of machine learning in medical image analysis?
   a) Calculating blood pressure
   b) Predicting patient demographics
   c) Diagnosing diseases from radiological images
   d) Identifying dietary habits
4. In biomedical signal processing, what is the purpose of feature extraction using machine learning?
   a) To increase signal amplitude
   b) To reduce signal complexity
   c) To amplify noise
   d) To improve signal transmission speed
5. Which of the following machine learning tasks is commonly used for classifying different stages of sleep-in polysomnography signals?
   a) Regression
   b) Clustering

c) Classification
d) Reinforcement learning

6. How is machine learning applied to analyze functional MRI data?
   a) Identifying genetic markers
   b) Predicting future medical conditions
   c) Classifying brain regions based on activation patterns
   d) Enhancing MRI image resolution
7. Which machine learning technique is effective in reducing noise and artifacts in biomedical signals?
   a) Principal component analysis (PCA)
   b) K-nearest neighbors
   c) Random forest
   d) Naive Bayes
8. What is the role of machine learning in CAD systems for medical imaging?
   a) Enhancing physician's intuition
   b) Automating surgical procedures
   c) Assisting in disease detection and diagnosis
   d) Analyzing patient demographics
9. Which machine learning approach is commonly used for time–frequency analysis of biomedical signals?
   a) Fourier transform
   b) Wavelet transform
   c) Laplace transform
   d) Radon transform
10. What is the main objective of using machine learning for image segmentation in medical imaging?
    a) Identifying color patterns
    b) Enhancing image brightness
    c) Locating and delineating structures or regions of interest
    d) Measuring image resolution

Chapter 4

Machine learning algorithms for cancer susceptibility, recurrence, and survival prediction

Viability, challenges, and survey on the state-of-the-art

4.1 INTRODUCTION TO RECENT TRENDS IN CANCER RESEARCH

In the year 2020, according to the World Health Organization (WHO) [1], cancer caused nearly 10 million deaths worldwide. The most common cancers were breast cancer (2.26 million cases), lung cancer (2.21 million cases), colon and rectal cancer (1.93 million cases), prostate cancer (1.41 million cases), skin cancer (nonmelanoma) (1.20 million cases), and stomach cancer (1.09 million cases). Cancer prevention is a global priority, but according to the historical evidence, the path to achieve this is full of roadblocks and detours. A wide range of tools and costly reagents are needed by researchers when they work to find the answers to the questions about the disease. Cancer investigation begins with three steps: imaging tests, biopsy, and tumor markers. Cancer is suspected based on individual's symptoms, based on the results of a physical examination, or on the results of screening tests. When a doctor first suspects cancer, some type of imaging study, for example, X-rays, ultrasonography (USG), or a computed tomography scan (CT scan), is done. Rarely, X-rays obtained for many other reasons, for example as an injury, may show abnormalities that are suspected to be a cancer. In the last decade, a lot of progress has been centered around computational tools for cancer imaging. Whether they are X-rays of whole organs or microscopic pictures of the cancer cells, doctors are using a multitude of imaging methods in order to find the cancer in its earliest stages, determine the stage of a tumor, analyze if treatment is progressive, and then monitor whether the cancer has recurred after the treatment or not. Confirmation that a cancer is present requires some diagnostic tests. After diagnosis, staging is a way of describing how advanced the cancer has become by examining how big it is and measuring its spread to its neighboring tissues. Confirmation of cancer is done by obtaining a small piece of the tumor using a needle or surgery and obtaining cancer cells on a microscopic examination of the sample taken from the suspected area. Tumor markers are substances secreted into the blood by certain tumors. When the prescribed examination outputs or

DOI: 10.1201/9781003503033-4

imaging test results show cancer using blood levels of tumor markers, the patient is prescribed medication and therapies for the treatment.

Artificial intelligence (AI) refers to the perception, interpretation, and synthesis of information demonstrated by machines, opposite to the intelligence demonstrated by animals and humans [2]. AI researchers and scientists have integrated a complete range of problem-solving techniques such as mathematical optimization, logic optimization, neural networks (NNs), statistics, and probability. Machine learning (ML) is a field of AI that allows machines to learn from past experiences or data without being programmed explicitly. Deep learning (DL) is a class of multilayer NNs, which is currently excelling at the problem of learning from big data compared to other ML algorithms. As a result of recent technological advances, in particular, the introduction of advanced medical imaging and computerized systems, radiation treatments for cancer have evolved rapidly in recent decades, leading to the advent of highly conformal and more precise treatments. Cancer research has witnessed massive development of AI tools in the last decade. There is a lot of hype around AI, and at the same time, there is a lot of research going into ML-based research in cancer, as was said recently by Stephanie Harmon, Ph.D., a well-known data scientist in the Molecular Imaging Branch of National Cancer Institute (NCI) in United States. For the purpose of disseminating authentic information, this chapter uses most of the resources from the Scopus database [3] and the biomedical PubMed Repository [4]. In Figure 4.1, barplot illustrates the number of publications on the most commonly occurring cancers, declared by NCI [5] and Figure 4.2 gives the use of AI techniques during different stages of a cancer patient. The number of publications in the last 20 years (2003–2023) was identified when considering searches of each type of cancer in the databases. The rest of the chapter is organized as follows:

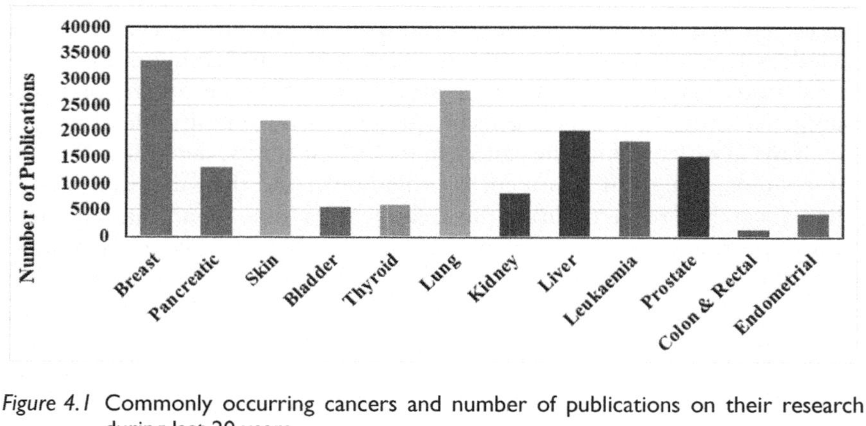

Figure 4.1 Commonly occurring cancers and number of publications on their research during last 20 years.

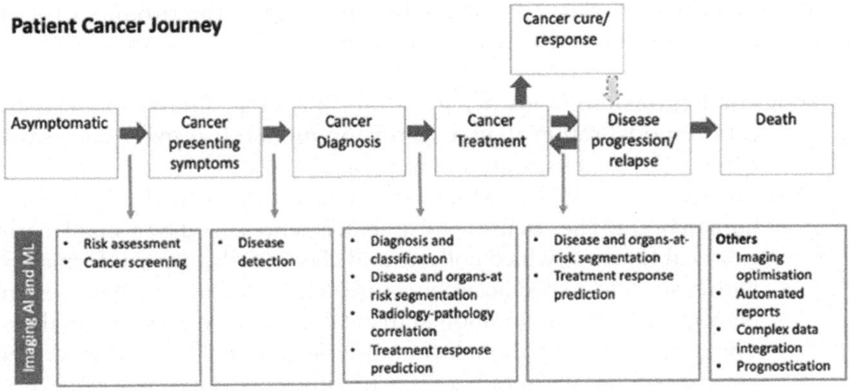

Figure 4.2 Use of AI techniques during different stages of a cancer patient.

Section 4.2 throws light on some preliminaries of ML algorithms. Section 4.3, in order to discuss the viability of AI in cancer, addresses the question in Section 4.3.1. Is ML an appropriate tool for cancer research? and discussion is carried out on the topic and success of supervised learning in cancer in Section 4.3.2. Sections 4.4, 4.5, and 4.6 demonstrate the state-of-the-art AI algorithms used in cancer susceptibility, cancer recurrence, and cancer survival. In Section 4.7, challenges of AI in cancer are discussed, while Section 4.8 concludes the chapter. Since ML tools belong to the AI, it can be noted that the term AI algorithms tools and techniques and ML algorithms tools and techniques may be used interchangeably throughout the chapter.

4.2 SOME PRELIMINARIES OF MACHINE LEARNING ALGORITHMS

AI is a science and has a subset called ML. In AI, algorithms are used to automate tasks such as problem-solving and pattern recognition. ML refers to self-improving algorithms [2]. This implies that explicit rules and steps are not prespecified but are learned by the algorithm through understanding of data. Essentially, ML algorithms mimic self-learning from humans, but at the same time, they are physically just the machines. Similarly, they not only interpret and learn from data, but they also improvise from experience. Here, "learning" means that with time, the

ML algorithms alter the ways of data processing, although they are not programmed explicitly for it. The four basic types of ML algorithms [6] are supervised learning algorithms, unsupervised learning algorithms, semisupervised learning (SSL) algorithms, and reinforcement learning algorithms.

In supervised learning, the dataset contains the output of given inputs, which means that to classify and predict the output, the training process involves analysis of both the inputs and outputs.

Logistic Regression: Logistic regression [7] is more similar to a classification model rather than a regression model. It is extensively used for healthcare, business, and industry.

Neural Networks: A NN [8] has a structure similar to the NN of the human brain. The "neuron" in an NN is represented by a small mathematical function which collects and classifies the input information with respect to a specific architecture. The NNs bear a strong resemblance to the most common statistical method, regression analysis. The connections of the neurons used in the artificial NNs (ANN) are denoted as weights between the nodes. A layer is a collection of neurons. The positive weight is an excitatory connection, and negative values refer to the inhibitory connections. An activation function is applied after each layer controls the value of the output. A simple NN with more than three layers is called a deep neural network (DNN). DNN processes the input data in complex ways by applying sophisticated modeling. Another very popular NN is the convolutional neural network (CNN) that contains convolutional layers. CNN contains a set of layers that are able to transform an image into a set of probabilities. The types of layers of DNN and CNN are convolutional, RELU, pooling, and fully connected layers.

Support Vector Machine (SVM): An SVM [9] is a popular algorithm, primarily used for classification as well as regression. The goal of the SVM is to form the most suitable line, which can separate data in space into classes that can easily make the new data point in different categories.

The Naive Bayes (NB): NB are probabilistic classifiers [10], suitable for binary and multiclass classification. NB is well suited for categorical input variables compared to numerical variables. NB is successful at making forecasting sample results based on previous results. Broadly, there are two ways in which unsupervised learning techniques are categorized:

Regression Algorithms: This technique involves identification [10] of the patterns in the sample input data, and then the predictions of continuous outcomes are produced.

In the unsupervised learning algorithms, we can use the unlabeled data. By the training process, the algorithm discovers specific patterns that help to solve the clustering or association problems.

Classification Algorithms: This technique involves labeling of input data according to the historical data samples, and therefore, it is manually trained

to recognize some particular type of objects. When the algorithm learns to completely recognize desired objects, it also becomes capable of categorizing these objects appropriately.
Other ways in which unsupervised learning techniques are categorized:

Clustering: The clustering technique [11] is exploited to categorize data into sensible groups called the "clusters". These clusters are created without any initial information about their credentials and are solely based on the specific internal pattern of each cluster. The identification of the cluster depends upon the similarities of some sample data objects and how they are distinct from the rest of the sample data objects.

Dimensionality Reduction: Dimensionality reduction [11] technique is used to discover a better and simpler representation of the given input data. By using this method, the input data is made free of the redundant information, or unnecessary information is removed, and at the same time, all the essential bits are retained.

Semisupervised learning (SSL): SSL [10] juxtaposes the best of both supervised and unsupervised algorithms. In SSL, a small set of labeled data is used for algorithm training to produce the desired results. Since it uses only a small amount of labeled data, it then creates an incomplete trained model, which assigns labels to the unlabeled data set. This gives rise to a unique algorithm, which is an amalgamation of labelled and partially labeled data sets. Thus, semisupervised algorithm is a combination of attributes of both supervised and unsupervised learning.

Reinforcement learning (RL): RL are self-sustained algorithms [12], which are able to improve themselves using cycles of trials and errors depending upon the combination and collision between the labeled available input and the incoming data. When the training process is started, rewards are generated if the algorithm can succeed in completion of a specific task. The rewards also define the next course of action. There are two types of reward signals: positive rewards, which are triggered when a specific sequence of action is to be continued. The negative rewards in which a penalty is imposed for performing certain tasks and require the modification of the algorithm before moving further.

4.3 VIABILITY OF AI IN THE CANCER DOMAIN

4.3.1 Is AI an appropriate tool for cancer research?

There are several significant outcomes of the clinical cancer management with a multitude of relevant outcomes of interest.

ML has potential advantages compared to pathologists. Undoubtedly, machines are able to work faster than humans. A biopsy which usually takes a pathologist 10 days to get a decision, a computer is able to perform hundreds of biopsies in a minute. Machines can replicate the same process and repeat it thousands of times, and not getting exhausted, which is something humans are not that good at. Machines can repeat a task thousands of times without getting exhausted. Although practice makes humans perfect, whatever the amount of practice, it cannot bring human results close to the efficiencies and computational speed of a computer. Figure 4.3 shows number of publications versus the types of ML algorithms used for cancer research in them.

In medicines, digitized techniques, such as imaging, were the early adopters of AI. Biomedical imaging [13] refers to the stepwise processes of image acquisition, image reconstruction, pattern interpretation, reporting, and the presentation of results, all of which use the digital domain. In particular, cancer imaging is an area where firstly AI and ML technologies were used by radiologists.

Radiomics [14] is a field in which computerized study of medical images is performed. The medical images can be categorized in various ways, but for imaging purposes, they are classified in terms of multiple dimensions, for example, two-dimensional X-rays, three-dimensional computed tomography (CT), and four-dimensional ultrasound images (USG).

In Figure 4.4, the selection of input image and sampling through a DNN for testing of radiomics features is illustrated to classify the cells as normal, benign, in situ, and invasive. Images taken from patients are first preprocessed and then transformed as inputs to develop the ML models and algorithms for ensuring data uniformity or conformity. These preprocessing

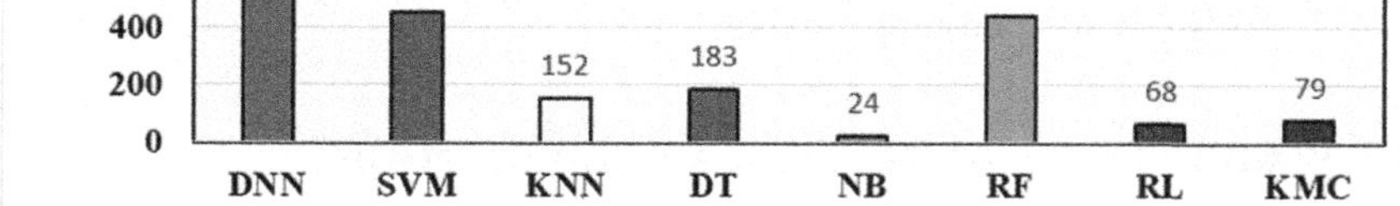

Figure 4.3 Number of publications versus types of machine learning algorithms used for cancer research in them (last 20 years (2003–2023)).

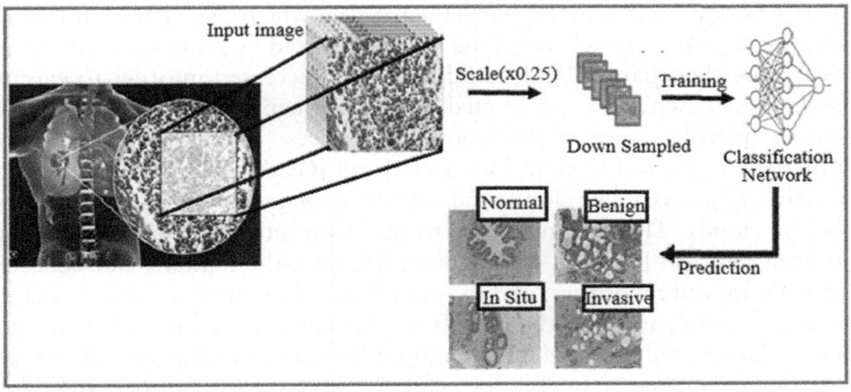

Figure 4.4 Classification of a lung cancer input sample using deep convolutional neural network.

steps are applied either to the mathematically derived features or to the features required by the radiologist. For the process of imaging, the input to every ML model is the images of equal image section thickness and of the same pixel dimensions. Some ML algorithms are more frequently applied than the others in imaging. Let us consider that x is an input variable, f is the mathematical function and y is the output variable. The most common algorithm is the prediction model, in which y is predicted based on learning $f(x)$. In the case of exploratory models, an attempt is made in order to link the input data x, for example an imaging feature with the output y, for example, a gene expression. In the case of continuous variables, imaging techniques rely upon important regression models, such as linear, Cox analysis, Lasso, Regression Trees, ElasticNet, and Ridge [15, 16].

ML algorithms commonly used for discrete models are NB, decision trees, SVMs, random forests (RF), generalized linear models, and k-nearest neighbors (KNN) [17]. These models have been used for cancer diagnosis, stratification, characterization, and treatment or survival outcomes. The success of an ML algorithm is related to the type of data, the computational power of the machine, and the parameters used in the algorithm. Moreover, the choice of the algorithm also depends on the data size. If smaller datasets are available, typically with less than a thousand samples, classical ML algorithms, for example, NB, decision trees, logistic regression, and SVMs, are applied. However, when the dataset is large, more recent and much complex ML models, for example, CNNs are used. The CNNs are extremely efficient in learning the features directly from images. Deep CNN (DCNN) models are very computationally intensive and require more power for execution on computing devices such as desktop or GPU.

In the present scenario, the number of healthcare organizations is increasing day by day, and some of them are moving to the high-performance computing (HPC) which are cloud and centralized facilities for hosting and exploiting their data. The demand for cloud increased in order to execute large models while having limited computing capabilities in hand. Cloud service providers such as Amazon Web Services (AWS), Microsoft Azure, Alibaba Cloud, and Google Cloud Platform (GCP), are organizations that provide access to public clouds and offer on-demand computing components on the clouds. This has given rise to the distributed or federated learning approaches also [18, 19]. In federated learning, the data are not collected in a centralized repository, and the models are circulated to various devices, near or remote, and then the models are trained using the local data at each site and share only the weights of a model between institutions. The proper use of cancer imaging technologies demands that the resources should be directed to the patients at greatest risk. In the United States, many states demand assessment of the breast density to calculate the risk for developing cancer. Recently, a DL technique demonstrated high accuracy in classifying the thresholds of breast density for providing consistent density notification to the patients for breast cancer screening [20, 21]. The use of the latest AI algorithms can improve the current risk models. For instance, a DNN model that used mammographic features with the traditional risk factors was able to determine the samples that are at the greatest risk of malignancy. The results of these algorithms are more effective than the conventional breast cancer risk models alone [22, 23]. Recently, excellent results were reported for breast cancer risk determination using the mammographic breast density, which was determined by a senior and a junior radiologist along with an AI software [24]. Studies have revealed the potential of AI in the identification and classification of major intracranial tumors, which included various high-grade and low-grade gliomas (malignant tumors), meningiomas, cerebral metastases, pituitary adenomas (benign tumors of the pituitary gland), and acoustic neuromas (benign tumors developed on the balance of hearing) [25].

4.3.2 The success of supervised learning in cancer

DNNs are supervised learning algorithms that have demonstrated significant improvements in cancer diagnosis and detection using fundamental image classification and pattern matching [26, 27]. The DNN technique, generally referred as deep learning (DL) architectures, is composed of multiple layers of neurons. It has been recently demonstrated that the application of DNNs on cancer outperforms other ML algorithms. Phenotype and genotype profiles are also exploited for cancer classification and treatment using the DNNs [28]. Transcriptomic study is the investigation of all ribonucleic acid (RNA) molecules in a cell. One significant resource of cancer transcriptomic profile is The Cancer Genome Atlas (TCGA) which consists of samples of more than 11,000 tumors taken from 33 types of the most commonly occurring cancers [29]. Literature shows a number of DL models that are developed for cancer diagnosis. Ahn et al. [30] designed a fully connected DL model that was trained using a diverse dataset of 6705 tumors and 6403 nontumor samples and also provided an assessment of individual's gene contribution to the ultimate Cancer classification. Lyu et al. [31] further improved this classification of individual tumor types.

4.4 CANCER SUSCEPTIBILITY

Positive output in the case of early prediction of cancer susceptibility involves higher survival rates and reduced mortality rates. Patients found susceptible to cancer need less complex medication regimens and lower hospital utilization, and consequentially lower healthcare costs. On the other hand, cancer detected at later stages needs difficult multimodal management, many cycles of very expensive medication over significant periods of time, resulting in a staggering requirement of money. Therefore, assessing the cancer susceptibility especially the early diagnosis is a process that cannot be overestimated [32–34]. Early prediction of the susceptibility of cancer has huge cost-saving benefits also. In the United States, within 2 years after diagnosis, cancer treatment costs are increased with stage such as 72000 US dollars for stage 0, 97000 for stages 1 and 2, 159000 for stage 3, and 182000 US dollars for stage 4 [35]. This corresponds to a saving of 26 billion US dollars per year in the United States alone [36]. Similarly, in the UK, the 10-year survival rate of patients for eight types of cancers (cervical, uterine, ovarian, breast, colorectal, testicular, malignant melanoma, bladder) is 80% when predicted in stages 1 and 2 compared to 26% when the cancers are detected at later stages [37]. In the UK, early prediction of several cancers, such as lung cancer, ovarian cancer (OC), and colorectal cancer can save more than 44 million Euros in England only, benefitting approximately 11000 patients [38].

An example can be localized breast cancer and OC in which the chances for survival for early prediction are 99% and 92%, respectively, compared to 27% and 29% for metastatic one, respectively [39]. Many publications reveal the effectiveness of ML models for prediction of cancer susceptibility. A comparison of ML models with a state-of-the-art prediction tool is made by Stark et al. [40]. This tool is the Breast Cancer Risk Prediction Tool popularly called BCRAT [41]. The factors used for prediction by this tool are number of first-degree relatives with breast cancer in their lifetime, age of the person at the time of tested, and at menarche, number of biopsies in the past, etc. AUC represents area under the ROC (region of converge curve), and it is a measure of the quality of how well the model predicts irrespective of the value of classification threshold. Stark et al. observed that the area under the ROC curve (AUC) for decision trees is 0.51 and 0.61 for linear regression, linear discriminant analysis, and NNs. The AUC value of BCRAT that uses features less broad than Stark et al. is 0.56. Therefore, the ML algorithms excelled in terms of AUC. For other metrics such as precision, sensitivity, and specificity, the values for ML algorithms are comparable with those of the BCRAT.

In [42], it is observed that the AUC of NNs is higher than logistic regression and linear discriminant analysis in spite of the great potential of NNs to analyze noisy data and nonlinear complex functions. This may be due to smaller or insufficient training data or fewer number of hyperparameters in [42]. Hundreds of annual researches publish their research work on lung cancer early prediction, treatment, and diagnosis. In [43], an advanced tool for early prediction of lung cancer is deployed. This tool is validated by testing on local medical cases, and feedbacks are used to find the accuracy of the scores achieved. Some of the ML algorithms are also employed for the analysis of 1000 patient records from a dataset for comparison. This tool is intended for computing the factors of risk for economically weaker sections of society who cannot afford to have regular checkups. OC is a common type of cancer in women. In the United States alone, it is estimated that 12,810 deaths can be caused by OC [44]. Accurate prediction of benign tumors has an important practical value. In [45], eight significant features were selected by using maximum relevance minimum redundancy (MRMR) which is an algorithm for feature selection. Decision trees are used to identify the two most important features, which are human epididymis protein-4 (HE4) and carcinoembryonic antigen (CEA). In [46], in order to pursue a model for future diagnosis of lung cancer based on the routine clinical and laboratory data using ML, a very small p-value is used, which is less than 0.00001. A novel ML algorithm is used and comparison of accuracy is made with the well-validated mPLCOm2012 trial risk model for ovarian, prostate, colorectal, and lung cancer screening. This model is more accurate for early diagnosis of lung cancer than the standard well-known mPLCOm2012, and therefore, has the potential for prevention of lung cancer deaths by providing precise early detection. Acute myeloid leukemia (AML) can be categorized as a genetically heterogenous blood cancer having a very poor prognosis, and the disease relapses very fast which is the primary cause of the treatment failure. The heterogeneity of AML arises from various genetic and nongenetic origins, one of which is the hierarchical structure having the leukemic stem cells (LSC) and certain types of progenitors. ML is capable of finding nontrivial patterns in high-dimensional 2D and 3D datasets and identify these rare subpopulations. In [47], a review of some recent ML algorithms is presented that applies to the single-cell data and could help in the disentanglement of the cell heterogeneity in AML. This is done by identifying the distinct core molecular structure of the available leukemic cell subsets in the patient's blood.

Traditional methods for understanding leukemia stem cells (LSCs) and their biological characteristics use the construction of cells similar to LSC cells and mouse models by using the transgenic or knock-in methods. The drawbacks of these methods are retroviral insertion mutagenesis, nonphysiological level gene expression and expansion, and the difficulty to build them. The researchers in [48] constructed the stemness index based on mRNA expression (mRNAsi) for detection of leukemia. The results of this research demonstrated that LSC-related genes based on mRNAsi had strong interactions as a cluster. These genes, precisely the RFC4 and RFC5, can be regarded as the formal therapeutic targets for the purpose of inhibiting stemness characteristics of AML. Long noncoding ribonucleic acids (lncRNAs) are recently one of the most useful factors in immunology for colorectal cancer. In [49], an ML-based integrative method is developed for constructing a consensus immune lncRNA.

Integrating AI algorithms and genetic evaluations has shown several promising results for signature (IRLS). IRLS may be considered as an independent risk parameter for the overall survival of colorectal cancer, and it displays stable performance, but IRLS has a limitation that it demonstrates limited prediction for relapse-free survival. Improved biomarkers of diagnoses are required to stratify the patients having early-stage colorectal cancer and for selection of the most suitable adjuvant therapy. The aim is to develop a biomarker of colorectal patient outcome by directly analyzing their conventional hematoxylin along with stained eosin using DL [50]. Table 4.1 shows some publications with ML algorithms applied to cancer susceptibility, under several heads, such as the algorithm used, datatype used as input, output metric, etc.

Colorectal cancer. AI models help to reduce the percentage of missed adenomas, and therefore, the risk of developing cancer is also reduced by improving the cancer screening outcomes [51, 52]. Based on genetic expression, simulation experiments are performed in [53] for classifying 53 colon cancer patients along with the Union for International Cancer Control (UICC). These patients were categorized into two groups: relapsed and no relapse postsurgery. Comparisons were made with the classification accuracy achieved by the S-Kohonen which is 91% for backpropagation, 66% for SVM, and 70% for NNs. It is concluded that the S-Kohonen NN is very effective for the classification of colon cancer. Using the SVM analyses, Xu et al. [54] conducted a research for the identification of differentially expressed genes for distinguishing the patients having a high risk of colon cancer recurrence. Moreover, they identified a signature of 15 genes that is expected to be useful for prediction of recurrence risk and will be used for prognosis of colon cancer patients. Ten-fold cross-validation is denoted by 10-fold CV in Table 4.1. Figure 4.5 shows SVM for classification of blood cells.

Table 4.1 Some publications with ML algorithms applied to cancer susceptibility

Publication	*AI algorithm (validation method)*	*Types of cancer*	*Types of data*	*Metrics (accuracy, Fi score, etc.)*	*Relevant features*	*Significant advancement*
[43]	DT, RF (NA)	Lung	1000 records and 23 attributes	Specificity = 90.47%, Accuracy = 93.33%, Sensitivity = 100%	Smoking, air pollution, genetic risk, and occupational hazards are responsible factors	LCPT tool is reusable so new risk factors can be added owing to the generalized LCRD equation. For prediction of lung cancer risk, the average time is 0.0159 s
[45]	Machine learning Minimum Redundancy Maximum Relevance (MRMR), DT (10-fold CV)	Ovarian	349 patients, 49 tumor feature markers	AUC of ROC for DT and ROMA on training data = 0.888 and 0.814, respectively, and on testing data are 0.949 and 0.943, respectively	HE4 and CEA are the two biomarkers that have the most significant prediction power	Using only CEA and HE4, the proposed simple decision tree model produces a better prediction result in both training and testing data compared to the state-of-the-art
[20]	CNN (NA)	Breast	22,000 images from digital mammogram imaging dataset	AUC = 0.9421	Breast density classifier, scattered density, heterogeneously dense	High accuracies between two very dissimilar breast density categories can be assessed by the radiologists
[55]	ANN (10-fold CV)	Breast	62219	AUC = 0.965	Age, mammographic findings	ANN shows superior discrimination (AUC = 0.965) compared to the radiologists (AUC = 0.939) for $p < .001$

[56]	SVM (LOO-CV)	Multiple myeloma	80	Accuracy = 71%	Snp739514	Performance better than radiologist
[57]	SVM (10-fold CV)	Breast	174	Accuracy = 69%	snpCY11b2	We have shown that multiple SNP sites from different genes over distant parts of the genome are better at identifying breast cancer patients than any one SNP alone
[58]	BN (K-fold CV)	Colon	53	AUC = 0.71	Primary tumor histology	Performance better than radiologist

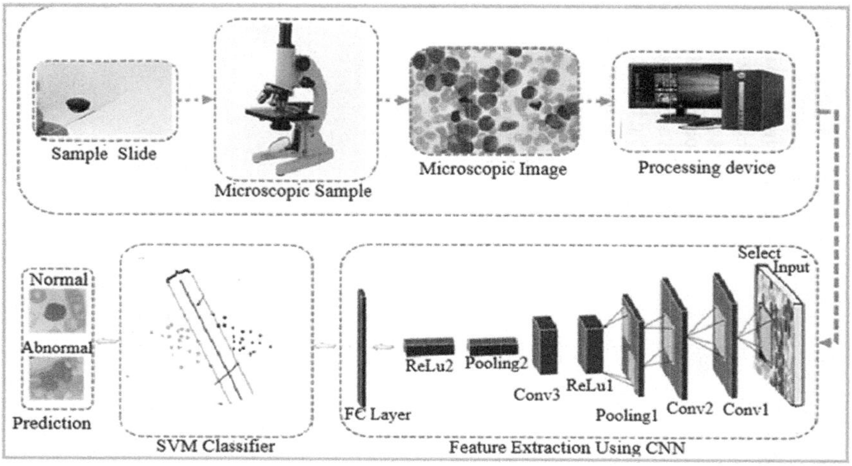

Figure 4.5 SVM for classification of blood cells.

4.5 CANCER RECURRENCE

The cancer may again come after the treatment of its previous stage called the cancer recurrence. In [59], the basis of oral squamous cell carcinoma (OSCC) is analyzed after cancer patient's remission by using a decision support system that is multiparametric. The datasets exploited are sources such as clinical data, data from imaging and genomic data. In order to predict the relapse of OSCC and its subsequent recurrence, the number of patients used is 86, in which 13 had the relapse and the remaining were free of disease. Cancer recurrence is the greatest fear for cancer survivors after having their apparently successful therapy. Metastasis is defined as the spread of cancer cells from the first site to other organs, and it accounts for nearly 60–70% of all cancer mortality around the world [60, 61]. Due to the advancements in medicine and methodologies, latest therapies, and improved chemotherapies, there is a significant improvement in the overall reduction of many types of cancer. Still, metastasis holds a share of approximately 90% of all the cancer mortality. Some cancers are more recurrent than others such as kidney cancer, breast cancer, nonsmall cell lung cancer (NSCLC), AML, melanoma, OC, prostate cancer, and osteosarcoma. Lung cancer is the primary cause of cancer deaths around the globe with NSCLC accounting for 90% of new cases [62], and these patients develop distant or locoregional recurrence. In 50% of melanoma patients, recurrence takes place after a decade or later [60]. Although prostate cancer is a slow growing tumor, showing biogenetic recurrence in low- and high-risk patients, it may begin some 4–5 years following a therapy. The curative intent of this recurrence is 25% of patients [63]. A high percentage of recurrence can be observed in the OC, with an estimated 85% of patients achieving full remission after the first treatment, which can be a surgery with adjuvant chemotherapy. The median survival rate of these patients is 1–2 years [64]. Breast cancer with over 274,000 cases in 2020 alone is the most common type of cancer in US after skin cancer. If the cancer cells arrive once at a new environment, they face different fates. A large portion of them undergo apoptosis process and face death instantly. The cells that successfully use adaptive behavior and try hard to survive enters a dormant condition. Some of these dormant cells may reside in solitude called the quiescent cells, also termed as cellular dormancy. Some of these also survive as tiny clusters of cells termed as quiescent cell groups. The remaining may stay as tiny indolent micrometastases, and this is where the cell proliferation is readily balanced by apoptosis. Some of the indolent micrometastases remain as dormant, and they form angiogenic signals. As reported in some recent publications, there are no known imaging moieties that can be used for finding the dormant micrometastases (quiescent and indolent) in patients. Moreover, owing to the quiescence of these micrometastases, the dormant disseminated tumor cells (DTCs) are now resistant to the traditional cancer prevention therapies. Hence, these dormant DTCs then stay in the body just like ticking time bombs and produce deadly breast cancer metastatic relapse [65–68].

Recurrence of liver cancer after the surgery is a common obstacle for improving the survival rate of liver cancer patients. In [69], a messenger RNA is a molecule that contains the instructions or recipe that directs the cells to make a protein using its natural machinery. The authors used random forest ML algorithm, which uses decision trees made by randomly selected samples. A series of bioinformatic analyses is performed on the genetic profiles of liver cancer patients, and 18mRNAs are selected as biomarkers for prediction of recurrence. A joint analysis of liver cancer recurrence risk was performed and found significant factors involved with the risk of postoperative liver cancer recurrence. These results are very helpful for the treatment of patients having liver cancer after the surgery to reveal the actual mechanism of recurrence of liver.

In [70], a breast cancer recurrence study is performed, and ML forecasting algorithms are used to compare the accuracy of cancer recurrence within 10 years after the surgery. This study also aims to identify significant predictors of recurrence. Data of breast cancer patients who underwent surgery was applied to a training dataset with 798 samples. The testing and validation samples are both taken equal to 171. The global sensitivity analysis is performed for the evaluation of selected predictors. Quality of care, demographic characteristics, clinical aspects, and the quality of life before the operation are the factors that were prominently associated with the recurrence in the duration of 10 years after the cancer surgery. p-value is the primary parameter of comparison. The p-value can be defined as the probability value, which tells us how likely is the occurrence of our data under the null hypothesis. The p-value chosen is less than 0.001, which indicates that the analysis is carried out very precisely. Overall five algorithms are used in this research, namely, ANN, KNN, SVM, Naive Bayes Classifiers (NBC), and COX models. It is observed by experiments that ANN has the highest values of metrics for accurate prediction of recurrence. In [71], genomical, demographic, and clinical data are integrated to construct more accurate portrait of NSCLC treatment using ML predictive models. A comparative analysis of these three methods demonstrates that CART tree models provide a good predictive performance and more advantageous in terms of understandable tree-like graphs. These graphs help in generation of rules to predict the LUSC recurrence and possible survivability. The if-then rules and major key factors demonstrated by the tree models are able to provide overall understanding of recurrence risk to the clinicians and survivability of premature stage NSCLC. Glioblastoma is the most common malignant brain tumor with more than 12000 cases every year in the United States with median survival rate of only 1 year after diagnosis. In [72], data of patients from thousands of hospitals across the United States are analyzed with many ML algorithms, and analysis perspective is focused plausibly more generalizable towards patients coming from diverse geographic regions and undergoing a variety of treatments for this disease. DT, SVM, MLP, NB, RF, and KNN algorithms are used to assess the interpretability, prediction, and computational efficiency of these algorithms. Table 4.2 shows some publications with ML algorithms applied to cancer recurrence. This study provides a framework for the development of prediction tools for cancer patients, as well as an online survival calculator for patients with GBM [72]. OC is the second most devastating gynecologic cancer, which is the leading cause of deaths in the world. More than 90% of women having OC reportedly had symptoms long before the diagnosis was made. A vast amount of research papers on this cancer demonstrate that recurrence can be predicted with regard to the personal risk factors following the clinical symptoms of the OC. In [73], ensemble learning, SVM, extreme learning machine (ELM), C5.0, multivariate adaptive regression splines (MARS), and RF were together integrated to rank the risk factors that have the ability to diagnose the recurrence of OC. The paper also presents the important influence of personality along with the clinical symptom representations with the complexities of the unique symptoms that are associated with OC in most of the phases of the recurrent trajectory.

4.6 CANCER SURVIVAL

A predictive algorithm is developed in [74] for the assessment of breast cancer patients' survival, and they discussed the significance of robustness in the developed algorithm's parameter variation. Three classification ML techniques such as SVMs, NNs, and SSL are discussed using the popular

Table 4.2 Some publications with ML algorithms applied to cancer recurrence

Publication	*AI algorithm (validation method)*	*Types of cancer*	*Types of data*	*Metrics (accuracy, Fi score, etc.)*	*Relevant features*	*Significant advancement*
[71]	DT, NN, SVM (10-fold CV)	Lung	NSCLC dataset, 275 early stage LUSC, 295 early stage LUAD	AUC = 0.767, 0.837, 0.815, respectively	Patients of white race have a lower recurrence and lower survival rate compared to patients of other races	EGFR and KRAS copy number variations can have large impact on survival rate. The mutation status of NF1, STK11, KEAP1 along with SMARCA4 can be important factors
[72]	DT,SVM, MLP, NB, RF, KNN (5-fold CV)	Brain (Glioblastoma)	20821 patients from US	Survival probability = 0.7, 0.7, 0.61, 0.69 and 0.67 for DT, SVM, MLP, RF, and KNN, respectively	Molecular markers IDH1 mutation and 1p19q codeletion impact survival in glioblastoma patients	Additional algorithms should be experimented with train on right-censored survival data, granularity of the population-specific registries
[73]	ensemble learning, SVM, extreme learning machine (ELM), C5.0, multivariate adaptive regression splines (MARS), RF (LOO CV)	Ovarian	Ovarian cancer dataset provided by the Chung Shan Medical University Hospital Tumor Registry 987 patients	Recurrence rate = 84.04% c5.0 87.23% mars, 27.13 % pure RF, 96.28% SVM, 96.28% PURE ELM	Assessing the predictor variables in the proposed scheme support that FIGO, pathologic M, age, and pathologic T were significantly related to the recurrence of ovarian cancer	To improve surveillance after treatment might lead to earlier detection of relapse, and provide decision-makers with the effective support for quality clinical decision-making

(*continued*)

Table 4.2 (Cont.)

Publication	*AI algorithm (validation method)*	*Types of cancer*	*Types of data*	*Metrics (accuracy, Fi score, etc.)*	*Relevant features*	*Significant advancement*
[86]	SVM (hold-out)	Breast	679	Accuracy = 89%	Histological grade, tumor size, number of metastatic lymph node, estrogen receptor, lymphovascular invasion, local invasion of tumor, and number of tumors	The BCRSVM evidenced substantially high sensitivity (0.89), specificity (0.73), positive predictive values (0.75), and negative predictive values (0.89)
[87]	Graph-based SSL algorithm (k-fold CV)	Colon	Gene Expression Omnibus (GEO) database,GSE2990, 125 samples	Accuracy = 76.7%	BRCA1, CCND1	sensitivity and specificity of most of the methods compared, higher classification sensitivity and specificity are better
[88]	SVM (Hold-out)	Cervical	168	Accuracy = 68%	Pathologic_S, Cell type target summary	Lymph node metastases (LNM) is critical to examine
[89]	SVM, DT, ANN (10-fold CV)	Breast	Iranian Center for Breast Cancer (ICBC).1189 records	Accuracy = 95.7%, 94.7%, and 93.6%	Effect of age at diagnosis and Menarche	SVM superior to ANNs, ANNs can improve if large dataset used

SEER database [75] for cancer. This dataset consists of 162,500 items and 16 essential (key) features. A new metric, 'survivability' is used, categorizing the survival or death of patients. The significant and informative categories are tumor size, amount of nodes, and the age of the patient at the time of cancer diagnosis. The corresponding accuracies of the three techniques SVM, ANN, and SSL are 51%, 65%, and 71%, respectively. Five-fold cross validation is used for the evaluation purpose. This study demonstrates that the SSL technique is a better method for survival analysis. Bladder cancer is one of the most common malignant tumors of the urinary system, having the fourth incidence among the male malignant tumors. In [76], ML-based diagnostic models are created for patients with bladder cancer. The slice images used are H&E-stained slice, and normal bladder tissues were randomly allocated to two computer-generated seeds in the R environment, which included training cohort and testing cohort. Table 4.3 shows some publications with ML algorithms applied to cancer survival.

4.7 CHALLENGES OF AI IN CANCER

While ML in cancer prognosis, diagnosis, and treatment is a promising technology in promoting care and treatment, latest researches demonstrate that AI in healthcare needs an evidence-based improvement and deployment approach. Using AI technologies in oncology and their integration into clinical practices raises technological challenges in the model development. Creation, organization, and maintenance of data sets to make them accessible to be used by researchers and sanitization process have reduced the bias in collection and management preventing subsequent errors during the ML training. The socioeconomic and legal aspects of these should be considered before the use of AI algorithms in medical techniques for the empowerment of doctors and clinicians. This will help in better prevention, diagnosis, treatment, and care in oncology. Also, the promise of AI in cancer research, the challenges of transparency, and reproducibility must be met. Although there are many opportunities for the success of AI and ML in cancer imaging, various challenges in this field are left to be addressed. Let us discuss some of the crucial clinical, technical, and professional challenges that must be encountered in the application of useful machine algorithms into broader clinical practice for the benefit of patient.

Clinical challenges

It is expected that the developers have a full understanding of the environment in which the AI tools are anticipated to operate. For this, we need to involve doctors during the development of the tool. The data for this need to be sourced from different places. For genomics, molecular pathology, and proteomics, a large amount of data is stored in the electronic health records.

Table 4.3 Some publications with ML algorithms applied to cancer survival

Publication	*AI algorithm*	*Types of cancer*	*Types of data*	*Metrics (accuracy, Fi score, etc.)*	*Relevant features*	*Significant advancement*
[76]	LASSO COX + Generalized ML Model (10-fold CV)	Bladder	108 BCa images and 53 normal bladder tissue images from Shanghai General Hospital	AUC = 0.767, 0.837, 0.815, respectively	Radiomics-based, prediction of lymph node metastasis in bladder carcinoma.	Patients with high-risk score and low-risk score presented significant overall survival differences among both TCGA and the general cohorts
[92]	NB, TRF, (1NN), AdaBoost (AD), (SVM), RBF Network (RBFN), MLP (10-fold CV)	Breast	900 patients in which 876 patients (97.3%) and 24 (2.7%) patients were females and males, respectively	Survival probability = 0.7, 0.7, 0.61, 0.69 and 0.67 for DT, SVM, MLP, RF and KNN, respectively	They try to exploit patterns and relationships among a large number of cases and predict the outcome of a disease using historical cases stored in datasets	Highest accuracy compared to state-of-the-art
[90]	ANN (k-fold CV)	Lung	440	Recurrence rate = 84.04% c5.0 87.23% mars, 27.13 % pure RF, 96.28% SVM, 96.28% PURE ELM	Availability of T_stage, N_ stage and ERBB2 genes, sex and age factors	excellent predictions given that patients in the high-risk group obtained a lower median overall survival compared with low-risk patients (log-rank test *P*-value < 0.00001)

[74]	Graph based SSL (5-fold CV)	Breast	162500	Accuracy = 89%	Age at diagnosis, size and number of nodes, size of tumor	Some models with a higher accuracy than others may be heavily dependent on parameter selection
[91]	SVM (k-fold CV)	Oral	69	Accuracy = 98%	Number of recurrences, TNM stage	Discriminant analysis. Recurrence, number of recurrences, and TNM stage have been identified as the most relevant prognosis factors with both used methods

Therefore, interdisciplinary knowledge and a collaborative environment are critical to success. The complicated and diverse information from the samples can potentially be integrated using the ML to support the personalized medicine for a particular illness [77]. Moreover, these large datasets have their own challenges for data science. AI can revolutionize cancer image analysis by the application of state-of-the-art ML and HPC. Cutting-edge AI methods have the potential to transform the organization-centric to the patient-centric healthcare organization [78]. To implement such a paradigm, there are prominent challenges that need better AI solutions to solve. Precision oncology is an area where AI could be transformative. Precision oncology is defined as the patients' therapy using the tumors molecular profile. Precision oncology can benefit from integrated diagnostics [79, 80].

Professional challenges

Professional challenges can shape the deployment and success of AI/ML in cancer imaging. Stimuli that promote the development of ML include the exceptional rise in the demand for imaging which, when collaborated with workforce shortages, can result in radiologist stress and burnout. To alleviate this, departments should consider updating or redesigning their IT and computing infrastructures. One more challenge is the perception of the radiological workforce to find the potential utility of AI/ML in the clinic.

"The Wizardry of Artificial Intelligence: AI and ML in Cancer Imaging" was the conference organized by International Cancer Imaging Society (ICIS) in 2019, from May 17–18 at the Champalimaud Foundation, Lisbon, Portugal [81]. In this conference, an online survey of 569 radiologists was conducted. These are from 36 countries that were included in the survey. The majority of these (more than 60%) accepted that the benefits of AI can outweigh its potential risks. Most of them agreed with the positive impacts of AI/ML in radiology because

- It can provide a huge help to the radiologists to mark and investigate abnormal findings.
- It can increase work efficiency.
- Making most probable diagnostic suggestions when the radiologist is not sure about the output.

While some of the respondents expressed their confidence that AI and ML are unlikely to be a threat to the job of a radiologist, the majority of them (more than 70%) expressed that it was crucial to prepare for the arrival of AI by investing in education, experimenting new tools, advancing in the curation of images and image annotation data, and collaborating with commercial vendors for the development of specific AI tools that can improve workflow.

Tool challenges

Required tools must focus on the following areas:

(1) Tools that automatically track tumors ranging multiple time points to evaluate their response to the treatment.
(2) Tools that drastically improve(high accuracy) automatic or semi-automatic segmentation of tumor.
(3) Tools supporting the proforma of annotation of the sample image to be captured prospectively.
(4) Tools that can help to extract the possibility of tumors throughout the body. Radiographers and technicians who have a better understanding of AI are required with systemic workflow management and image acquisition capabilities.

Technical challenges

A substantial number of state-of-the-art AI techniques based on DNN are achieving outstanding performance [82]. The main reasons behind their success are the strong ability of DL models to learn from details and the accessibility of large-scale precisely annotated datasets. However, in biomedical research, collecting these accurate annotations is a very expensive and comparatively time-consuming process, as the need for domain expert knowledge is always required [83]. When certain AI models that have bounding boxes encompassing an area of interest beyond precise outlining, or image-level labeling rather than specific image feature labeling have a drawback. These models are successful on rough annotations and weak supervision and have been attracting much attention [84].

Moreover, it is essential that with the availability of samples, the data quality and sample diversity should also be considered for collecting and preparing balanced datasets. This situation can be improved by using domain adaptation and transfer learning techniques. Studies that have been published using samples of as few as 10 patients are highly questionable owing to the potential overfitting effects that may negatively impact the generalizability of the findings. Sparse datasets and nonstandardized clinical approaches are other important challenges when it comes to developing integrative ML models, but there is hope that data acquisition can facilitate these cases of AI91.

The explainability of the AI models addresses a sensitive issue that concerns patient safety, more effectively in a clinical decision-support systems [85]. Whenever a domain expert is involved in the AI model development, the resultant models are more robust and reproducible and are trustworthy for the end-users. Evaluation of the overall performance of the AI technology, much more importantly than accuracy, is a mandatory requirement in the clinical pathway setting for cancer disease. This would also include testing the real-world implementation of these models for ascertaining their viability, trustworthiness, and cost-effectiveness.

4.8 CONCLUSION

In the last decade, rapid developments in AI technologies can be observed, having a broad range of disease diagnosis, prognosis, and treatment applications welcomed by a majority of clinicians and radiologists. AI techniques in cancer witnessed a huge revolution in the detection and treatment of cancer using computational techniques. This chapter presents the suitability of AI techniques at various stages of cancer. A systematic overview of the latest techniques in the diagnosis of several cancers that affect the human body is presented. If cancer is diagnosed early, the treatment can proceed with radiotherapy or surgery but treatment from these methods becomes increasingly difficult as the stages of cancer increase. Therefore, it is inevitable to find the cancer susceptibility. In this chapter, discussions on AI algorithms applied firstly to assess the susceptibility of various cancers are done. Later, recurrence of cancer and survival possibilities of the cancer patient are discussed with a plethora of research papers presented in the last 10 years on these topics. Publications discussed in the susceptibility, recurrence, and survival showcase the most successful domains of ML-based oncological applications. The chapter focuses on the review, analysis, categories, and methodologies of a multitude of cancers and uncovers existing limitations. In this chapter, the case for each of cancer susceptibility, cancer recurrence, and cancer survival by using ML algorithms is discussed. Only selected publications that used distinguishable ML techniques are mentioned. The chapter provides details on the multifaceted application of AI models, discussing the robustness and explainability of a variety of algorithms employed in the healthcare systems.

The success of the state-of-the-art AI/ML techniques is mostly constrained by the available data for cancer imaging. The chapter presents the clinical, professional, tool, and technical challenges of application of AI to the clinical domain of cancer disease. For the development of AI tools in the cancer analysis and treatment, there is a need for systematic evaluation that often undergo just a limited amount of testing prior to the release. At the same time, it is vital to empower all stakeholders, clinicians and radiologists, imparting sufficient knowledge and understanding.

REFERENCES

[1] J. Ferlay, M. Ervik, F. Lam, M. Colombet, L. Mery, M. Piñeros, et al. *Global cancer observatory: Cancer today*. Lyon: International Agency for Research on Cancer, 2020. https://gco.iarc.fr/today, accessed February 2021.

[2] S. Marinai, M. Gori, and G. Soda. "Artificial neural networks for document analysis and recognition." *IEEE Trans. Pattern Anal. Mach. Intell.*, vol. 27, no. 1, pp. 23–35, 2005. doi:10.1109/TPAMI.2005.4

[3] D. Trapani et al.. "An international survey on the knowledge, attitudes and clinical patterns of use of medical cannabis for cancer care: The TASMAN study." *Eur. J. Cancer*, vol. 215, 115158, 2025.

[4] I. Ahmad and F. Alqurashi. "Early cancer detection using deep learning and medical imaging: A survey." *Crit. Rev. Oncol. Hematol.*, vol. 204, 104528, 2024. doi: 10.1016/j.critrevonc.2024.104528.

[5] J. C. Zhang, N. Chambwe, J. S. Damrauer, T. A. Knijnenburg, A. G. Robertson, et al. "Comprehensive analysis of genetic ancestry and its molecular correlates in cancer." Cancer Cell, vol. 37, no. 5, pp. 639–654. e6, 2020. doi: 10.1016/j.ccell.2020.04.012

[6] M. Bkassiny, Y. Li and S. K. Jayaweera. "A survey on machine-learning techniques in cognitive radios." *IEEE Commun. Surv. Tutor.*, vol. 15, no. 3, pp. 1136–1159, 2013. doi:10.1109/SURV.2012.100412.00017

[7] K. Kosmelj and K. Vadnal. "Comparison of two generalized logistic regression models; a case study." In Proceedings of the 25th International Conference on Information Technology Interfaces, 2003. ITI 2003., pp. 199–204, 2003. doi:10.1109/ITI.2003.1225345

[8] J. J. Hopfield. "Neural networks and physical systems with emergent collective computational abilities". *Proc. Natl. Acad. Sci. U.S.A*, vol. 79, no. 8, pp. 2554–2558, 1982.

[9] N. Cristianini and J. Shawe-Taylor. An introduction to support vector machines and other kernel-based learning methods. Cambridge University Press, 2000.

[10] R. Caruana and A. Niculescu-Mizil. An empirical comparison of supervised learning algorithms. In *Proceedings 23rd International Conference on Machine Learning*, 2006.

[11] M. R. Bakrania, I. J. Rae, A. P. Walsh, D. Verscharen, and A. W. Smith. "Using dimensionality reduction and clustering techniques to classify space plasma regimes." *Front. Astron. Space Sci.*, vol. 7, p. 593516, 2020. doi:10.3389/fspas.2020.593516

[12] L. P. Kaelbling, M. L. Littman, and A. W. Moore. "Reinforcement Learning: A Survey." *J. Artif. Intell. Res.*, vol. 4, pp. 237–285, 1996. doi:10.1613/jair.301

[13] E.V. Spînu-Popa, D. Cioni, and E. Neri. "Radiology reporting in oncology—oncologists' perspective." *Cancer Imag*, vol. 21, article no. 63, 2021. https://doi.org/10.1186/s40644-021-00431-5

[14] J. van Timmeren, D. Cester, S. Tanadini-Lang *et al.* "Radiomics in medical imaging—"how-to" guide and critical reflection." *Insights Imag*, vol. 11, article no. 91, 2020. https://doi.org/10.1186/s13244-020-00887-2

[15] F. Dankers, A. Traverso, L. Wee, and S. M. J. van Kuijk. In *Fundamentals of clinical data science*. P. Kubben, M. Dumontier, and A. Dekker, editors, pp. 101–120, 2019. Cham: Springer. https://doi.org/10.1007/978-3-319-99713-1

[16] A. Traverso, F. Dankers, B. Osong, L. Wee, and S. M. J. van Kuijk. In Fundamentals of clinical data science. P. Kubben, M. Dumontier, and A. Dekker, editors, pp. 121–133, 2019. Cham: Springer. https://doi.org/10.1007/978-3-319-99713-1

[17] C. Parmar et al. "Radiomic machine-learning classifiers for prognostic biomarkers of head and neck cancer." *Front. Oncol.*, vol. 5, p. 272, 2015.
[18] N. Rieke et al. "The future of digital health with federated learning." *NPJ Digit. Med.*, vol. 3, p. 119, 2020.
[19] M. Kirienko et al. "Distributed learning: a reliable privacy-preserving strategy to change multicenter collaborations using AI." *Eur. J. Nucl. Med. Mol. Imag.*, vol. 48, pp. 3791–3804, 2021. https://doi.org/10.1007/s00259-021-05339-7
[20] A. A. Mohamed et al. "A deep learning method for classifying mammographic breast density categories." *Med. Phys.*, vol. 45, pp. 314–321, 2018.
[21] A. Arieno, A. Chan, and S. V. Destounis. "A review of the role of augmented intelligence in breast imaging: from automated breast density assessment to risk stratification." *Am. J. Roentgenol.*, vol. 212, pp. 259–270, 2019.
[22] A. Yala, C. Lehman, T. Schuster, T. Portnoi, and R. Barzilay. "A deep learning mammography-based model for improved breast cancer risk prediction." *Radiology*, vol. 292, pp. 60–66, 2019.
[23] K. Dembrower et al. "Comparison of a deep learning risk score and standard mammographic density score for breast cancer risk prediction." *Radiology*, vol. 294, pp. 265–272, 2020.
[24] M. Le Boulc'h et al. "Comparison of breast density assessment between human eye and automated software on digital and synthetic mammography: Impact on breast cancer risk." *Diagn. Interv. Imag.*, vol. 101, pp. 811–819, 2020.
[25] S. Chakrabarty et al. "MRI-based identification and classification of major intracranial tumor types by using a 3D convolutional neural network: a retrospective multi-institutional analysis." *Radiol. Artif. Intell.*, vol. 3, p. e200301, 2021.
[26] D. Baptista, P. G. Ferreira, and M. Rocha, "Deep learning for drug response prediction in cancer." *Brief. Bioinform.*, vol. 22, pp. 360–379, 2021.
[27] Esteva A, Robicquet A, Ramsundar B, Kuleshov V, DePristo M, Chou K, et al. "A guide to deep learning in healthcare." *Nat. Med.*, vol. 25, no. 1, 24–29, 2019.
[28] A. Echle, N. T. Rindtorff, T. J. Brinker, T. Luedde, A. T. Pearson, and J. N. Kather. "Deep learning in cancer pathology: A new generation of clinical biomarkers." *Br. J. Cancer*, vol. 124, no. 4, pp. 686–696, 2021.
[29] R. L. Grossman, A. P. Heath, V. Ferretti, H. E. Varmus, D. R. Lowy, W. A. Kibbe, and L. M. Staudt. "Toward a shared vision for cancer genomic data." *N. Engl. J. Med.*, vol. 375, no. 12, pp. 1109–1112, 2016.
[30] T. Ahn, T. Goo, C.-h. Lee, S. Kim, K. Han, S. Park, and T. Park. Deep learning-based identification of cancer or normal tissue using gene expression data. In 2018 *IEEE International Conference on Bioinformatics and Biomedicine (BIBM): IEEE*, p. 1748–1752, 2018.
[31] B. Lyu and A. Haque. Deep learning based tumor type classification using gene expression data. In *Proceedings of the 2018 ACM International Conference on Bioinformatics, Computational Biology, and Health Informatics: ACM*. p. 89–96, 2018.
[32] World Health Organization. Early detection of Cancer, 2016. Available at www.who.int/Cancer/detection/en/

[33] World Health Organization. Early Cancer diagnosis saves lives, cuts treatment costs, 2017. Available at www.who.int/news-room/detail/03-02-2017-early-Cancer-diagnosis-saves-lives-cuts-treatment-costs
[34] J. Phallen, M. Sausen, V. Adleff, et al. "Direct detection of early-stage cancers using circulating tumor DNA." *Sci. Transl. Med.*, vol. 9, p. 403, 2017. doi:10.1126/scitranslmed.aan2415
[35] H. Blumen, K. Fitch and V. Polkus. "Comparison of treatment costs for breast cancer, by tumor stage and type of service." *Am. Health Drug Benefits*, vol. 9, pp. 23–32, 2016.
[36] Z. Kakushadze, R. Raghubanshi, and W. Yu. "Estimating cost savings from early cancer diagnosis." *Data*, vol. 2, p. 30, 2017. doi:10.3390/data2030030
[37] Cancer Research UK. Saving lives, averting costs, 2014. Available at www.Cancerresearchuk.org/sites/default/files/saving_lives_averting_costs.pdf
[38] R. L. Siegel, K. D. Miller, and A. Jemal. "Cancer statistics." *CA Cancer J. Clin.*, vol. 69, pp. 7–34, 2019. doi:10.3322/caac.21551
[39] Cancer Research UK. Why is early diagnosis important? 2018. Available at www.Cancerresearchuk.org/about-Cancer/Cancer-symptoms/why-is-early-diagnosis-important
[40] G. F. Stark, G. R. Hart, B. J. Nartowt, et al. "Predicting breast cancer risk using personal health data and machine learning models." *PLoS One*, vol. 14, p. e0226765, 2019. doi:10.1371/journal.pone.0226765
[41] M. A. Schonberg, V. W. Li, A. H. Eliassen, R. B. Davis, A. Z. LaCroix, E. P. McCarthy et al., Performance of the breast cancer risk assessment tool among women age 75 years and older. *J. Natl Cancer Inst.*, vol. 108, no. 3, djv348, 2015. https://doi.org/10.1093/jnci/djv348.
[42] A. C. Lorena, L. F. O. Jacintho, M. F. Siqueira, et al. "Comparing machine learning classifiers in potential distribution modelling." *Expert Syst. Appl.*, vol. 38, pp. 5268–5275, 2011. doi:10.1016/j.eswa.2010.10.031 [CrossRef] [Google Scholar]
[43] S. Ahmad and A. M. Mayya. "A new tool to predict lung cancer based on risk factors." *Heliyon*, vol. 6, no. 2, e03402, 2020. https://doi.org/10.1016/j.heliyon.2020.e03402.
[44] Y. Wu, S. Xu, S., Cheng, S. et al. "Clinical application of PARP inhibitors in ovarian cancer: From molecular mechanisms to the current status." *J. Ovarian. Res.*, vol. 16, p. 6, 2023. https://doi.org/10.1186/s13048-023-01094-5
[45] M. Lu, Z. Fan, B. Xu, L. Chen, X. Zheng, J. Li, Q. M. TaiebZnati and J. Jiang. "Using machine learning to predict ovarian cancer." *Int. J. Med. Inform.*, vol. 141, p. 104195, 2020. https://doi.org/10.1016/j.ijmedinf.2020.104195
[46] M. K. Gould, B. Z. Huang, M. C. Tammemagi, Y. Kinar, and R. Shiff. "Machine learning for early lung cancer identification using routine clinical and laboratory data." *Am. J. Respir. Crit. Care Med.*, vol. 204, no. 4, pp. 445–453, 2021. doi:10.1164/rccm.202007-2791OC
[47] Y. E. Sánchez-Corrales, R. V. C. Pohle, S. Castellano, and A. Giustacchini. Taming cell-to-cell heterogeneity in acute myeloid leukaemia with machine learning. *Front. Oncol.*, 2021. https://doi.org/10.3389/fonc.2021.666829
[48] Y. Zhang, D. Liu, F. Li, Z. Zhao, X. Liu, D. Gao, Y. Zhang, and H. Li. "Identification of biomarkers for acute leukemia via machine

learning-based stemness index." *Gene*. vol. 804, p. 145903, 2021. doi:10.1016/j.gene.2021.145903

[49] Z. Liu, L. Liu, S. Weng et al. "Machine learning-based integration develops an immune-derived lncRNA signature for improving outcomes in colorectal cancer." *Nat. Commun.*, vol.13, p. 816, 2022. https://doi.org/10.1038/s41467-022-28421-6

[50] O.-J. Skrede, S. De Raedt, A. Kleppe, T. S. Hveem, K. Liestøl, J. Maddison, et al., "Deep learning for prediction of colorectal Cancer outcome: a discovery and validation study." *The Lancet*, 2020. https://doi.org/10.1016/S0140-6736(19)32998-8

[51] Y. Mori, S.-E. Kudo, T. M. Berzin, M. Misawa and K. Takeda "Computer-aided diagnosis for colonoscopy." *Endoscopy*, vol. 49, pp. 813–819, 2017.

[52] R. M. Jiménez-Rodríguez, M. Rubio-Dorado-Manzanares, J. M. Díaz-Pavón, M. L. Reyes-Díaz, J. M. Vazquez-Monchul, A. M. Garcia-Cabrera, J. Padillo, and F. De la Portilla. "Learning curve in robotic rectal cancer surgery: Current state of affairs." *Int. J. Colorectal Dis.*, vol. 31, pp. 1807–1815, 2016.

[53] H. Hu, Z. Niu, Y. Bai, and X. Tan. "Cancer classification based on gene expression using neural networks." *Genet. Mol. Res.*, vol. 14, pp. 17605–17611, 2015.

[54] G. Xu, M. Zhang, H. Zhu, and J. Xu. "A 15-gene signature for prediction of colon Cancer recurrence and prognosis based on SVM." *Gene*, vol. 604, pp. 33–40, 2017.

[55] T. Ayer, O. Alagoz, J. Chhatwal, J. W. Shavlik, C. E. Jr Kahn and E. S. Burnside. "Breast cancer risk estimation with artificial neural networks revisited: Discrimination and calibration." *Cancer*, vol. 116, no. 14, pp. 3310–3321, 2010. doi:10.1002/cncr.25081

[56] M. Waddell, D. Page, and J. Shaughnessy. Predicting cancer susceptibility from single-nucleotide polymorphism data: a case study in multiple myeloma. In *Proceedings of the 5th international workshop on Bioinformatics (BIOKDD '05)*. Association for Computing Machinery, New York, NY, USA, 21–28, 2005. https://doi.org/10.1145/1134030.1134035]

[57] J. Listgarten, S. Damaraju, B. Poulin, L. Cook, J. Dufour, A. Driga, et al. "Predictive models for breast Cancer susceptibility from multiple single nucleotide polymorphisms." *Clin. Cancer Res.*, vol. 10, pp. 2725–2737, 2004.

[58] A. Stojadinovic, A. Nissan, J. Eberhardt, T. C. Chua, J. O. W. Pelz and J. Esquivel. "Development of a Bayesian belief network model for personalized prognostic risk assessment in colon carcinomatosis." *Am. Surg.*, vol. 77, pp. 221–230, 2011.

[59] K. P. Exarchos, Y. Goletsis and D. I. Fotiadis. "Multiparametric decision support system for the prediction of oral cancer reoccurrence." *IEEE Trans. Inf. Technol. Biomed.*, vol. 16, pp. 1127–1134, 2012.

[60] H. Dillekas, M. S. Rogers and O. Straume. "Are 90% of deaths from cancer caused by metastases?" *Cancer Med.*, vol. 8, no. 12, pp. 5574–5576, 2019. doi:10.1002/cam4.2474

[61] G. P. Gupta and J. Massague. "Cancer metastasis: Building a framework." *Cell*, vol. 127, no. 4, pp. 679–695, 2006. doi:10.1016/j.cell.2006.11.001

[62] J. A. Barta, C. A. Powell and J. P. Wisnivesky. "Global epidemiology of lung cancer." *Ann. Glob. Health*, vol. 85, no. 1, pp. 1–16, 2019. doi:10.5334/aogh.2419

[63] S. Ginzburg, T. Nevers, I. Staff, J. Tortora, A. Champagne, S. S. Kesler, et al. "Prostate cancer biochemical recurrence rates after robotic-assisted laparoscopic radical prostatectomy." *JSLS*, vol. 16, no. 3, 443–450, 2012. doi:10.4293/108680812X13462882736538

[64] C. Della Pepa, G. Tonini, C. Pisano, M. Di Napoli, S. C. Cecere, R. Tambaro, et al. "Ovarian cancer standard of care: Are there real alternatives?" *Chin. J. Cancer*, vol. 34, no. 1, pp. 17–27, 2015. doi:10.5732/cjc.014.10274

[65] L. Holmgren, M. S. O'Reilly, and J. Folkman. "Dormancy of micrometastases: balanced proliferation and apoptosis in the presence of angiogenesis suppression." *Nat. Med.*, vol. 1, no. 2, pp. 149–153, 1995. doi:10.1038/nm0295-149

[66] A. F. Chambers, A. C. Groom and I. C. MacDonald. "Dissemination and growth of cancer cells in metastatic sites." *Nat. Rev. Cancer,* vol. 2, no. 8, pp. 563–572, 2002. doi:10.1038/nrc865

[67] J. A. Aguirre-Ghiso. "Models, mechanisms and clinical evidence for cancer dormancy." *Nat. Rev. Cancer*, vol. 7, no. 11, pp. 834–846, 2007. doi:10.1038/nrc2256

[68] D. Barkan and A. F. Chambers. Prevention of conversion of tumor dormancy into proliferative metastases. New York: New York Springer, 2016. doi:10.1007/ 978-1-4939-3363-1_7

[69] X. Qian, H. Zheng, K. Xue, Z. Chen, Z. Hu, L. Zhang and J. Wan. "Recurrence risk of liver cancer post-hepatectomy using machine learning and study of correlation with immune infiltration." *Front. Genet.*, vol. 12, p. 733654, 2021. doi:10.3389/fgene.2021.733654

[70] S. J. Lou, M. F. Hou, H. T. Chang, C. C. Chiu, H. H. Lee, S. J. Yeh, and H. Y. Shi. "Machine learning algorithms to predict recurrence within 10 years after breast cancer surgery: A prospective cohort study." *Cancers (Basel*). vol. 12, no. 12, p. 3817, 2020. doi:10.3390/Cancers12123817

[71] Y. Yang, L. Xu, L. Sun, P. Zhang, and S. S. Farid. "Machine learning application in personalised lung cancer recurrence and survivability prediction." *Comput. Struct. Biotechnol. J.*, vol. 20, pp. 1811–1820, 2022. https://doi.org/10.1016/j.csbj.2022.03.035

[72] J. T. Senders, P. Staples, A. Mehrtash, D. J. Cote, M. J. B. Taphoorn, D. A. Reardon, W. B. Gormley, T. R. Smith, M. L. Broekman, and O. Arnaout. "An online calculator for the prediction of survival in glioblastoma patients using classical statistics and machine learning." *Neurosurgery*, vol. 86, no. 2, pp. E184–E192, 2020. doi:10.1093/neuros/nyz403

[73] C. J. Tseng, C. J. Lu, C. C. Chang, G. D. Chen, and C. Cheewakriangkrai. "Integration of data mining classification techniques and ensemble learning to identify risk factors and diagnose ovarian cancer recurrence." *Artif. Intell. Med.*, vol. 78, pp. 47–54, 2017. doi:10.1016/j.artmed.2017.06.003

[74] K. Park, A. Ali, D. Kim, Y. An, M. Kim, and H. Shin. "Robust predictive model for evaluating breast cancer survivability." *Engl. Appl. Artif. Intell.*, vol. 26, pp. 2194–2205, 2013.

[75] N. Howlader, A. Noone, M. Krapcho, J. Garshell, N. Neyman, and S. Aletkruse. SEER cancer statistics review, 1975–2010, *National Cancer Institute*. Bethesda, MD: National Cancer Institute, 2013.

[76] S. Chen, L. Jiang, X. Zheng, J. Shao, T. Wang, E. Zhang, F. Gao, X. Wang, and J. Zheng. "Clinical use of machine learning-based pathomics signature

for diagnosis and survival prediction of bladder cancer." *Cancer Sci.*, vol. 112, no. 7, pp. 2905–2914, 2021. doi:10.1111/cas.14927

[77] E. J. Topol. "High-performance medicine: the convergence of human and artificial intelligence." *Nat. Med.*, vol. 25, pp. 44–56, 2019.

[78] A. A. Seyhan and C. Carini. "Are innovation and new technologies in precision medicine paving a new era in patients centric care?" *J. Transl. Med.*, vol. 17, p. 114, 2019.

[79] M. Bukowski et al. "Implementation of eHealth and AI integrated diagnostics with multidisciplinary digitized data: Are we ready from an international perspective." *Eur. Radiol.*, vol. 30, pp. 5510–5524, 2020.

[80] S. K. Mun, K. H. Wong, S. B. Lo, Y. Li and S. Bayarsaikhan. "Artificial intelligence for the future radiology diagnostic service." *Front. Mol. Biosci.*, vol. 7, p. 614258, 2020.

[81] W. L. Bi MD et al. "Artificial intelligence in cancer imaging: Clinical challenges and applications." *CA Cancer J. Clin.*, vol. 69, pp. 127–157, 2019. https://doi.org/10.3322/caac.21552

[82] Y. LeCun, Y. Bengio, and G. Hinton. "Deep learning." *Nature*, vol. 521, pp. 436–444, 2015.

[83] G. Litjens et al. "A survey on deep learning in medical image analysis." *Med. Image Anal.*, vol. 42, pp. 60–88, 2017.

[84] M. Rajchl et al. "DeepCut: Object segmentation from bounding box annotations using convolutional neural networks." *IEEE Trans. Med. Imag.* vol. 36, pp. 674–683, 2017.

[85] E. H. Shortliffe and M. J. Sepulveda. "Clinical decision support in the era of artificial intelligence." *JAMA*, vol. 320, pp. 2199–2200, 2018.

[86] W. Kim, K. S. Kim, J. E. Lee, D.-Y. Noh, S.-W. Kim, Y. S. Jung, et al. "Development of novel breast cancer recurrence prediction model using support vector machine." *J. Breast Cancer*, vol. 15, pp. 230–238, 2012.

[87] C. Park, J. Ahn, H. Kim, and S. Park. "Integrative gene network construction to analyze cancer recurrence using semi-supervised learning." *PLoS One*, vol. 9, p. e86309, 2014.

[88] C.-J. Tseng, C.-J. Lu, C.-C. Chang, and G.-D Chen. "Application of machine learning to predict the recurrence-proneness for cervical cancer." *Neural Comput. Appl.*, vol. 24, pp. 1311–1316, 2014.

[89] A. T. Eshlaghy, A. Poorebrahimi, M. Ebrahimi, A. R. Razavi, and L. G. Ahmad. "Using three machine learning techniques for predicting breast cancer recurrence." *J. Health Med. Inform.*, vol. 4, p. 124, 2013.

[90] Y.-C. Chen, W.-C. Ke, and H. -W. Chiu. Risk classification of cancer survival using ANN with gene expression data from multiple laboratories. *Comput. Biol Med.*, vol. 48, pp. 1–7, 2014.

[91] P. Rosado, P. Lequerica-Fernández, L. Villallaín, I. Peña, F. Sanchez-Lasheras, J. C. de Vicente. Survival model in oral squamous cell carcinoma based on clinicopathological parameters, molecular markers and support vector machines. *Expert Syst. Appl.*, vol. 40, pp. 4770–4776, 2013.

[92] M. Montazeri, M. Montazeri, M. Montazeri, and A. Beigzadeh. "Machine learning models in breast cancer survival prediction." *Technol. Health Care*, vol. 24, no. 1, pp. 31–42, 2016. doi:10.3233/THC-151071

Chapter 5

AI technologies for diagnosis, prognosis, and survival of neurological, cardiovascular, and infectious diseases

State-of-the-art analysis

5.1 INTRODUCTION

The integration of advanced machine learning (ML) and deep learning (DL) algorithms [1] has ushered in a new era of precision medicine in the healthcare sector, providing unprecedented insights into the complex mechanisms of various medical conditions [2–4]. Neurological disorders, ranging from Parkinson's disease (PD) to Alzheimer's, present significant challenges for patients and healthcare professionals [5]. The incorporation of artificial intelligence (AI) technology has demonstrated a substantial impact on early disease detection, accurate prognosis, and prediction of patient survival outcomes through the utilization of neuroimaging data and sophisticated algorithms [6, 7]. Cardiovascular health remains a global priority, and AI is at the forefront of revolutionizing diagnostic and treatment approaches for this condition. The integration of state-of-the-art ML and DL algorithms [8] has ushered in a new era of precision medicine in the healthcare sector [9], yielding unprecedented insights into the intricate dynamics of various medical conditions [10]. Neurological disorders, encompassing a spectrum from Parkinson's to Alzheimer's disease (AD), pose significant challenges for both patients and healthcare providers. The incorporation of AI technology has demonstrated remarkable efficacy in early disease detection, prognostic accuracy, and patient survival prediction through the analysis of neuroimaging data and complex algorithmic processes [11]. Cardiovascular health continues to be a global priority, with AI spearheading transformative approaches to diagnosis and treatment. AI is facilitating a paradigm shift towards proactive and personalized cardiovascular care, enabling early identification, tailored treatment strategies, and survival forecasts through the examination of intricate cardiac imagery and continuous patient data monitoring via wearable devices [12]. In the wake of global health crises, swift and precise interventions are imperative for combating infectious diseases [13]. AI technologies play a pivotal role in the expeditious diagnosis, prognosis, and survival prediction of infectious diseases such as COVID-19, malaria, and tuberculosis, leveraging

DOI: 10.1201/9781003503033-5

diverse medical data sources. This chapter explores the dynamic interplay between AI and infectious diseases, emphasizing its potential to revolutionize pandemic response strategies and enhance patient outcomes. As the demarcations between medical specialties become increasingly blurred, this chapter presents interdisciplinary perspectives on the application of AI in neurological, cardiovascular, and infectious disorders.

Figure 5.1 sheds light to some of the AI-assisted key processes used in the advanced treatment of neurological diseases. By examining shared methodologies, challenges, and advancements, the analysis aims to unveil the synergies that can be harnessed to create a more holistic and integrated healthcare approach. Through a state-of-the-art analysis, the chapter navigates the current landscape of AI technologies, shedding light on their transformative potential and paving the way for a future where precision medicine becomes a cornerstone in the battle against complex and pervasive diseases. In this exploration of AI technologies, this chapter endeavors to offer a nuanced understanding of how cutting-edge advancements are reshaping the landscape of diagnosis, prognosis, and survival prediction, ultimately propelling healthcare into an era of unprecedented precision and effectiveness.

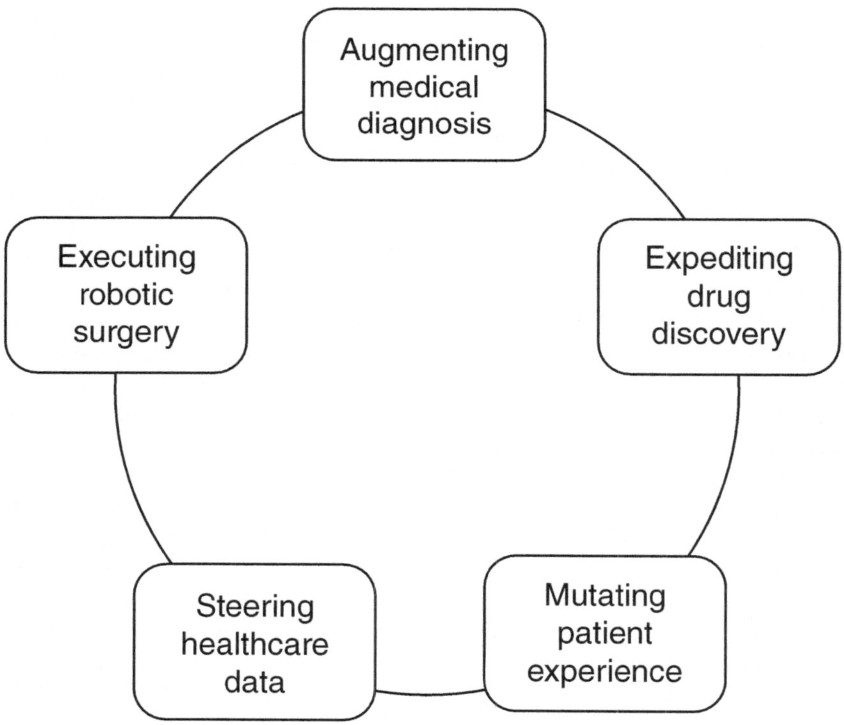

Figure 5.1 Role of AI in advanced treatment of neurological diseases.

5.2 ASSESSMENT OF AI METHODS IN DIAGNOSIS AND PREDICTION

The complexity and heterogeneity of neurological disorders pose significant challenges. AI-driven technologies have enhanced patient care, provided novel insights, and fundamentally transformed the diagnosis and treatment of neurological conditions. In the analysis of neuroimaging data, including magnetic resonance imaging (MRI) and computed tomography (CT) scans [1], AI algorithms—particularly DL models—have demonstrated remarkable accuracy. These models exhibit high sensitivity and specificity in identifying subtle abnormalities indicative of conditions such as multiple sclerosis, PD, and AD. Furthermore, natural language processing (NLP) tools can analyze unstructured clinical notes to identify neurological patterns and symptoms. Predicting the progression of neurological disorders is crucial for treatment planning and patient counseling [14].

Cardiovascular diseases (CVDs) remain the leading cause of mortality worldwide, necessitating accurate risk assessment and diagnosis. AI-powered solutions, utilizing big data analytics and ML algorithms, offer innovative approaches to address these challenges. AI algorithms analyze various cardiovascular imaging modalities, including cardiac MRI, echocardiography, and angiography, to identify structural abnormalities and assess cardiac function. These tools facilitate early intervention and risk mitigation by detecting subtle changes indicative of arrhythmias, heart failure, and ischemic heart disease [15]. The optimization of treatment plans and preventative measures necessitates the capacity to predict the probability of adverse cardiovascular events. AI-powered risk assessment models predict a patient's likelihood of experiencing events such as myocardial infarction, stroke, or sudden cardiac death by integrating clinical data, biomarkers, and imaging results. These models facilitate individualized care plans and targeted interventions by stratifying individuals according to their cardiovascular risk profiles. Regarding survival prediction, AI technologies enhance the monitoring and care of CVD patients, enabling timely interventions to prevent negative outcomes. AI-enabled remote monitoring systems analyze physiological data, including blood pressure readings and electrocardiogram (ECG) signals to detect indicators of cardiac arrhythmias or decompensation. These technologies enable proactive management of high-risk patients and early intervention.

The global health landscape is significantly impacted by infectious diseases, underscoring the critical need for expeditious and precise diagnostic methodologies to manage outbreaks and guide therapeutic interventions. AI-based approaches offer promising avenues for the diagnosis, prognosis, and survival prediction of infectious diseases. These advanced algorithms enhance the efficiency and accuracy of pathogen detection through the examination of various clinical specimens, including hematological samples, respiratory tract swabs, and histological biopsies [16]. ML models, trained on comprehensive datasets to recognize characteristic microbial signatures, facilitate rapid responses and containment strategies. Furthermore, AI-enhanced diagnostic platforms, such as next-generation sequencing technologies and polymerase chain reaction assays, enable swift and scalable screening for infectious agents. The capacity to forecast the clinical progression of infectious diseases plays a pivotal role in optimizing resource allocation and patient stratification. AI-based predictive models assess the likelihood of disease progression and adverse outcomes in patients by integrating clinical observations, laboratory findings, and epidemiological factors [17–19]. These advanced systems enable healthcare providers to tailor therapeutic approaches based on anticipated results and prioritize interventions for individuals at elevated risk. AI-powered technologies facilitate continuous patient surveillance in cases of infectious diseases, enabling prompt identification of complications and clinical deterioration [20]. Sophisticated remote monitoring platforms utilizing AI analyze physiological parameters, biomarkers, and clinical manifestations to identify patients at heightened risk of mortality, organ dysfunction, or sepsis development [21, 22]. During infectious disease outbreaks, these systems enhance patient care delivery and improve survival rates by facilitating early intervention and targeted therapeutic strategies [23–25]. In summation, the advent of AI technologies has heralded a transformative era in healthcare innovation, offering unprecedented capabilities for diagnosing, prognosticating, and predicting survival outcomes across infectious, neurological, and cardiovascular disorders [26, 27]. By leveraging big data, ML algorithms, and sophisticated analytical tools, AI-driven solutions empower healthcare practitioners to deliver care that is more tailored, efficacious, and resource-efficient [28, 29]. This paradigm shift not only enhances patient outcomes but also propels advancements in medical practice. As these technologies continue to mature, they exhibit remarkable potential to tackle the multifaceted challenges associated with diverse medical conditions and to fundamentally reshape the landscape of global healthcare delivery in the years to come [30]. Figure 5.2 shows the basic steps that are adopted for the AI-based treatment of neurological and CVDs.

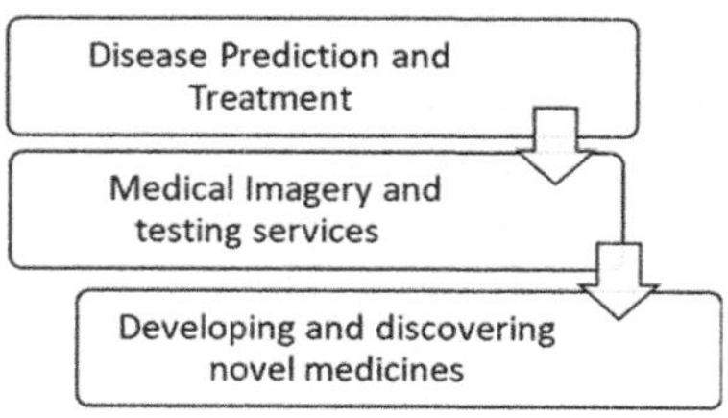

Figure 5.2 Steps of AI based treatment of neurological and cardiovascular diseases.

5.3 STATE-OF-THE-ART AI TECHNIQUES FOR DIAGNOSIS AND TREATMENT OF DISEASES

5.3.1 Implications of AI algorithms in the diagnosis and treatment of motor neuron diseases (MND)

Motor neuron diseases (MNDs) are a collection of long-term neurological disorders marked by the progressive degeneration of the motor system. These conditions arise due to the gradual breakdown of motor neurons (MNs), which are classified into two types based on their location within the central nervous system (CNS): upper and lower MNs. Upper MNs are found in the motor cortex, whereas lower MNs reside in the brainstem and spinal cord. MNs are essential for controlling skeletal muscle contractions. As motor nerve axons deteriorate, the muscles they supply lose functionality, leading to impaired motor control. This degeneration contributes to several well-known MNDs, including amyotrophic lateral sclerosis, spastic paraplegia, bulbar palsy, polytopic paralysis, primary lateral sclerosis, postpolio syndrome, and spinal muscular atrophy. Since no definitive cures currently exist for these disorders, there is an urgent demand for innovative diagnostic and therapeutic approaches. Enhancing diagnostic accuracy and management strategies is crucial for reducing the global burden of MNDs and ensuring timely, effective patient care [31]. However, early detection remains a challenge due to the extensive clinical variability among different types of MNDs and the absence of reliable biomarkers. As a result, patients often experience delays in diagnosis, ranging from 9 to 27 months. Therefore, refining methods for analyzing clinical data is imperative to improve disease classification, accelerate diagnosis, and minimize the overall impact on affected individuals.

AI has gained significant traction in the healthcare sector for its applications in medical data interpretation, image analysis, health monitoring, disease detection, drug discovery, and treatment protocol development [32]. The integration of AI into MND diagnosis holds promise for enhancing accuracy and efficiency, enabling earlier detection and better patient outcomes. By recognizing subtle patterns and intricate relationships within complex datasets, AI-driven algorithms facilitate the early and precise identification of various medical conditions, including neurological disorders, cancer, CVDs, and infectious illnesses. In particular, deep neural networks (DNNs) present a range of opportunities to improve the understanding, diagnosis, and treatment of MND [33, 34]. The following discussion explores the role of DNNs in advancing MND-related research and clinical applications.

Disease Prediction and Diagnosis: DNNs can analyze diverse datasets, including genetic data, clinical notes, medical imaging scans (such as MRI and CT scans), and patient demographics, to predict the risk of developing

MND or assist in early diagnosis. By identifying patterns and biomarkers associated with the condition, DNNs can aid medical professionals in early diagnosis of MND, when treatment options may be more efficacious, or identify individuals at high risk of developing the disease.

Disease Progression Monitoring: DNNs can analyze longitudinal data from individuals with MND, including clinical evaluations, biomarker measurements, and disease progression metrics, to monitor the course of the disease over time [35]. By tracking changes in motor function, disease severity, and other clinical indicators, DNNs can provide insights into the progression of MND and assist medical professionals in optimizing supportive care and treatment plans.

Treatment Response Prediction: DNNs have the capability to predict individual patient responses to various MND treatment modalities by analyzing data from clinical trials and real-world patient populations. By identifying parameters associated with treatment response, such as genetic markers, disease subtype, or demographic characteristics, DNNs can assist clinicians in selecting personalized treatment plans tailored to the specific needs and characteristics of each patient [36].

Biomarker Discovery: DNNs can analyze multimodal data, including genetic, genomic, proteomic, and imaging data, to identify novel biomarkers associated with the etiology, progression, and treatment response of MND [37]. Through the identification of MND-specific molecular signatures and disease signatures, DNNs enhance our understanding of the disease mechanisms and facilitate the development of precision medicine approaches and targeted therapies.

Drug Development and Discovery: DNNs can analyze extensive datasets, including molecular interaction networks, chemical compound libraries, and drug screening data, to accelerate drug development and discovery for MND [38, 39]. By utilizing DNNs to predict the efficacy, safety, and pharmacokinetic properties of potential drug candidates, researchers can prioritize promising compounds for preclinical and clinical testing, potentially identifying novel treatments for MND. A comprehensive analysis of the implications of DNNs for MND research is provided in [40–42]. Following are step-by-step applications of explanation of how DNNs can be applied in MND diagnosis:

Data Collection: The initial phase involves collecting various datasets pertinent to diagnosing MND. This may encompass patient information, clinical records, symptomatology, physical exam results, genetic data, and neuroimaging results like MRI and CT scans.

Data Preprocessing: The amassed information requires processing to ensure uniformity and suitability for analysis. This might involve data cleansing, addressing missing information, and scaling or normalizing numerical variables. For neuroimaging data, preparation may include aligning images, standardizing, and isolating relevant anatomical features.

Model Architecture Design: DNNs are composed of multiple tiers of interconnected nodes, or artificial neurons, arranged hierarchically. The DNN's structure, including the number of tiers, activation function types, and neuronal connections, is devised based on the intricacy of the diagnostic task and the nature of the input data.

Model Training: After data preparation and DNN structure definition, the model is educated using labeled examples of MND cases and healthy subjects. During this process, the DNN learns to recognize patterns and characteristics in the input data associated with MNDs. This involves adjusting neuronal weights and biases to minimize discrepancies between predicted outcomes and actual labels.

Model Evaluation: Trained DNN models are tested using separate validation datasets to gauge their ability to differentiate between MND and non-MND cases. Performance metrics such as accuracy, sensitivity, specificity, area under the receiver operating characteristic curve (AUC-ROC), and precision-recall curve are employed to measure the model's effectiveness.

Clinical Integration: Upon validation, DNN models are incorporated into clinical procedures to aid healthcare professionals in MND diagnosis. They may function as decision support tools, offering clinicians probabilistic evaluations or risk scores based on patient information and medical imaging results.

Iterative Refinement: DNN models may undergo repeated refinement and validation using additional datasets to enhance their performance and applicability. Ongoing feedback from medical professionals and updates to the model structure or training data may be necessary to improve diagnostic precision and reliability. DNNs provide robust tools for MND diagnosis by examining complex clinical data and medical imaging studies to identify patterns indicative of these conditions. By integrating DNN-based diagnostic approaches into medical practice, healthcare providers can potentially improve diagnostic accuracy, enable earlier intervention, and enhance patient outcomes in MNDs.

5.3.2 Implications of DNN in diagnosis and treatment of epilepsy

Epilepsy, a neurological disorder characterized by recurrent seizures, manifests as abnormal electrical discharges in the brain. These seizures exhibit a spectrum of presentations, ranging from brief alterations in consciousness or muscular contractions to severe convulsive episodes. The underlying causes of epilepsy are diverse and may encompass genetic predispositions, traumatic brain injuries, infections, or other neurological conditions. The diagnostic process for epilepsy presents significant challenges due to the heterogeneous nature of seizure manifestations and the absence of definitive diagnostic tests. A comprehensive evaluation typically includes a detailed medical history, physical examination, and neurological assessment, complemented by diagnostic modalities such as electroencephalography (EEG), neuroimaging techniques (MRI or CT scans), and hematological analyses. Despite these diagnostic tools, epilepsy may remain undetected or misclassified in certain cases, potentially resulting in delayed intervention and management strategies. Pharmacological management of epilepsy often involves the administration of antiepileptic medications, which aim to modulate abnormal neuronal activity and mitigate seizure occurrence. However, the process of identifying optimal medication regimens and dosages for individual patients can be complex, given the considerable variability in treatment responses. In cases of drug-resistant epilepsy or focal seizures originating from specific brain regions, surgical interventions may be considered to resect or disconnect the epileptogenic focus. Despite advancements in epilepsy research and therapeutic approaches, significant challenges persist in effectively managing this disorder. These include the development of reliable seizure prediction and prevention methods, minimization of medication-related adverse effects, addressing comorbid conditions such as depression and cognitive impairment, and improving accessibility to specialized epilepsy care, particularly in underserved populations.

Epilepsy poses significant challenges in both diagnosis and treatment, requiring a collaborative approach that includes neurologists, epileptologists, neurosurgeons, and other healthcare specialists. Advancing research on the underlying mechanisms of epilepsy, alongside the development of innovative diagnostic tools and treatment options, is crucial for enhancing patient outcomes and quality of life. The causes of epilepsy vary among individuals and may stem from factors such as genetic susceptibility, brain injuries (including head trauma or stroke), infections like meningitis or encephalitis, developmental disorders, or structural brain abnormalities. However, in many cases, the exact cause remains unknown, a condition referred to as idiopathic epilepsy. Diagnosing epilepsy involves a thorough medical history review, physical examination, and neurological assessment, complemented by diagnostic procedures such as EEG, brain imaging (MRI or CT scans), and blood tests. Treatment approaches commonly include antiepileptic medications, which help regulate abnormal electrical activity in the brain to control seizures. In cases where seizures are resistant to medication, surgical intervention may be an option to remove or disconnect the affected brain region, particularly for individuals with focal epilepsy. Living with epilepsy presents various challenges, including an increased risk of injury during seizures, limitations on certain activities such as driving or swimming, and potential social stigma or discrimination. However, with accurate diagnosis, effective treatment, and proper management, many individuals with epilepsy can lead fulfilling and independent lives. It is essential for patients to collaborate closely with healthcare providers to create a personalized treatment plan and access necessary support services, such as educational resources, counseling, and community assistance. Continued research into the causes, mechanisms, and treatment of epilepsy remains vital to further improving patient care and overall quality of life for those affected by the condition.

DNNs enable personalized seizure prediction models tailored to individual patient profiles, facilitating early intervention and improved patient outcomes. Additionally, DNNs aid in surgical planning by analyzing neuroimaging data, enhancing localization of epileptogenic foci for respective surgery. Overall, the integration of DNNs in epilepsy care holds promise in revolutionizing diagnosis, treatment, and management strategies, ultimately improving the quality of life for epilepsy patients. Mentioned below are a few ways in which DNN can impact epilepsy management:

Seizure Detection and Prediction: DNNs can analyze electroencephalogram (EEG) data to detect and predict seizures with high accuracy. Through the analysis of patterns indicative of seizure activity from labeled EEG recordings, DNNs can automatically detect epileptic events in real time, facilitating early intervention and timely medical assistance for patients.

Personalized Seizure Prediction Models: DNNs can develop individualized seizure prediction models by incorporating patient-specific data, including EEG recordings, clinical history, medication usage, and lifestyle factors. These models can identify patient-specific seizure patterns and initiate personalized alerts or interventions to mitigate seizure risk, thereby enhancing patient safety and quality of life.

Medication Response Prediction: DNNs can predict individual patient responses to antiepileptic medications through the analysis of clinical data, genetic information, and EEG features. By identifying biomarkers associated with medication response or resistance, DNNs can assist clinicians in selecting optimal treatment regimens tailored to each patient's needs, thus optimizing seizure control and minimizing adverse effects.

Identifying Biomarkers and Disease Mechanisms: DNNs can elucidate biomarkers and disease mechanisms underlying epilepsy through the analysis of large-scale datasets, including genetic profiles, neuroimaging studies, and clinical records. By identifying genetic variants, imaging biomarkers, and physiological abnormalities associated with epilepsy subtypes, DNNs contribute to a more comprehensive understanding of the disease pathophysiology and facilitate the development of targeted therapies.

Image Analysis for Surgical Planning: DNNs can analyze neuroimaging data, such as MRI and positron emission tomography (PET) scans, to assist in surgical planning for epilepsy patients undergoing resective surgery. By accurately delineating epileptogenic lesions, cortical dysplasia, and functional brain regions, DNNs enable neurosurgeons to precisely localize seizure foci and optimize surgical outcomes, potentially leading to improved seizure control and reduced postoperative complications.

Remote Monitoring and Telemedicine: DNNs support remote monitoring and telemedicine initiatives for epilepsy management through the analysis of wearable sensor data, including accelerometers and gyroscopes, to detect seizure-related movements and physiological changes. By providing real-time seizure detection and monitoring outside traditional healthcare settings, DNNs enhance patient safety and enable timely interventions, particularly for individuals with refractory epilepsy or high seizure frequency.

DNNs demonstrate significant potential in advancing epilepsy diagnosis and treatment by enabling accurate seizure detection and prediction, personalized medication management, identification of disease biomarkers, and optimization of surgical interventions. By leveraging AI-driven approaches, clinicians can potentially improve patient outcomes, enhance quality of life, and advance the understanding of epilepsy as a complex neurological disorder. Studies proposed by Singh et al. [43] illustrate the diagnosis of epileptic seizures, using two key segments: user segment and cloud segment.

User Segment: This segment encompasses the interface and components accessible to the end-user, such as patients or healthcare providers. It may include wearable devices equipped with sensors for monitoring physiological signals, such as EEG data, heart rate, and movement patterns. The user segment interfaces with the individual experiencing seizures, providing real-time data collection and feedback on seizure activity. The wearable device may feature an intuitive user interface for ease of use and may provide alerts or notifications to the user or caregiver when seizure-like activity is detected.

Cloud Segment: The cloud segment handles the storage, processing, and analysis of data gathered from the user segment. This typically involves cloud-based servers or platforms designed to securely manage and store large volumes of physiological data. Advanced ML models and algorithms deployed in the cloud analyze this data to identify patterns associated with epileptic seizures. Additionally, the cloud segment supports remote

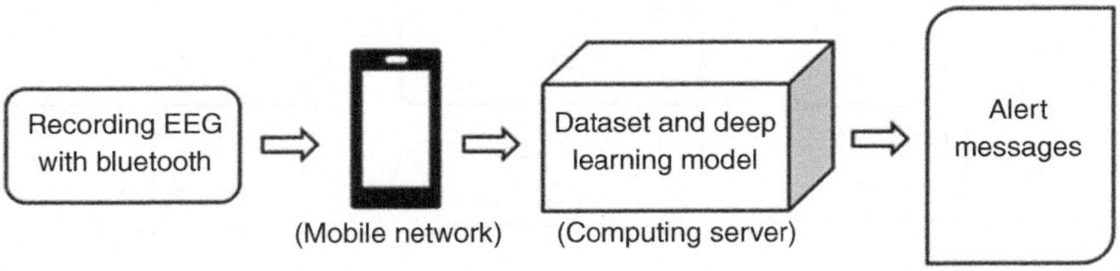

Figure 5.3 Block diagram illustrating an epileptic seizure detection system utilizing deep learning methods with EEG signals.

monitoring and facilitates seamless data sharing among patients, caregivers, and healthcare providers, promoting collaborative and efficient epilepsy management.

Integration between the user segment and the cloud segment allows for seamless data collection, analysis, and feedback in the diagnosis and management of epileptic seizures. By leveraging wearable technology and cloud computing, this utilitarian product aims to enhance the accessibility, accuracy, and timeliness of seizure detection, ultimately improving the quality of life for individuals living with epilepsy. Figure 5.3 illustrates a block diagram of an epileptic seizure detection system utilizing DL methods with EEG signals.

Advancements in hardware technology have significantly improved seizure detection strategies. Hospitals can integrate predictive models into cloud-based platforms, allowing mobile applications, handheld devices, and wearables to incorporate these models while cloud servers handle the computational processing. By leveraging predictive analytics, these devices can provide early warnings to patients, helping them take preventive measures.

Upon detecting a seizure, real-time alerts can be sent to family members, caregivers, hospitals, and healthcare providers via mobile or wearable devices, ensuring timely medical intervention. Additionally, EEG signals can be captured using a cap embedded with EEG electrodes and transmitted to a cloud-based model for immediate analysis. Early detection during the interictal phase of EEG signals enables rapid administration of medication, potentially preventing the onset of a seizure. A novel technique introduced by Glory et al. [44] combines a DNN with an adaptive Haar wavelet-based binary grasshopper optimization algorithm (AHW-BGOA). This hybrid model optimizes hyperparameters while selecting the most relevant features to improve classification accuracy. To extract features, the researchers applied the discrete wavelet transform (DWT) to decompose EEG signals into subbands. A diverse set of features, including nonlinear properties, the Hurst exponent, and entropy-based measures, was then extracted. Figure 5.4 visually represents the application of ML methods in EEG signal analysis.

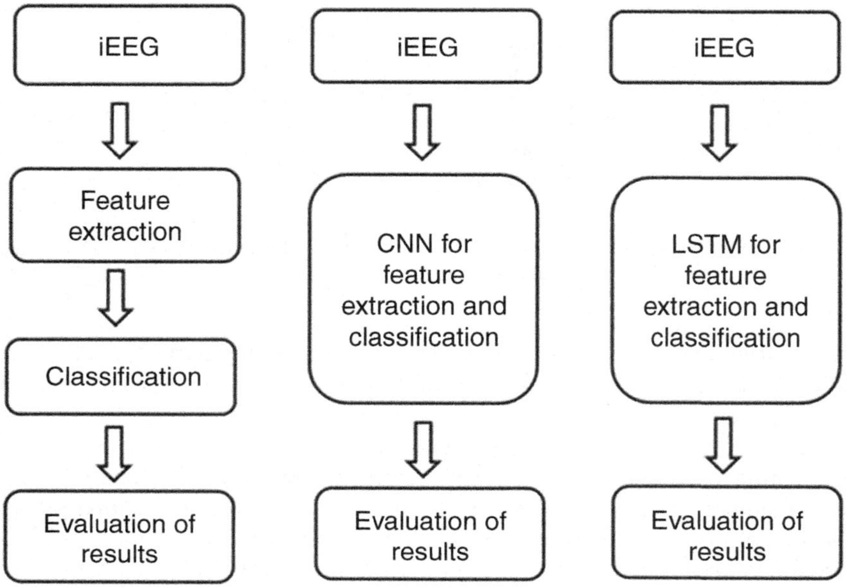

Figure 5.4 Schematic of conducted research depicts implementation of machine learning approaches in EEG analysis.

Kołodziej et al. [45] proposed an advanced approach that focused on selecting high-quality intracranial electroencephalography (iEEG) recordings with precise labeling to ensure effective feature comparison. They divided the iEEG signals into shorter segments, generating an extensive dataset for training and testing DL models. The study compared traditional ML techniques, including feature extraction and classification, with DL methods such as convolutional neural networks (CNN) and long short-term memory (LSTM) networks.

A range of feature extraction techniques was employed, including spectral analysis, autocorrelation, energy-based features, chaos theory-related metrics, Lyapunov exponents, attractor dimensions, wavelet analysis, higher-order statistical measures, and empirical mode decomposition (EMD). The support vector machines (SVM) algorithm was utilized to classify signals containing epileptic seizures. The study aimed to comprehensively compare AI-driven approaches—both traditional ML and DL—in seizure detection. The evaluation of extracted features was conducted using performance metrics such as accuracy, sensitivity, precision, and specificity. Additionally, the authors applied gradient-weighted class activation mapping (Grad-CAM) to highlight the signal segments that significantly contribute to seizure detection when using CNN models.

Feature extraction plays a crucial role in EEG-based seizure detection as it helps reduce data dimensionality, making signal processing more efficient.

Moreover, it facilitates the identification of critical signal patterns linked to seizures, aiding in accurate classification and detection by ML models. Extracted features also assist in distinguishing between various seizure types, thereby improving diagnostic precision.

The EMD method assumes that any signal can be broken down into intrinsic mode function (IMF) components, which must fulfill two criteria: they should be smooth at every point, and the number of extrema (maxima and minima) should be equal or differ by at most one. The EMD process involves the following steps:

1. Detecting all local maxima and minima within the signal.
2. Computing the average value between each adjacent pair of maxima and minima for a given IMF component.
3. Deriving the first IMF component by subtracting this computed average from the input signal.
4. Assessing whether the extracted IMF component meets smoothness and extrema count criteria. If it does, it is accepted as an IMF component; otherwise, the process is repeated for the remaining signal.
5. Repeating steps 2–4 until all IMF components are obtained.

Once EMD is applied, the signal is divided into IMF components representing different frequencies and amplitudes within the original signal. These components enable detailed analysis, providing insights into the signal's characteristics at various time scales. Feature extraction from EEG signals using EMD follows a similar approach to wavelet transformation; however, instead of computing features directly from the raw signal, features are extracted from each successive IMF component. This process allows for multiresolution signal characterization, offering a deeper understanding of the signal's dynamics at different levels.

The design of CNN layers for discrete signals requires careful consideration of the unique properties of the signals and the specific objectives of the analysis. Critical factors such as filter size, stride, padding, and activation functions must be carefully optimized to enhance model performance. Moreover, customizing the network architecture, including the integration of fully connected layers, is essential for effective signal processing and classification. CNNs are widely adopted for EEG-based seizure detection due to their ability to automatically extract key features from signals, eliminating the need for manual feature engineering. By leveraging convolutional layers, CNNs can effectively identify characteristic wave patterns and amplitude variations in EEG signals that indicate seizures. These networks excel at detecting changes in signal structure, such as distinct wave sequences and amplitude fluctuations, making them highly effective tools for seizure detection in clinical and research settings.

CNNs create hierarchical data representations, allowing them to model complex relationships between EEG signal features. The initial convolutional layers extract fundamental patterns, such as wave shapes, while deeper layers combine these elements to form more abstract representations. This progressive approach enables the network to recognize increasingly intricate patterns, ultimately enhancing seizure detection. By employing CNNs for EEG-based seizure identification, an automated and unbiased method is achieved, potentially improving the efficiency of algorithms and enabling rapid epileptic seizure detection.

The search for an optimal CNN architecture involved evaluating multiple factors, including the number of convolutional layers (ranging from 2 to 5), the quantity of filters (ranging from 3 to 10), and filter sizes (tested at 2, 4, 8, 16, 32, 64, and 128). Rather than relying on domain-specific expertise in iEEG signal processing, the optimal network configuration was determined through an automated exploration of the best layer count, filter number, and filter dimensions. Ultimately, a relatively simple CNN architecture with three convolutional layers was selected. Rectified linear unit (ReLU) activation functions were applied after each convolutional layer, with the final convolutional and ReLU layers consisting of 128 filters.

The Adam optimization algorithm was used to train the CNN, with an initial learning rate of 0.001. This learning rate controlled the rate at which the network updated its weights during training. The training process was capped at 50 epochs, meaning the model could iterate over the entire dataset a maximum of 50 times. To improve generalization, the training data were randomized before each epoch. Additionally, approximately 10% of the training data was randomly designated as a validation set, ensuring continuous performance evaluation throughout the training process.

LSTM networks are crucial for effectively modeling sequential data, which is essential in epileptic seizure detection. During seizures, brain signals display characteristic patterns of changes that require time series data analysis [1]. LSTM networks possess internal memory, enabling them to retain information from previous states and use it to predict future changes. The memory cell is the cornerstone of an LSTM network, storing an internal state that can be updated and accessed by gates. These gates regulate the flow of information within the network, determining which data should be kept and which should be discarded. By concentrating on relevant information while filtering out noise and irrelevant details, LSTM networks are particularly adept at analyzing sequential data, such as EEG signals used in seizure detection [1]. When applying LSTM networks to epileptic seizure detection, the network is trained using EEG data representing both seizure and normal brain activity. The LSTM network acquires the ability to identify epileptic seizure patterns and differentiate them from regular brain activity through its training process. After training, the network can evaluate EEG signals in real-time and predict whether they exhibit seizure-like characteristics based on the input data. The research explored the impact of varying hidden units (from 5 to 30) to determine the optimal LSTM configuration for accurate seizure detection in EEG data. In assessing epileptic seizure detection systems, understanding metrics like sensitivity and precision is essential. Sensitivity measures the system's ability to correctly identify actual seizures, aiming for maximum detection. Precision, equally crucial, represents the proportion of correctly identified seizures among all signals classified as such, minimizing false alarms. Striking a balance between high sensitivity and precision is critical for these systems to ensure accurate seizure identification while reducing false positives. This balance is vital for the system's effectiveness in clinical settings, providing timely and accurate seizure alerts without unnecessary alarms.

Yogarajan et al. [46] introduced an approach combining DL and swarm intelligence to enhance classification accuracy, specificity, and sensitivity in epileptic seizure detection. The system employs a DNN for classification and a binary dragonfly algorithm for feature selection, aiming to achieve superior detection accuracy and computational efficiency. Incorporating a feature selection mechanism into the proposed EEG-based epileptic seizure detection system presents an opportunity to further improve its performance through DL.

The main contributions of this work include as follows:

1. Developing a lightweight DNN framework specifically designed for detecting seizures from EEG signals. This framework is optimized to process EEG data efficiently and extract relevant features for accurate seizure detection.
2. Introducing a binary version of the dragonfly algorithm, a swarm intelligence-based optimization technique, for robust and optimal feature selection from various EEG signal subbands. This feature selection process aims to identify discriminative features that effectively distinguish seizure signals from non-seizure signals, enhancing the overall performance of the seizure detection system.
3. The proposed approach incorporates a feature reduction component into the DNN framework to enhance the efficiency and speed of seizure onset detection in patients. This integration ensures the DNN utilizes only the most crucial features, resulting in improved classification accuracy and faster detection times.

The process begins with the collection and preprocessing of EEG signals from the human brain. These signals are then subjected to stationary wavelet transform (SWT), which decomposes them into multiple sub-bands up to level 4. From each coefficient within these sub-bands, various statistical features are extracted, including mean absolute value, standard deviation, skewness, kurtosis, root mean square (RMS) power, the ratio of mean absolute values between adjacent subbands, and multiple Hjorth parameters.

These extracted features offer a detailed representation of the EEG signals. To refine the feature selection process, the binary dragonfly algorithm is employed, ensuring that only the most relevant and distinguishing features are retained. This optimization step enhances the classification model's efficiency by reducing redundant information and improving accuracy. The selected optimal features are then fed into a DNN for training. By utilizing only the most informative features, the computational overhead of the network is minimized, leading to a more efficient and accelerated training process. Once trained, the DNN model is used to classify incoming EEG signals as either seizure or normal, relying on learned patterns from the training data to make accurate predictions. The effectiveness of this approach is assessed using key performance metrics, including accuracy, sensitivity, specificity, and F1 score. These metrics provide a comprehensive evaluation of the model's ability to differentiate between seizure and normal EEG signals, ensuring its reliability in practical applications. Figure 5.5 illustrates the proposed epileptic seizure detection framework, which integrates a hybrid approach combining ML techniques with swarm intelligence for improved diagnostic performance.

The process begins with the decomposition of EEG signals into distinct sub-bands using SWT, followed by the extraction of various features. A binary dragonfly algorithm is then utilized to carefully select optimal and robust features essential for detecting seizures. The selected features are subsequently used to train a DNN model, employing a nature-inspired heuristic algorithm to differentiate between ictal and interictal EEG signals compared to normal EEG signals. This approach improves classification accuracy and speeds up both training and detection processes. Experimental results demonstrate the system's outstanding performance, achieving perfect scores (100%) in classification accuracy, sensitivity, specificity, F1 score, and average Fischer score, while using only 13% of the features compared to existing methods. The system's integration with hospitals through the Internet of Medical Things supports precision medicine, allowing healthcare professionals to more effectively diagnose and treat epilepsy patients. Future

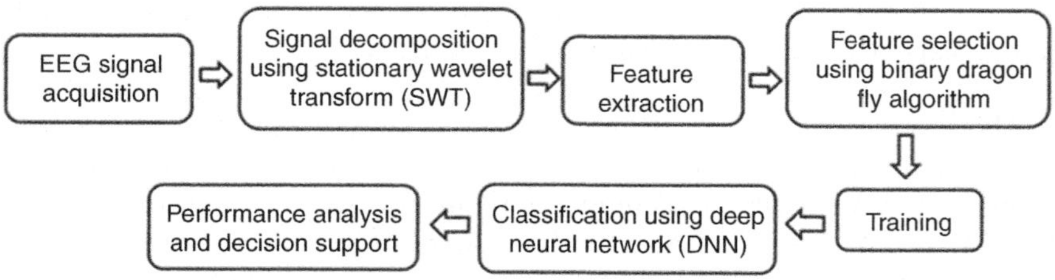

Figure 5.5 Epileptic seizure detection model, integrating a hybrid approach that combines ML techniques with swarm intelligence.

work includes developing an edge device for detecting seizure onset and alerting medical staff and family members to initiate prompt medication, as well as evaluating the proposed approach on various EEG datasets.

Singh et al. [47] propose a novel approach for the automatic prediction of epileptic seizures using long-term multichannel EEG signals, as illustrated in Figures 5.6 and 5.7. Specifically, the approach employs a spectral feature-based two-layer LSTM network model, utilizing spectral power and mean

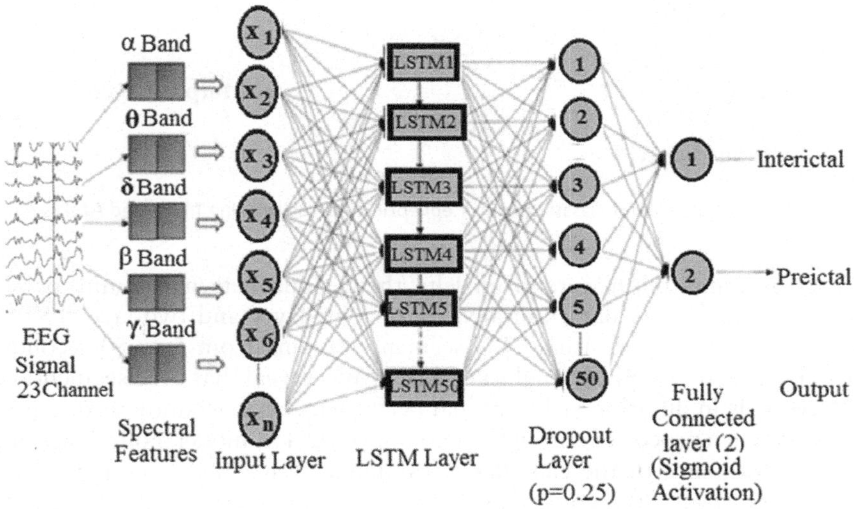

Figure 5.6 Single-layer LSTM (1L-LSTM) model for epileptic seizure prediction.

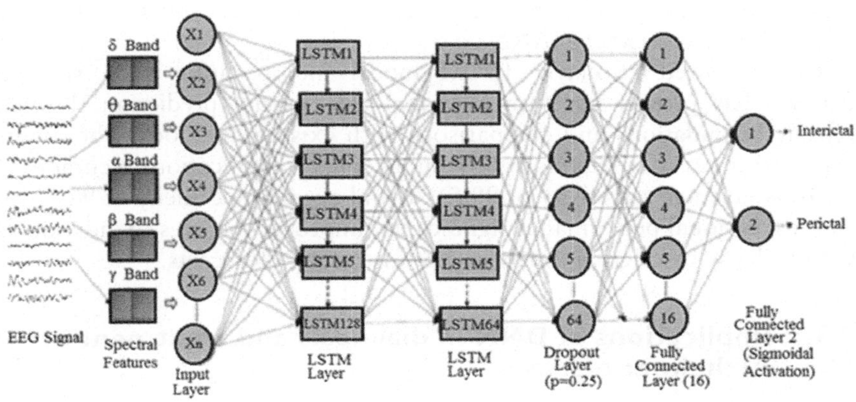

Figure 5.7 Two-layer LSTM (2L-LSTM) model for epileptic seizure prediction.

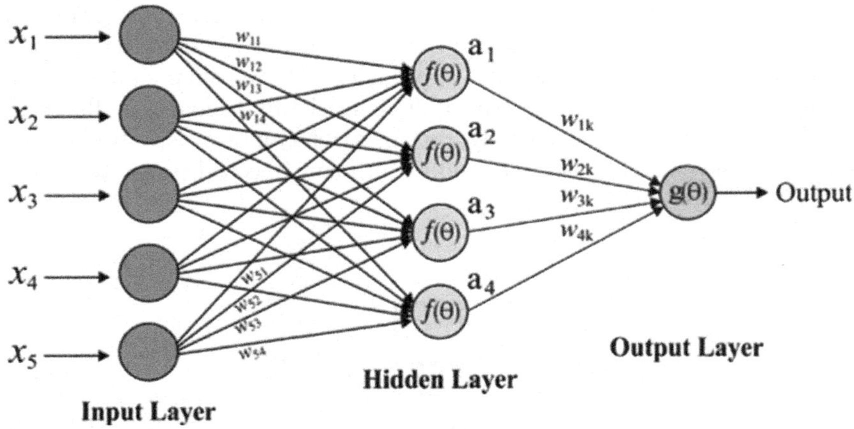

Figure 5.8 Detection and classification of epileptic seizures utilizing ML-based ANNs.

spectrum amplitude features from delta, theta, alpha, beta, and gamma bands of 23-channel EEG data. Initially, both single-layer and two-layer LSTM models are evaluated using EEG segments ranging from 5 to 50 seconds, recorded from 24 epileptic subjects. The results reveal that EEG segments of 30 seconds in duration yield optimal performance for accurate seizure prediction when processed through the two-layer LSTM model. Following this, the performance of the classifier is validated by feeding spectral features extracted from 30-second EEG segments into various ML classifiers, including random forest, decision tree, K-nearest neighbors (KNN), SVM, and Naive Bayes. The parameter estimation for these classifiers is facilitated by grid search, ensuring optimal settings. Figure 5.8 demonstrates the process of detection and classification of epileptic seizures utilizing ML-based artificial neural networks (ANNs).

The proposed two-layer LSTM model incorporating EEG spectral features has proven its efficacy in real-time seizure prediction through repeated simulations and comparisons with existing methods. The model achieves impressive results, with an average classification accuracy of 98.14%, average sensitivity of 98.51%, and average specificity of 97.78%. This exceptional performance significantly improves the lives of individuals with epilepsy by offering timely and precise seizure forecasts.

5.3.3 Implications of DNN in diagnosis and treatment of Alzheimer disease

AD is a degenerative neurological condition marked by a decline in cognitive abilities and loss of memory [48]. It stands as the primary cause of dementia, a condition that impacts memory, cognition, behavior, and the capacity to carry out daily activities. The disease worsens gradually, affecting various cognitive functions including memory, language skills, decision-making abilities, and personality traits. It is linked to the buildup of abnormal protein deposits in the brain, specifically beta-amyloid plaques and tau tangles, which interfere with neural communication and ultimately lead to cell death. Over time, brain tissue diminishes, particularly in areas responsible for memory, thinking, and other cognitive processes. Figures 5.9 and 5.10 illustrate the differences between a healthy brain and one affected by Alzheimer's. Initial symptoms typically manifest as mild memory loss and difficulty recalling recent events or conversations. As the condition advances, individuals may experience disorientation, confusion, language difficulties, mood or behavioral changes, and challenges with reasoning and decision-making. In later stages, patients may require assistance with everyday tasks and struggle to recognize familiar faces or places. While the exact cause of AD remains unclear, it is believed to result from a combination of genetic, environmental, and lifestyle factors. The most significant

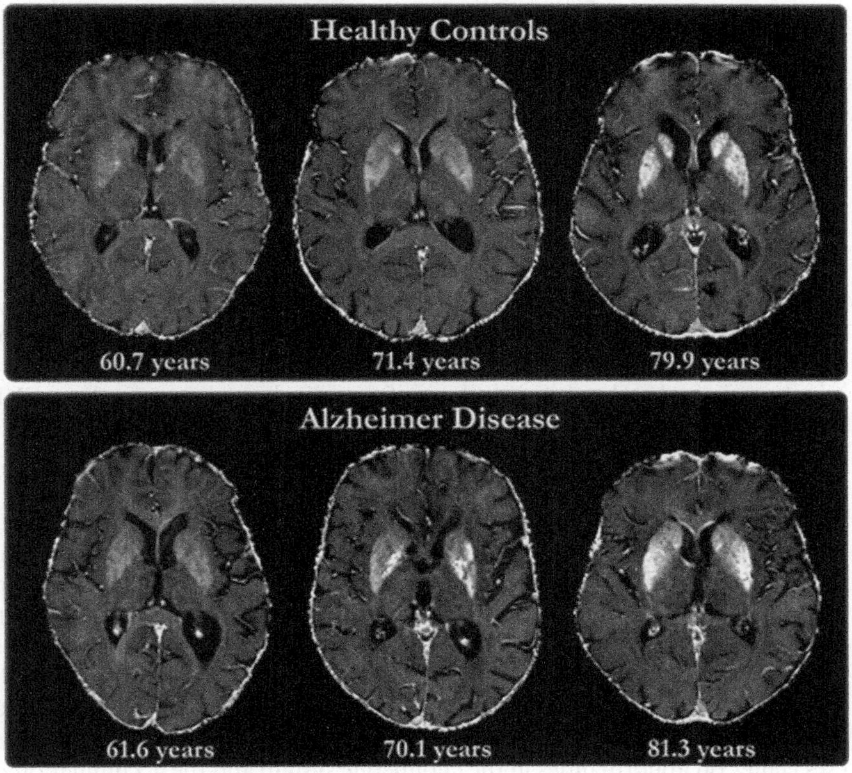

Figure 5.9 Brain imaging of healthy controls and Alzheimer disease.

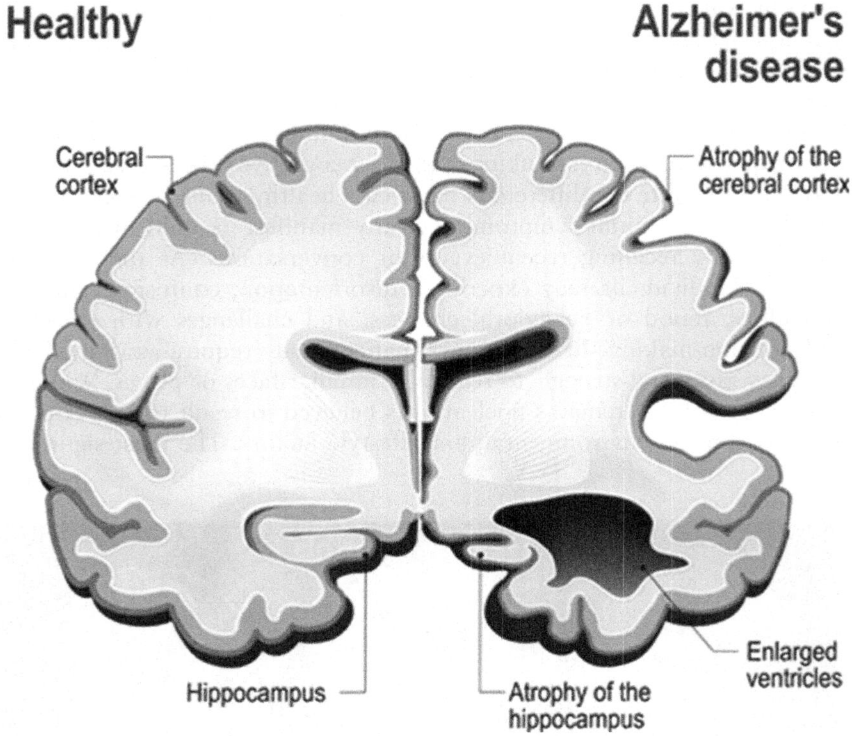

Figure 5.10 Difference between healthy brain and brain effected with AD.

risk factor is age, with the likelihood of developing Alzheimer's increasing as one gets older. Additional risk factors include family history, certain genetic mutations, head trauma, and specific medical conditions such as CVD and diabetes. Figure 5.11 depicts potential risk factors associated with this disease. Although there is currently no cure, treatments are available to manage symptoms and slow the disease's progression.

AD management often involves pharmacological interventions aimed at enhancing cognitive performance, controlling behavioral manifestations, and supporting overall health. Ongoing scientific endeavors seek to uncover potential treatments and preventive measures for Alzheimer's, with the ultimate goals of refining diagnostic techniques, enhancing therapeutic approaches, and eventually discovering a cure for this devastating neurological condition. The cholinergic and amyloid hypotheses represent two primary theories proposed to elucidate the underlying mechanisms of AD [49]. These hypotheses center on abnormalities in the cholinergic system and the accumulation of beta-amyloid plaques within the brain, respectively. While AD is commonly

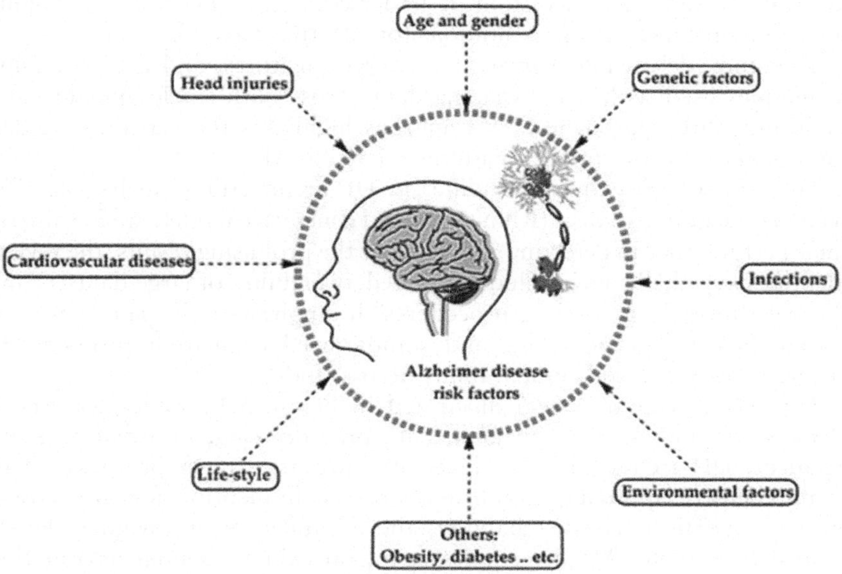

Figure 5.11 Risk factors for Alzheimer's disease.

associated with progressive cognitive decline, various other factors can contribute to similar impairments. These include toxic exposures, infections, cardiopulmonary abnormalities leading to cerebral hypoxia, nutritional deficits, vitamin B12 deficiency, neoplasms, and other cerebral disorders. When evaluating cognitive deterioration in individuals, it is essential to consider this diverse array of potential causes, as each may require a distinct approach to diagnosis and management. Currently, only two classes of medications have received approval for AD treatment: cholinesterase inhibitors and N-methyl-D-aspartate (NMDA) receptor antagonists. These drugs help alleviate symptoms but do not offer a cure or prevent disease progression. Contemporary research efforts are directed towards elucidating AD pathology by targeting various mechanisms, including aberrant tau protein metabolism, beta-amyloid accumulation, inflammatory processes, and cholinergic and oxidative damage. The objective is to develop therapeutic interventions capable of halting or modifying AD progression, ultimately leading to more effective treatment strategies.

5.3.4 Application of DNN in diagnosis and treatment of Alzheimer's disease

Alsubaie et al. [50] conducted a systematic literature review to assess the current landscape of AD detection using DL techniques. The review emphasizes the potential of DL models, particularly in neuroimaging, to facilitate accurate AD detection. It underscores the importance of highly discriminative feature representations for effective detection.

The study delves into various biomarkers, features, and pre-processing techniques used with neuroimaging data across both single-modality and multi-modality approaches. This analysis highlights the versatility of DL models in capturing complex patterns related to AD.

The review also investigates different DL architectures, such as CNNs, recurrent neural networks (RNNs) [2], and generative models, and evaluates their performance in detecting AD. Despite the promising results, the review identifies key challenges, including limited availability of large datasets and the need for robust training procedures. It emphasizes the significance of having benchmark platforms and standardized evaluation protocols to ensure consistency and comparability across studies.

The AD detection system illustrated in Figure 5.12 integrates crucial elements, including neuroimaging, data preprocessing, information management, DL architectures, and performance assessment protocols. This comprehensive approach establishes a robust foundation for the system, ensuring its effectiveness, reliability, and accuracy. Neuroimaging plays a central role in the AD detection system, providing essential information about the structural and functional changes associated with AD.

The system employs multiple neuroimaging modalities, such as MRI, PET, and diffusion tensor imaging (DTI), to acquire detailed brain images. MRI utilizes magnetic fields and radio waves to produce high-resolution images that reveal brain anatomy. PET requires the administration of a radioactive tracer to highlight specific brain regions implicated in AD pathology. DTI measures water molecule movement in brain tissue, allowing for the visualization of white matter pathways and evaluation of neuronal connectivity integrity. These imaging techniques serve as primary data sources in the AD detection system, capturing individual brain characteristics. Subsequent preprocessing steps enhance data quality and reliability by registering scans to a standardized reference space and reducing noise through methods such as Gaussian filtering. Motion correction algorithms compensate for head movements, ensuring accurate representation of brain features.

Effective data management is a fundamental component of AD detection systems, involving the structured organization and processing of vast

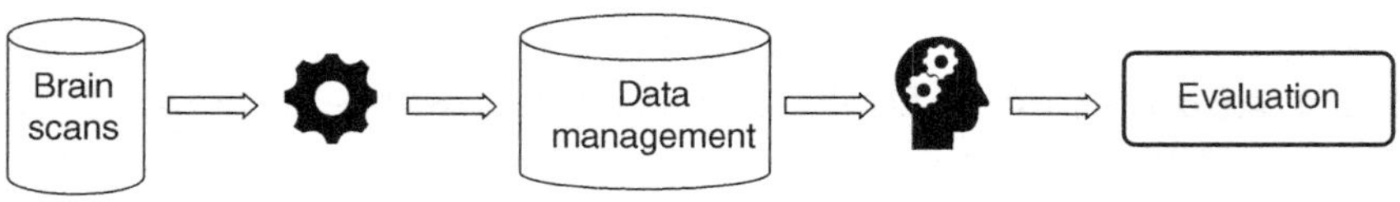

Figure 5.12 Comprehensive framework designed to facilitate efficient detection of AD.

imaging and clinical datasets. The data acquisition phase entails gathering imaging and clinical information using standardized protocols and validated instruments to ensure consistency and reliability. Large-scale datasets are efficiently handled through storage solutions such as relational and NoSQL databases, which provide secure storage and facilitate seamless data retrieval. To uphold data integrity, quality control procedures, including data cleaning and validation checks, are implemented to detect and correct inconsistencies. Furthermore, adherence to ethical and privacy regulations is critical for protecting participant confidentiality and ensuring data security. This includes obtaining informed consent and applying de-identification techniques to comply with regulatory standards.

DL models have demonstrated remarkable capabilities in AD detection by extracting complex patterns from extensive neuroimaging datasets. This section examines the application of DL in AD classification, discussing model architectures, training approaches, and performance assessment. CNNs have emerged as a widely used method in AD research due to their effectiveness in analyzing spatial relationships in brain images. These networks consist of multiple convolutional layers that extract hierarchical features, followed by pooling layers that reduce dimensionality while preserving essential information. The final classification stage involves fully connected layers, enabling the model to distinguish between AD and healthy brain images.

Training DL models necessitates access to well-annotated datasets. Prominent resources such as the Alzheimer's Disease Neuroimaging Initiative (ADNI), the Open Access Series of Imaging Studies (OASIS), and the Australian Imaging, Biomarkers, and Lifestyle (AIBL) study have been instrumental in advancing DL techniques for AD detection by providing high-quality neuroimaging data for model training and validation.

The effectiveness of these models is typically measured using key evaluation metrics, including accuracy (the percentage of correctly classified cases), sensitivity (the true positive rate), specificity (the true negative rate), and the area under the receiver operating characteristic curve (AUC-ROC), which is a crucial indicator of overall model performance. These metrics ensure the reliability and robustness of DL models in AD detection. Figure 5.13 presents the DL-based AD classification framework, illustrating the network architecture, training process, and evaluation methodology.

Cross-validation and independent test sets play a crucial role in evaluating the generalization capability of DL models used for AD detection. Cross-validation involves dividing the dataset into multiple subsets (or folds), training the model on a portion of these subsets while testing it on the remaining ones. This process ensures that every data point contributes to both training and validation, offering a more comprehensive assessment of the model's ability to generalize to new data. Conversely, independent test sets consist of an entirely separate dataset used exclusively for testing, providing an unbiased evaluation of the model's performance on unseen cases.

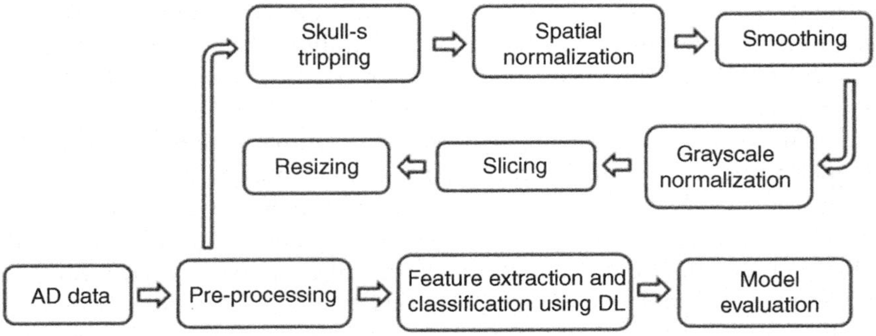

Figure 5.13 DL-based AD classification framework.

Another effective technique in AD detection is transfer learning, which is particularly beneficial when working with limited labeled data. By leveraging pre-trained models originally developed on large-scale image datasets such as ImageNet, researchers can fine-tune these models to analyze AD-related brain imaging data. This approach enables the model to apply previously acquired knowledge from the general image domain to the specific task of AD classification. Transfer learning minimizes the need for extensive labeled datasets, improving model performance and accuracy even when data availability is constrained. The evaluation process is a critical step in determining the effectiveness of AD detection models. Various assessment methodologies and metrics are used to gauge model performance, ensuring accurate and reliable detection outcomes. In AD classification, commonly used evaluation metrics include accuracy, sensitivity, specificity, and the area under the receiver operating characteristic curve (AUC-ROC). Accuracy measures the overall proportion of correctly classified cases, while sensitivity and specificity assess the model's ability to detect AD cases and differentiate them from healthy samples, respectively. AUC-ROC provides a comprehensive evaluation of the model's discriminatory power, reflecting its capability to distinguish between positive and negative cases across different threshold settings. These evaluation techniques help validate the reliability of DL-based AD detection systems, ensuring their applicability in clinical and research settings.

Accuracy represents the overall correctness of a system's predictions, while sensitivity and specificity evaluate its effectiveness in identifying positive and negative cases, respectively. The area under the receiver operating characteristic curve (AUC-ROC) provides a comprehensive measure of the model's ability to distinguish between classes by balancing the true positive rate and false positive rate. Cross-validation is a widely adopted technique for assessing the generalization capability of AD detection models.

In k-fold cross-validation, the dataset is divided into *k* subsets, and the model undergoes training and testing *k* times, ensuring that each subset serves as the test set once. This method improves performance estimation by utilizing the entire dataset for validation, reducing bias and variance in results. Independent test sets also play a crucial role in model evaluation, as they consist of entirely separate datasets not used during training. These test sets provide an objective assessment of the system's ability to handle unseen data, offering valuable insights into its real-world applicability. Additionally, comparing the proposed AD detection model's performance with baseline models and state-of-the-art techniques is essential for demonstrating advancements in the field. Such comparisons help researchers identify the strengths and limitations of their approach, ensuring continuous improvement and innovation in AD diagnosis.

Future research should focus on enhancing discriminative feature representations and refining model architectures and training strategies to boost the performance and generalizability of DL models in AD detection. Figure 5.14 illustrates the AD detection process using DL. While DL has the potential to improve diagnostic accuracy, its integration with clinical data and diagnostic tools is crucial for achieving a more comprehensive and precise detection framework. Despite its promise, further advancements in models and methodologies are necessary to address current challenges. By overcoming these limitations and promoting collaboration and standardization, DL can play a pivotal role in developing practical diagnostic solutions for AD. This can facilitate earlier detection and intervention, ultimately leading to better patient outcomes. The application of DL techniques in AD diagnosis involves multiple strategies, including multimodal data fusion [14], optimization methods, regularization techniques, and appropriate preprocessing selection. Effective utilization of these approaches can significantly enhance the accuracy and efficiency of AD detection.

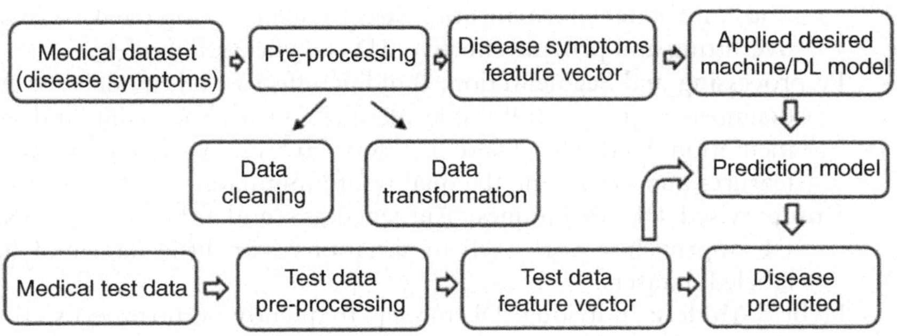

Figure 5.14 Detection system of AD using DL techniques.

Performance Superiority: When diagnosing AD, DL approaches typically perform better than traditional ML techniques. In particular, DNN architectures typically perform better than shallow neural network topologies.

Assistance from Conventional Techniques: Although DL models are strong on their own, they can be helped with feature selection and discrimination by using traditional ML approaches like random forest, KNN, and SVMs.

Multimodal Fusion: Multimodal [14] classification models typically perform better than single-modal settings because they incorporate data from various sources, including MRI, PET, and neurophysiological data. The effectiveness of AD classification models is increased by combining various modalities.

Initialization and Optimization Techniques: DL model parameters, such as learning rate, drop-out rate, number of hidden layers, and number of nodes in each layer, can be effectively initialized using strategies like greedy layer-wise pre-training and Bayesian approaches.

CNN Advantages: For medical image processing, CNNs are especially well-suited because of their scale-invariant and shift-invariant characteristics. CNN models with Max pooling functions and leaky ReLU activation functions frequently produce the best results.

Transfer Learning and Data Augmentation: Techniques for data augmentation and transfer learning are useful for preventing overfitting in DL models, particularly when working with small datasets.

Importance of Brain Regions: Hippocampal atrophy is a significant determinant in the diagnosis of AD, and the hippocampus is an essential region of interest (ROI) for AD diagnosis. DL models frequently concentrate on finding anomalies in this area.

Regularization Techniques: Drop-out regularization, data augmentation, and batch normalization are frequently employed to avoid overfitting and provide effective AD classification models.

Preprocessing and Segmentation: Building effective DL models for AD diagnosis requires careful consideration of preprocessing and segmentation methods. These methods aid in extracting pertinent features and improving the quality of input data.

Unsupervised DL Techniques: Autoencoders and other unsupervised DL approaches work well in situations with little data and few labeled datasets.

Hybrid Models: Individual DL models frequently perform worse than hybrid DL models, which integrate DL with other approaches or mix different DL architectures.

5.3.5 Implications of DNNs in diagnosis and treatment of stroke and hypertension

Hypertension and stroke are intimately connected, with high blood pressure being the most common risk factor for cerebrovascular events. Globally, stroke ranks second in mortality and third in disability causes. It presents in three primary forms: ischemic, intracerebral, and subarachnoid hemorrhage. The prevalence of hypertension in stroke patients, at approximately 64%, emphasizes its crucial role in stroke development. The diverse origins of stroke and its varying hemodynamic effects across different subtypes and presentations make blood pressure (BP) control challenging in affected individuals. Precise diagnosis and well-defined treatment objectives are crucial for successful management. Postischemic stroke, BP often elevates due to various factors, including psychological stress, pain, increased intracranial pressure, urinary retention, and hypoxemia. Impaired autoregulation or compensatory mechanisms to maximize blood flow to ischemic brain regions may also contribute to elevated BP after stroke. Although most acute ischemic stroke patients experience a temporary hypertensive response, BP typically decreases naturally over time. This fluctuation highlights the dynamic nature of poststroke BP regulation and the complexities involved in its management. Effective strategies must consider these BP variations while addressing individual patient needs and optimizing cerebral perfusion to reduce further neurological damage. The approach to treating stroke patients varies based on the type and severity of the cerebrovascular event. Timely medical intervention is crucial to minimize brain damage and enhance outcomes, particularly in ischemic stroke cases where rapid action can significantly improve recovery prospects. Figure 5.15 illustrates the pathogenetic connections between hypertension and stroke. Broadly, strokes are categorized into two main types: ischemic and hemorrhagic, each requiring a distinct treatment approach.

1. **Ischemic Stroke:**
   Thrombolytic Therapy: Blood clots that cause ischemic stroke are broken up by giving clot-dissolving drugs such tissue plasminogen activator (tPA). The best time to provide this medicine is in the initial hours following the development of stroke symptoms.
   Mechanical Thrombectomy: Mechanical thrombectomy is a minimally invasive procedure that may be used when a big blood clot is the cause of the ischemic stroke. This entails extracting the clot straight from the clogged blood vessel using a catheter.
2. **Hemorrhagic Stroke:**
   Surgical Intervention: Surgery may be required in certain hemorrhagic stroke instances in order to remove extra blood from the brain or repair damaged blood arteries.

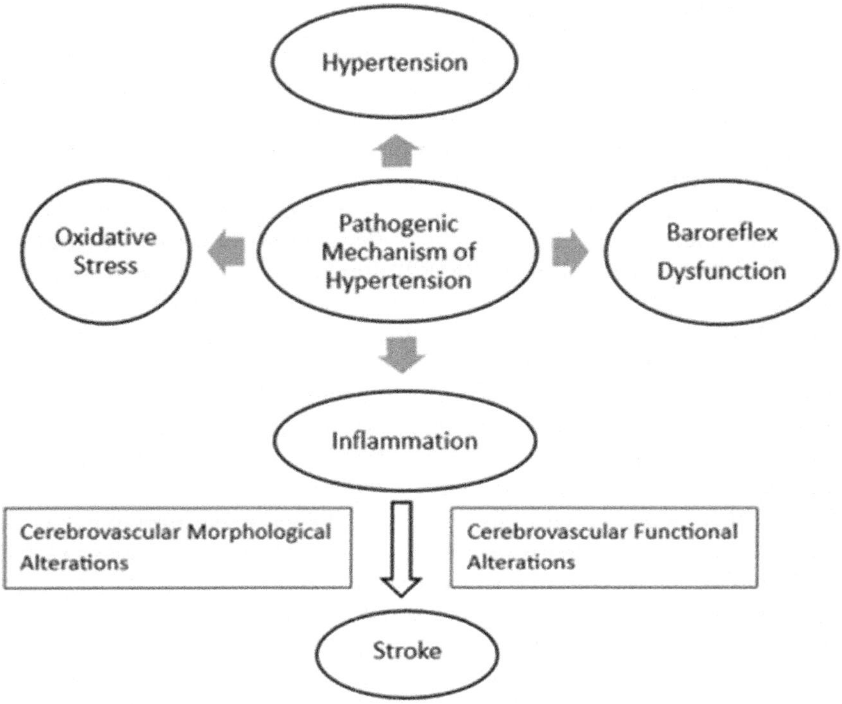

Figure 5.15 Pathogenetic links between hypertension and stroke.

Medications: Medication for blood pressure can be used to assist reduce blood pressure and stop more bleeding. Both anticonvulsant drugs and drugs to lessen brain edema may potentially be taken in order to prevent seizures.

In both types of strokes, supportive care is essential to manage symptoms and prevent complications. This may include as follows:

- Oxygen therapy to ensure adequate oxygenation of the brain
- Monitoring and controlling blood pressure
- Rehabilitation therapy to help regain lost function and improve quality of life
- Speech therapy, physical therapy, and occupational therapy to address speech and language difficulties, mobility issues, and activities of daily living
- Medications to prevent blood clots and reduce the risk of future strokes

AI has demonstrated significant potential in predicting stroke risk, as illustrated in Figure 5.16, which outlines the factors involved in AI utilization for this purpose. ML algorithms, a key component of AI, excel at analyzing extensive patient datasets to identify stroke-related patterns and risk factors. The application of AI in stroke risk prediction offers substantial benefits for improving early detection, prevention, and management strategies. By employing advanced data analytics and ML techniques, AI enables healthcare professionals to identify high-risk individuals, implement targeted interventions, and ultimately reduce the burden of stroke on both patients and healthcare systems.

The pivotal role of AI in stroke risk prediction lies in its capacity to leverage sophisticated algorithms and computational methods for analyzing vast patient information datasets. AI models, utilizing ML and DL algorithms, can discern patterns and correlations among diverse risk factors, including medical histories, lifestyle habits, genetic predispositions, and demographic characteristics. These models generate predictive frameworks to assess an individual's likelihood of experiencing a stroke within a specified timeframe. Through the analysis and interpretation of complex data

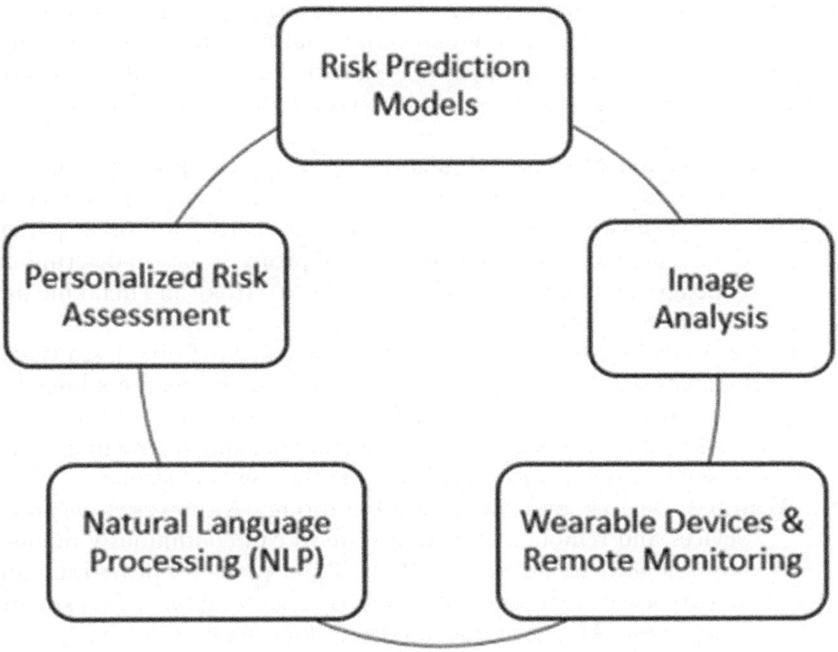

Figure 5.16 Utilization of AI for stroke risk prediction.

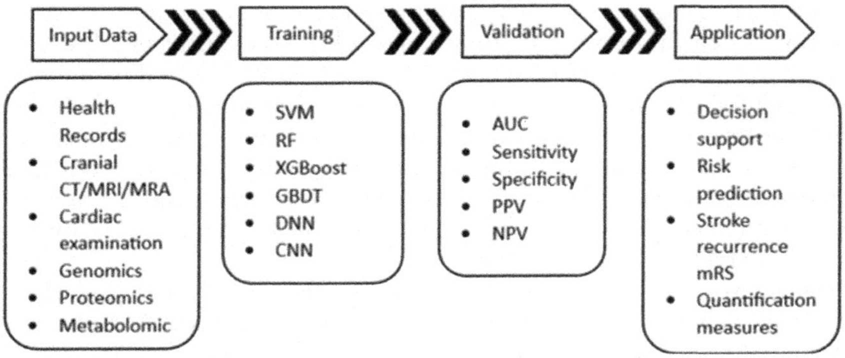

Figure 5.17 Application of AI techniques in predicting stroke risk. The list shows technique or algorithm used at the particular step.

patterns, AI algorithms provide clinicians with valuable insights into stroke risk factors, facilitating early intervention and targeted preventive measures. Furthermore, AI-powered risk prediction tools enable personalized risk assessments, leading to more tailored approaches in stroke prevention and management for individual patients. The promising potential of AI in enhancing stroke risk prediction accuracy and improving patient outcomes through proactive risk management strategies is evident. Figure 5.17 delineates the various steps involved in applying AI techniques for predicting stroke risk.

Risk Prediction Models: ML algorithms can create predictive models for stroke risk by analyzing genetic information, lifestyle factors, medical imaging data, electronic health records, and other patient data. These models can assist medical professionals in determining which patients may be more susceptible to stroke and in taking preventative action.

Image Analysis: Medical imaging data, such as MRI or CT scans, can be analyzed using AI techniques like DL to find markers linked to an increased risk of stroke or to detect early signs of stroke. AI systems, for instance, can examine brain imaging to find indications of small vessel disease, which frequently results in stroke.

Wearable Devices and Remote Monitoring: AI-powered wearable devices and remote monitoring systems can continuously monitor physiological parameters, such as blood pressure, heart rate, and activity levels, to assess stroke risk. By analyzing these data streams in real-time, AI algorithms can detect abnormalities or changes that may indicate an increased risk of stroke.

Natural Language Processing (NLP): NLP techniques can extract valuable information from unstructured clinical notes, medical records, and research literature to identify stroke risk factors, symptoms, and comorbidities. By analyzing text data on a large scale, AI can uncover new insights and associations related to stroke risk.

Personalized Risk Assessment: AI-driven risk prediction models can provide personalized risk assessments for individual patients based on their unique characteristics, medical history, and genetic profile. These personalized risk assessments can help guide preventive interventions and treatment decisions tailored to each patient's needs.

The current healthcare landscape is experiencing a proliferation of clinically significant data, encompassing biomedical imagery, physiological indicators, and digital patient records. However, the overwhelming volume and complexity of this information challenge human capacity to effectively discern its predictive value for clinical decision-making.Neuroimaging is crucial in the treatment of stroke patients, a leading cause of global morbidity and mortality. Despite the potential advantages of cutting-edge neuroimaging techniques in acute stroke care, their optimal utilization is impeded by factors such as temporal constraints, clinician-to-clinician variability, and the lack of systematic clinical data integration. Recent progress in DL offers innovative approaches to harness computational analysis of medical images, aiding decision-making in acute stroke scenarios. While imaging is essential for stroke patient assessment, concerns persist regarding time-intensive brain scans. Some experts discourage advanced imaging modalities like CT perfusion or MRI, citing extended acquisition and processing times compared to noncontrast CT and CT angiography. Although MRI protocols require less than 10 minutes of scan time, comprehensive screening and patient transfer prolong the process. Consequently, expediting MRI scans remains vital, given DWI's superior tissue contrast and specificity for irreversibly damaged tissue.AI-based techniques show promise in enhancing medical image quality, enabling faster acquisition or reduced doses.

In this field, reconstruction algorithms, especially those utilizing deep CNNs, have shown exceptional performance. For example, a CNN can reduce noise in MR brain perfusion images using arterial spin labeling, enabling shorter scan times and facilitating the creation of diagnostic images. CNNs have the ability to analyze spatial relationships between various pixel areas within an image. These networks employ convolutional layers, which are composed of filter sets, to transmit information from one layer to the next. Another relevant category is RNNs, which feature interconnected nodes forming a directed graph along a temporal sequence. RNNs utilize their internal state, or "memory," to process inputs of varying lengths and consider historical information.

5.3.6 Implications of DNNs in diagnosis and treatment of chronic heart disease

Cardiovascular events such as heart attacks and strokes can be triggered by various underlying conditions, including coronary artery disease, high blood pressure, and atherosclerosis. These acute incidents occur when blood circulation to the heart or brain is impeded, potentially resulting in tissue damage or death if not treated promptly.

The term "heart diseases" encompasses a wide array of conditions affecting the heart, while CVDs specifically pertain to disorders involving the blood vessels that supply the heart, brain, and other organs. CVD, commonly known as heart disease, is a primary cause of mortality worldwide and includes conditions that impact the heart's blood vessels, muscle, valves, or electrical conduction system. Figure 5.18 depicts various types of heart diseases. Risk factors for heart disease include hypertension, elevated cholesterol levels, smoking, diabetes, obesity, physical inactivity, poor dietary habits, excessive alcohol consumption, and family history. Prevention and management approaches often involve lifestyle modifications (such as maintaining a balanced diet and engaging in regular physical activity), medication regimens, and in some cases, surgical or medical interventions. Early identification and treatment are crucial for enhancing patient outcomes and reducing the likelihood of complications associated with heart disease.

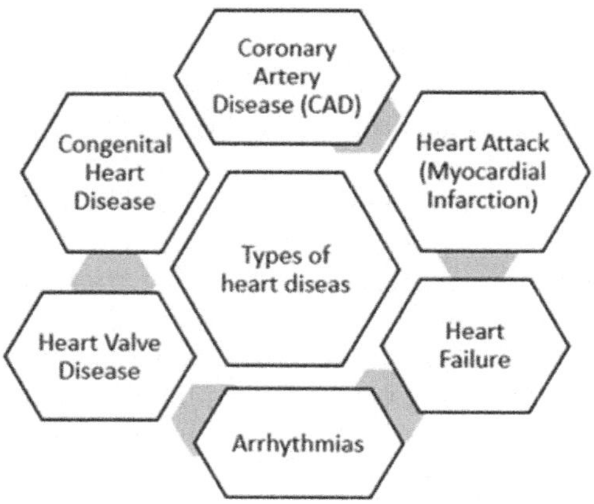

Figure 5.18 Types of heart disease.

Coronary Artery Disease (CAD): This condition arises when the arteries responsible for supplying oxygen-rich blood to the heart become narrowed or blocked due to plaque buildup (atherosclerosis). As a result, individuals may experience chest pain (angina), heart attacks, or other serious complications.

Heart Attack (Myocardial Infarction): A heart attack occurs when blood flow to a section of the heart is obstructed, often due to a blood clot. This blockage deprives the heart muscle of essential oxygen and nutrients, potentially leading to tissue damage or cell death.

Heart Failure: This condition develops when the heart is unable to pump sufficient blood to meet the body's demands. It can occur due to weakened heart muscles (systolic heart failure) or stiffened heart muscles (diastolic heart failure), leading to circulation problems and organ dysfunction.

Arrhythmias: These are irregular heart rhythms caused by disruptions in the electrical signals that regulate heartbeats. They can lead to an excessively fast heartbeat (tachycardia), an abnormally slow heartbeat (bradycardia), or erratic rhythms such as atrial fibrillation, affecting overall heart function.

Heart Valve Disease: This condition occurs when one or more of the heart's valves fail to function correctly, either not opening fully (stenosis) or not closing completely (regurgitation). These issues can significantly disrupt normal blood circulation within the heart.

Congenital Heart Disease: A group of structural heart abnormalities present from birth, congenital heart disease can impact both the form and function of the heart. These defects may result in abnormal blood circulation within the heart and throughout the body, potentially leading to long-term complications.

The broad category of heart disease also encompasses other conditions such as cardiomyopathy (disorders affecting the heart muscle), pericardial disease (affecting the protective sac surrounding the heart), and vascular diseases (disorders of the blood vessels). DNNs offer significant potential for advancing the diagnosis and treatment of chronic heart disease (CHD) through their ability to process complex data sets and identify meaningful patterns. These advanced computational models have the capacity to facilitate early detection, personalized treatment planning, and predictive analytics in CHD management. However, the successful implementation of DNNs in clinical settings relies on the availability of high-quality data, robust model development, and seamless integration into existing healthcare frameworks.

Early Detection and Diagnosis: DNNs can analyze various types of medical data, including ECGs, echocardiograms, and medical images, to detect subtle signs of CHD at an early stage. By identifying patterns indicative of heart disease, DNNs can assist healthcare providers in making timely and accurate diagnoses.

Risk Prediction and Stratification: DNNs can analyze a wide range of patient data, including demographic information, medical history, and biomarkers, to predict the risk of developing CHD or experiencing adverse cardiovascular events. By stratifying patients based on their risk levels, DNNs can help healthcare providers personalize treatment plans and interventions.

Image Analysis and Interpretation: In medical imaging, DNNs can analyze cardiac images such as MRI scans, CT scans, and angiograms to identify anatomical abnormalities, assess cardiac function, and quantify the extent of coronary artery disease. This enables clinicians to obtain detailed insights into the structural and functional aspects of the heart, guiding treatment decisions.

Personalized Treatment Planning: DNNs can analyze large datasets containing information about patients' genetic profiles, medical history, lifestyle factors, and treatment responses to identify optimal treatment strategies for individual patients. By considering multiple factors simultaneously, DNNs can assist clinicians in tailoring treatment plans to meet each patient's specific needs and preferences.

Drug Discovery and Development: DNNs can analyze molecular and genetic data to identify novel biomarkers associated with CHD and potential therapeutic targets. Additionally, DNNs can analyze large-scale clinical trial data to evaluate the efficacy and safety of new drugs or interventions for treating CHD.

Remote Monitoring and Predictive Analytics: DNNs can analyze data from wearable devices, remote monitoring systems, and electronic health records to monitor patients' cardiac health in real-time and predict impending cardiovascular events. By providing early warnings of deteriorating cardiac health, DNNs can help prevent adverse outcomes and improve patient outcomes.

DNNs are instrumental in diagnosing and treating chronic heart conditions by utilizing their capacity to examine intricate patterns within medical information. Figure 5.19 illustrates how DNNs function in predicting and managing CHD. These networks offer robust solutions for enhancing the identification and treatment of chronic cardiac ailments by employing sophisticated ML methods to examine complex medical data. Through the provision of precise diagnoses, individualized risk evaluations, tailored treatment strategies, and ongoing monitoring, DNNs have the potential to improve patient outcomes and lessen the impact of CVD. DNNs can scrutinize various forms of medical data, including electronic health records, cardiac imaging (such as echocardiograms and cardiac MRI scans), and

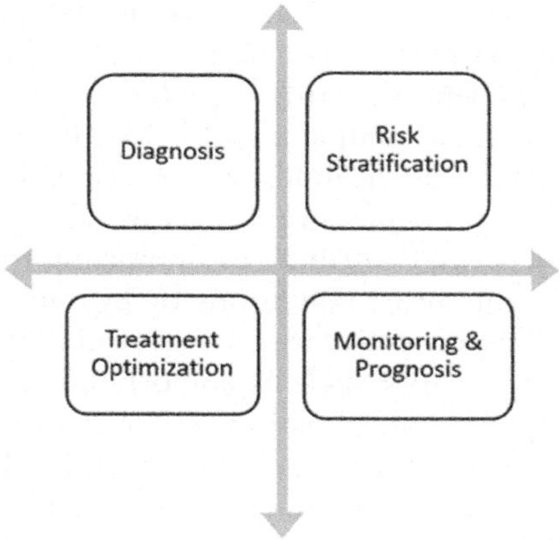

Figure 5.19 Working of DNNs in predicting and treatment of chronic heart disease.

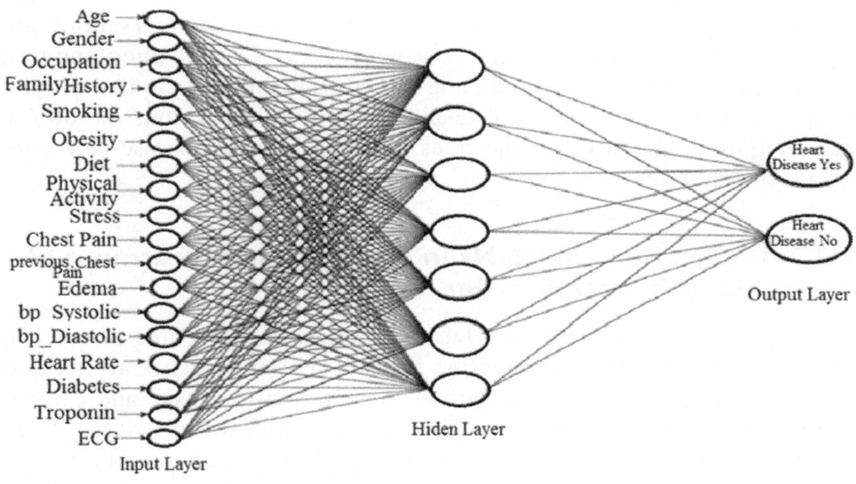

Figure 5.20 Application of DNNs technique predicting heart disease.

physiological measurements (like ECGs), to assist in diagnosing chronic heart conditions. This process is depicted in Figure 5.20. These networks can be trained to identify patterns and irregularities indicative of specific cardiac issues, including coronary artery disease, heart failure, arrhythmias, and valvular heart disease. By processing vast amounts of medical information, DNNs can support healthcare professionals in accurately diagnosing patients and identifying individuals at risk of developing heart diseases. In assessing the likelihood of developing chronic heart conditions, DNNs can analyze various risk factors, such as demographic data, medical history, lifestyle choices, and biomarkers. These networks can forecast the probability of an individual experiencing cardiovascular events, like heart attacks or strokes, based on their unique risk profile. By categorizing patients according to their risk levels, healthcare providers can implement targeted interventions and preventive measures to reduce the risk of future cardiovascular events. DNNs can contribute to optimizing treatment approaches for patients with chronic heart conditions by examining patient data and predicting individual responses to various treatment options. These networks can take into account factors such as comorbidities, medication history, genetic factors, and physiological parameters to customize treatment plans to each patient's specific requirements. By leveraging ML algorithms, DNNs can identify optimal treatment regimens that maximize effectiveness while minimizing adverse effects and complications. For patients with chronic heart conditions, DNNs can provide ongoing monitoring by analyzing longitudinal data and detecting changes in disease progression or treatment response. These networks can identify early indicators of disease exacerbation, complications, or adverse events, enabling timely intervention and adjustment of treatment strategies. Furthermore, DNNs can offer long-term prognostic assessments by predicting patient outcomes, such as mortality, hospitalizations, and functional decline, based on continuous monitoring data. Figure 5.21 illustrates the steps involved in heart disease prediction using AI techniques.

5.3.7 Implications of DNNs in diagnosis and treatment of neurophysical disorder

AI's core components, ML and DL techniques, have become essential in numerous commercial and scientific fields. These approaches are particularly adept at processing large datasets, generating forecasts, and categorizing information, especially in environments characterized by "big data." Their adaptability and effectiveness have resulted in widespread adoption across various sectors, including healthcare, where they are increasingly influencing diverse applications. In the realm of AI research, ANNs have emerged as a notable success story. They have shown the capacity to achieve performance levels that range from matching to surpassing human capabilities in various domains. This accomplishment contrasts with conventional AI methodologies, which typically relied on symbolic information processing and logical reasoning. ANNs, drawing inspiration from the organization and operation of biological neural networks, have demonstrated unmatched effectiveness in tasks such as image recognition, NLP, and game playing, among others. Their ability to discern intricate patterns and relationships within data has propelled them to the forefront of AI research

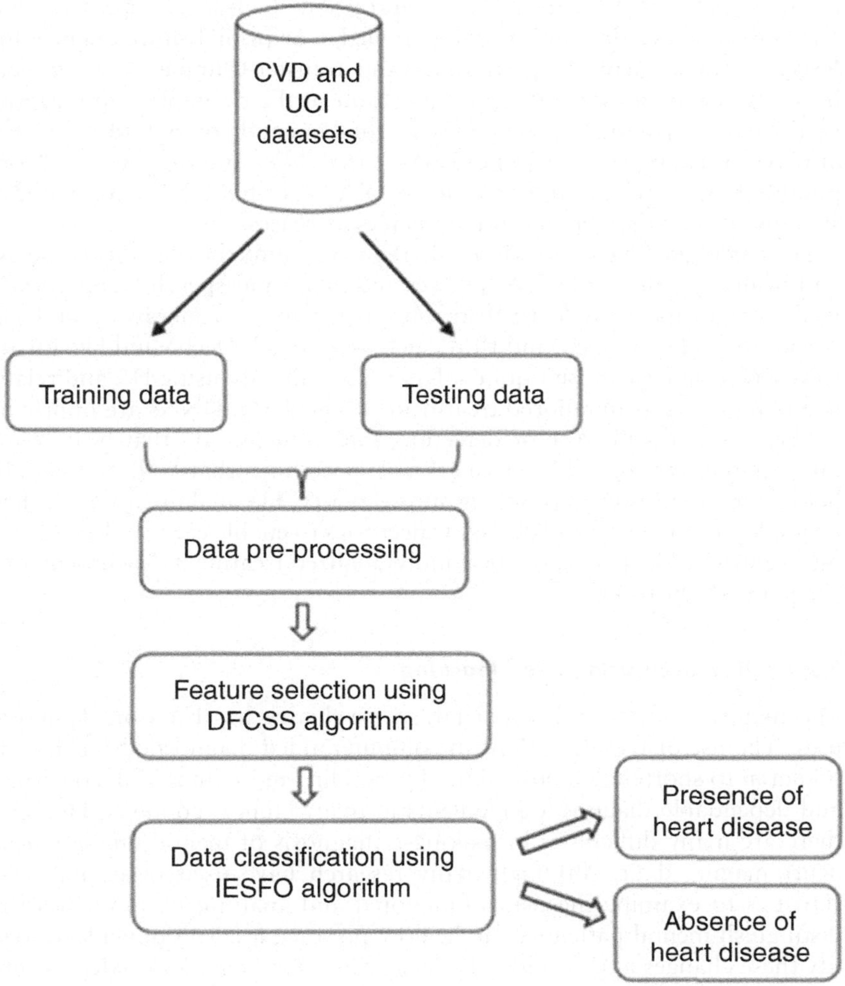

Figure 5.21 Heart disease prediction using AI technique.

and application, succeeding where traditional approaches had stagnated or progressed slowly for many years.

In the fields of psychiatry and neuroscience, traditional statistical and ML approaches for nonlinear regression and classification, such as SVMs, kernel methods, and basic neural networks, have been utilized extensively. However, DL algorithms, which are the focus of this brief review, frequently surpass these earlier ML techniques by significant margins. The reasons for this superior performance are not yet fully elucidated. One possible explanation is that DNNs can deduce appropriate high-level representations without extensive domain-specific knowledge or prior feature engineering. Recent improvements in pretraining and transfer-training methodologies have also enabled more efficient navigation of their complex optimization landscapes. Furthermore, there may be fundamental computational factors at play: for example, the compositional capabilities and the range of "computable functions" expand at a much faster rate for DNNs compared to shallow ones as the number of parameters increases.

DL techniques have quickly made their way into (bio-)medical research and healthcare due to DNNs' prowess in image and speech recognition as well as their capacity to learn abstract representations from raw input. Large corporations like Google and IBM, such as Google's DeepMind Health and IBM's Watson (which isn't quite a DNN), are already using DL and related techniques to inform tailored treatment. Particularly, DNNs are improving medical domains like tumor detection and segmentation that heavily rely on image processing. This has sparked expectations that DNNs could also help address unresolved problems in psychiatry, like making accurate diagnoses, forecasting risk and disease trajectories to enable early and preventive interventions, identifying the best individualized treatments, or finding possible new medications.

5.3.7.1 Research using deep learning

The majority of research using DL in psychiatry has been on diagnostic uses. The use of DL algorithms in computer-aided diagnostic tools has the potential to shorten diagnosis times by enabling more impartial, consistent, and dependable diagnostic judgments in many clinical contexts. However, there are many difficulties in making a diagnosis of mental illnesses using neuroimaging data. Although many research have used mass univariate statistics to examine the neuro-functional and anatomical anomalies that distinguish mental patients from healthy persons, it is still difficult to identify these changes at the individual level. The characteristics needed for precise individual categorization are probably complicated and might not be visible in a single imaging modality. Furthermore, since cross-modal feature combinations and interactions might only appear at abstract levels of analysis, finding them is considerably more difficult. A DNN model for classifying schizophrenia and bipolar disorder is displayed in Figure 5.22.

Because DNNs can effectively capture higher-order statistical correlations, they are well-suited to tackle these issues. In contrast to shallow architectures, their multi-layered architecture uses fewer parameters to extract complex nonlinear interactions among input characteristics. Through the integration of data from many imaging modalities, including PET, structural MRI (sMRI), and functional MRI (fMRI), DL-based systems can give clinicians

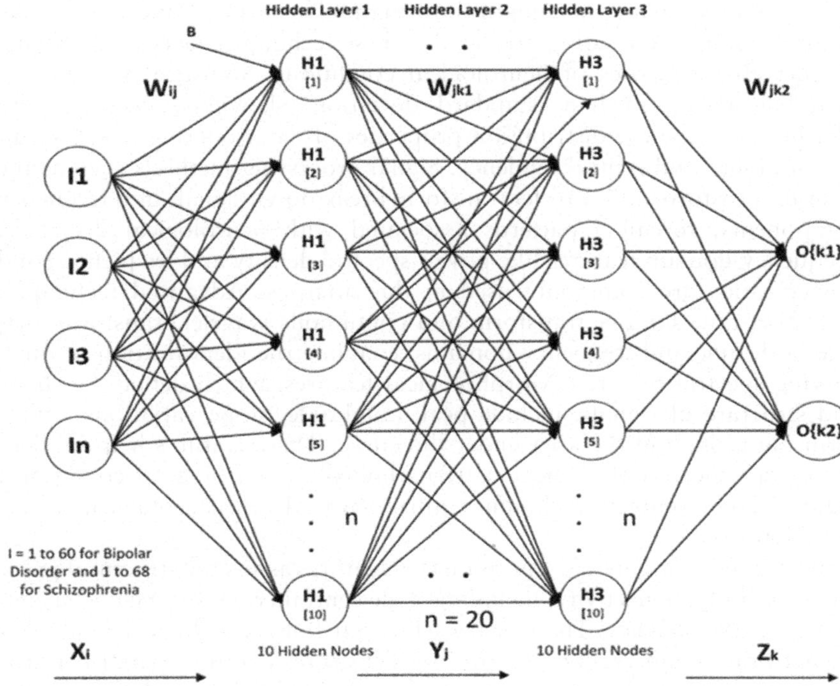

Figure 5.22 DNN model for bipolar disorder and schizophrenia classification.

important insights that are difficult to obtain using conventional techniques. Additionally, its capacity to interpret raw neuroimaging data directly removes the need for time-consuming and error-prone preprocessing stages, potentially streamlining diagnostic workflows in the future. Global rates of morbidity and mortality are greatly influenced by mental illnesses. DL has a lot of potential to enhance risk assessment and mental health diagnosis. There have been no new therapeutic approaches in recent years, and the treatment of mental illnesses is palliative rather than disease-modifying. DL techniques generate knowledge and enhance practice by identifying common principles and patterns in large datasets. More specific and relevant hypotheses for the identification, validation, and treatment of mental illnesses can be prepared using these techniques. These techniques can offer commensurate, objective measurements as well as noteworthy insights into disease prediction techniques. Stated differently, the application of DL techniques to extract insights from unprocessed data can help speed up diagnosis and treatment. ANN are essential to DL. There have been reports of probabilistic neural networks in the literature. These structures have the capacity to accurately classify a wide range of NLD.

Feature extraction techniques play a vital role in detecting neurological disorders by deriving meaningful information from raw data sources like brain imaging or physiological signals. These techniques help in identifying distinct characteristics of neurological conditions. Statistical parameters, including mean, median, standard deviation, skewness, kurtosis, and entropy, describe the distribution properties of data, offering insights into its variability and central tendency. Signal processing methods such as the Fourier transform and wavelet transform break down signals into frequency components, revealing patterns associated with neurological disorders. Frequency-domain features like power spectral density and frequency band power ratios are commonly used in this analysis. Advanced techniques like short-time Fourier transform and continuous wavelet transform analyze both time and frequency domains, enabling the identification of time-varying spectral features. Morphological features, which define the shape and structure of signals, include peak amplitude, slope variations, waveform duration, and the area under the curve. These features help in identifying specific morphological patterns linked to neurological conditions. Figure 5.23 presents the techniques utilized by CAD for neurological disease detection.

In brain network analysis, graph-based features assess the structural properties of brain connectivity, including node centrality, clustering coefficient, and network efficiency. These metrics illustrate how neurological conditions impact brain connectivity. Texture-based features capture spatial patterns within imaging data and are commonly extracted using methods like the gray-level co-occurrence matrix and local binary patterns. Such features highlight subtle structural abnormalities in tissues. Functional connectivity measures assess the strength and coordination of interactions between brain regions, using metrics such as correlation, coherence, or mutual information. These features provide insights into changes in brain network dynamics

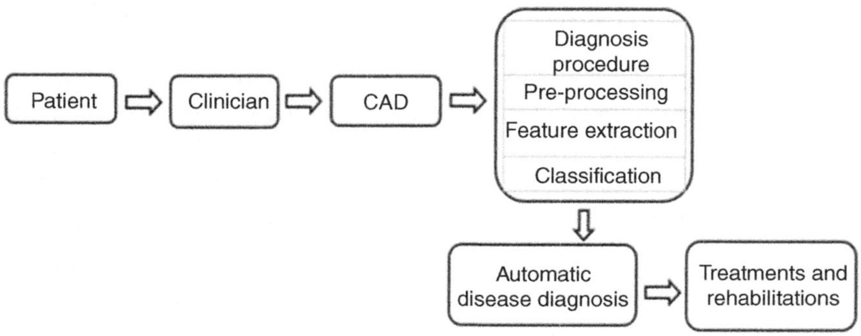

Figure 5.23 Techniques used by CAD for neurological diseases.

related to neurological disorders. Dimensionality reduction techniques, such as principal component analysis (PCA) and independent component analysis (ICA), help retain relevant information while reducing data complexity. By projecting high-dimensional data into a lower-dimensional space, these methods enhance feature extraction, improving the effectiveness of disease detection models. The use of these feature extraction techniques enables researchers to characterize neurological conditions effectively and develop diagnostic models with higher accuracy and clinical significance.

DL, a specialized branch of ML, has emerged as a powerful tool in AI, particularly in computer science applications. DL focuses on developing models that can identify complex patterns within high-dimensional datasets. It has gained significant attention in fields such as image analysis due to its ability to capture intricate relationships within data. CNNs, a key DL architecture, have shown exceptional performance in tasks involving computer vision and pattern recognition. Their breakthrough came in 2012 during the ImageNet competition, although the concept dates back to 1989. CNNs stand out because they can autonomously extract important spatial features from raw data, eliminating the need for manual feature selection. The architecture of CNNs consists of three main layers: convolutional, pooling, and fully connected layers. These networks have outperformed traditional algorithms when applied to large datasets containing millions of images across thousands of classifications. Inspired by the human visual system, CNNs excel in tasks such as MRI image analysis, identification of symptomatic patterns, and disease classification. The convolutional layer utilizes filters or kernels with trainable parameters to extract features, forming a feature map. The pooling layer then reduces the feature map's dimensionality, helping to minimize computational complexity and prevent overfitting. Due to this efficient design, CNNs can extract multiple hierarchical features while maintaining a manageable number of trainable parameters. Unlike conventional DL approaches, CNNs are particularly effective at thoroughly extracting features from complex data, making them a robust choice for medical image analysis and disease detection.

Implications of DLs in diagnosis and treatment of Parkinson's disease

PD is a progressive neurodegenerative condition that primarily impacts movement. It develops gradually, often beginning with mild symptoms that intensify over time. The disorder mainly targets the substantia nigra, a brain region responsible for dopamine production. Dopamine, a key neurotransmitter, plays a crucial role in regulating movement, and its depletion leads to motor impairments. The main symptoms of PD include as follows:

Tremors: Involuntary shaking, usually beginning in the hands or fingers.

Bradykinesia: Slowness of movement, making simple tasks difficult and time-consuming.

Rigidity: Stiffness or inflexibility of the limbs and trunk, leading to decreased range of motion.

Postural instability: Impaired balance and coordination, increasing the risk of falls.

Additional symptoms of PD may involve alterations in speech, handwriting, and facial expressions. Some individuals also experience freezing episodes, where they momentarily feel unable to move. Since Parkinson's is a progressive disorder, its symptoms tend to worsen over time.

Beyond these primary motor symptoms, the disease can also lead to various non-motor symptoms, such as:

- Changes in speech, such as softness, slurring, or monotone voice.
- Writing changes, including smaller handwriting (micrographia) or difficulty with fine motor control.
- Reduced facial expressions, known as facial masking, giving the face a fixed or expressionless appearance.
- Freezing episodes, where individuals feel temporarily unable to initiate or continue movement, often described as feeling "stuck" to the ground.

The precise cause of PD remains unclear, but it is believed to result from a combination of genetic predisposition and environmental influences. Although there is no definitive cure, various treatment options—including medications, physical therapy, and lifestyle adjustments—can help manage symptoms and enhance the quality of life for those affected. In certain cases, surgical procedures like deep brain stimulation may be suggested to provide symptom relief. Early diagnosis and timely intervention play a vital role in optimizing treatment outcomes and slowing disease progression.

The identification of PD is not immediate, as no single test, such as a blood test or ECG, can conclusively determine whether an individual has the condition. Instead, patients are often required to read specific content, which is recorded and analyzed for emotional and auditory patterns. Voice signal analysis is one of the simplest and most effective methods for diagnosing PD since most patients experience speech impairments. Various diagnostic tools have been applied to assess PD, including the multidimensional voice program and other voice-based indicators such as electromyography and speech analysis.

Deep belief networks (DBNs) have shown promise in accurately classifying and predicting the subcortical structures of PD patients due to their strong classification abilities, even with limited data. Neuroimaging techniques are frequently used to enhance diagnostic accuracy, and some studies have employed DL models to detect specific patterns in patient data. In ML applications for data analysis, effective feature extraction and representation are crucial for achieving reliable classification. ANNs are a class of ML models that mimic the structure of the human neural network and are designed to identify patterns in data.

DBN: A DBN is a generative model in ML that falls under the category of DNNs. It consists of multiple layers of hidden units, with connections between layers but not within each layer itself. DBNs can handle both binary and continuous data at the visible level, depending on how they are configured. Introduced by Geoffrey Hinton and his team in 2006, DBNs were developed to overcome the limitations of earlier neural network models. Considered the fourth generation of ANNs, DBNs represent a DL architecture where layers learn hierarchical representations of data. These networks integrate neural structures with efficient learning mechanisms, making them a state-of-the-art approach in various ML research domains. Figure 5.24 illustrates data mining techniques used for PD detection. DBNs can extract features from brain morphometry data, which involves measuring the external shapes and structures of biological organisms or other objects. Studies have explored DBN performance in distinguishing between healthy individuals and PD patients. Additionally, DBNs can be utilized for generative pre-training of DNNs by leveraging their learned weights as initial parameters for further training.

Classification Methods for PD Detection: Imam et al. [51] introduced a modified PCA-KNN classifier to diagnose PD. The proposed methodology was simulated using MATLAB 2012, a software toolbox containing various data mining functions. A comparative analysis of the modified method against existing approaches was performed using accuracy and precision metrics. The simulation results demonstrated that the proposed approach achieved an accuracy of 96.92%, surpassing previous methods. This suggests that the PCA-KNN classifier is more effective in PD diagnosis

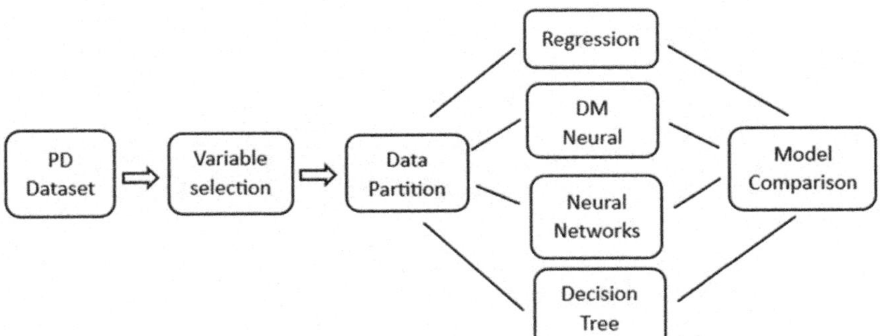

Figure 5.24 Data mining methods for PD recognition.

compared to earlier techniques. The researchers employed multiple classification algorithms to detect patterns in PD datasets. The classification process involved key steps such as feature extraction, feature selection, and classification. Additionally, data partitioning was used in the proposed technique to prepare the dataset. If a dataset was not classified correctly, it was further refined through additional preprocessing steps. Figure 5.25 illustrates the block diagram representing the process of determining accuracy using the PCA-KNN classifier. Several techniques and algorithms have been applied in the field of PD detection, including ML approaches such as KNN, PCA, random forest, DBNs, and neural networks. The study concluded that the

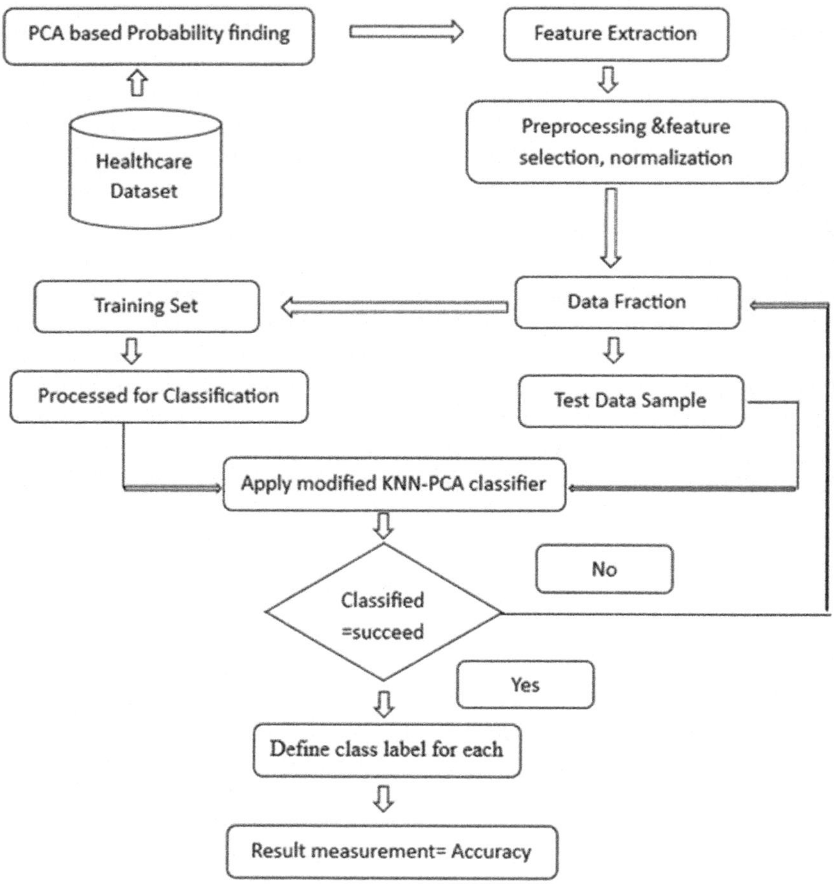

Figure 5.25 Block diagram illustrating process of determining accuracy using KNN-PCA classifier.

KNN classifier provided the highest accuracy, effectively classifying datasets based on given attributes.

5.4 CONCLUSION

AI-driven prognostic models leverage various data sources, such as genetic information, imaging scans, and clinical parameters, to predict disease progression and outcomes. By evaluating longitudinal patient data, these models can classify individuals based on their risk levels, enabling personalized treatment plans. AI technologies also facilitate real-time monitoring of neurological patients, allowing for the early detection of complications and disease deterioration.

Wearable devices integrated with AI algorithms can continuously track vital signs, gait dynamics, and cognitive performance, providing timely alerts to healthcare professionals about potential health crises. Additionally, AI-powered decision support systems assist clinicians in refining treatment strategies, ultimately enhancing patient outcomes and survival rates.

REFERENCES

[1] Y. Kumar, A. Koul, R. Singla, and M. F. Ijaz. "Artificial intelligence in disease diagnosis: a systematic literature review, synthesizing framework and future research agenda." *J. Ambient Intell. Humaniz Comput.*, vol. 14, no. 7, pp. 8459–8486, 2023. doi:10.1007/s12652-021-03612-z

[2] N. Ghaffar Nia, E. Kaplanoglu, and A. Nasab. "Evaluation of artificial intelligence techniques in disease diagnosis and prediction." *Discov. Artif. Intell.*, vol. 3, no. 1, p. 5, 2023. doi:10.1007/s44163-023-00049-5

[3] F. Jiang, Y. Jiang, H. Zhi, et al. "Artificial intelligence in healthcare: past, present and future." *Stroke Vasc. Neurol.*, vol. 2, e000101, 2017. doi:10.1136/svn-2017-000101

[4] M. Anjali, M. Maria Dominic, R. ShinojRober et.al. "An overview of deep learning." *J. Comput. Intell. Syst.*, 2017.

[5] M. Ene. Neural network based approach to discriminate healthy people from those with Parkinson's disease. *Ann. Univ. Craiova,* 35, 2008.

[6] C. Y. Chien, S. W. Hsu, T. L. Lee, P. S. Sung, and C. C. Lin. "Using artificial neural network to discriminate Parkinson's disease from other Parkinsonisms by focusing on putamen of dopamine transporter SPECT images." *Biomedicines*, vol. 9, no. 1, p. 12, 2020. doi:10.3390/biomedicines9010012

[7] F. Soleimanian Gharehchopogh and P. Mohammadi. "A case study of Parkinson disease using artificial neural network." *IJCA*, vol. 73, pp. 1–6, 2013.

[8] A.-R. Mohamed, G. E. Dahl, and G. Hinton. "Acoustic modeling using deep belief networks." *IEEE Trans. Audio Speech Lang. Process.*, vol. 20, pp. 14–22, 2012. doi:10.1109/TASL.2011.2109382

[9] R. Srivastava. "Applications of artificial intelligence in medicine." *Explor. Res. Hypothesis Med.*, vol. 9, no.2, pp. 138–146, 2023. doi:10.14218/ERHM.2023.00048

[10] C. J. Kelly, A. Karthikesalingam, M. Suleyman et al. "Key challenges for delivering clinical impact with artificial intelligence." *BMC Med.*, vol. 17, p. 195, 2019. https://doi.org/10.1186/s12916-019-1426-2

[11] D. Kumar, P. Kumar, M. I. Ahmad, and S. Singh. Integrating artificial intelligence in disease diagnosis, treatment, and formulation development: A review. *Asian J. Pharm. Clin. Res.*, vol. 16, p. 1–8, 2023. doi:10.22159/ajpcr.2023v16i11.48193

[12] Subbiah, V. "The next generation of evidence-based medicine." *Nat. Med.*, vol. 29, pp. 49–58, 2023. https://doi.org/10.1038/s41591-022-02160-z

[13] J. Kashyap, O. A. Olanrewaju, K. Mahar et al. "Neurological manifestations of infectious diseases: Insights from recent cases." *Cureus*, vol. 15, no. 12, p. e51256, 2023. doi:10.7759/cureus.51256

[14] J.N. Acosta, G. J. Falcone, P. Rajpurkar et al. "Multimodal biomedical AI." *Nat. Med.*, vol. 28, pp. 1773–1784, 2022. https://doi.org/10.1038/s41591-022-01981-2

[15] N. K. Tran, S. Albahra, L. May, S. Waldman, S. Crabtree, S. Bainbridge, and H. Rashidi. "Evolving applications of artificial intelligence and machine learning in infectious diseases testing." *Clin. Chem.*, 68. 125–133, 2021. doi:10.1093/clinchem/hvab239

[16] S. Mukherjee, S. Vagha, and P. Gadkari. Navigating the future: A comprehensive review of artificial intelligence applications in gastrointestinal cancer." *Cureus*, vol. 16, no. 2, p. e54467, 2024. doi:10.7759/cureus.54467

[17] K. R. Dasegowda, M. Y. Kavyasree, H. Prabhavathi, M. Rambabu, K. Vasudevan, and M. A. Kareem. "Applications of artificial intelligence, machine learning, and deep learning in diagnosis and treatment of rheumatoid arthritis." In K. Raza, S. Singh, editors. Artificial intelligence and autoimmune diseases. Studies in Computational Intelligence, vol. 1133. Springer, Singapore, 2024. https://doi.org/10.1007/978-981-99-9029-0_12

[18] P. Date, V. Pimprale, and S. Mandke. "Explorative study on potential of machine learning and artificial intelligence for improved healthcare diagnosis and treatment." *J. Autonom. Intell.*, vol. 7, 2023. doi:10.32629/jai.v7i3.1084

[19] P. Mathur, S. Srivastava, X. Xu, and J. L. Mehta. "Artificial intelligence, machine learning, and cardiovascular disease." *Clin. Med. Insights Cardiol.*, vol. 14, 2020. doi:10.1177/1179546820927404

[20] X. Xi, X. Meng, L. Yang, X. Nie, G. Yang, H. Chen, X. Fan, Y. Yin, and X. Chen. "Automated segmentation of choroidal neovascularization in optical coherence tomography images using multi-scale convolutional neural networks with structure prior." *Multimed. Syst.*, vol. 25, no. 2, p. 95, 2019.

[21] Y. Rizk, N. Hajj, N. Mitri, and M. Awad. Deep belief networks and cortical algorithms: a comparative study for supervised classification." *App. Comput. Inform.*, vol. 15, no. 2, p. 81, 2019.

[22] C. Bhatt, I. Kumar, V. Vijayakumar, K. U. Singh, and A. Kumar. "The state of the art of deep learning models in medical science and their challenges." *Multimed. Syst.*, vol. 27, no. 4, p. 599, 2021.

[23] K. Jain. Artificial intelligence applications in handling the infectious diseases. *Prim. Health Care*, vol. 10, no. 5, p. 351, 2020.

[24] M. M. Ahsan, S. A. Luna, and Z. Siddique. Machine-learning-based disease diagnosis: A comprehensive review. *Healthcare (Basel)*, vol. 10, no. 3, p. 541, 2022. doi:10.3390/healthcare10030541

[25] G. Briganti and O. Le Moine. "Artificial intelligence in medicine: today and tomorrow." *Front. Med.*, vol. 7, p. 27, 2020.

[26] G. S. Lodwick. Computer-aided diagnosis in radiology: A research plan. *Investig. Radiol.*, 1, no. 1, pp. 72–80, 1966.

[27] M. R. Maurya, N. U. Riyaz, M. Reddy, H. C. Yalcin, H. M. Ouakad, I. Bahadur, S. Al-Maadeed, and K. K. Sadasivuni. "A review of smart sensors coupled with internet of things and artificial intelligence approach for heart failure monitoring." *Med. Biol. Eng. Comput.*, vol. 59, no. 11, pp. 2185–2203, 2021.

[28] S. Shamshirband, M. Fathi, A. Dehzangi, A. T. Chronopoulos, and H. Alinejad-Rokny. "A review on deep learning approaches in healthcare systems: taxonomies, challenges, and open issues." *J. Biomed. Inform.*, vol. 113, p. 103627, 2021.

[29] M. S. Hossain and G. Muhammad. "Deep learning based pathology detection for smart connected healthcare." *IEEE Netw.*, vol. 34, no. 6, p. 120–125, 2020.

[30] M. Bakator and D. Radosav. "Deep learning and medical diagnosis: a review of literature." *Multimodal Technol. Interact.*, vol. 2, no. 3, p. 47, 2018.

[31] F. Piccialli, V. Di Somma, F. Giampaolo, S. Cuomo, and G. Fortino. "A survey on deep learning in medicine: Why, how and when?" *Inform. Fusion*, vol. 66, pp. 111–137, 2020. https://doi.org/10.1016/j.inffus.2020.09.006

[32] N. Shahid, T. Rappon, and W. Berta. "Applications of artificial neural networks in health care organizational decision-making: A scoping review." *PLoS One*, vol. 14, no. 2, p. e0212356, 2019. doi:10.1371/journal.pone.0212356

[33] R. Miotto, F. Wang, S. Wang, X. Jiang, and J. T. Dudley. "Deep learning for healthcare: review, opportunities and challenges." *Brief Bioinform.*, vol. 19, no. 6, pp. 1236–1246, 2018. doi:10.1093/bib/bbx044

[34] S. Shamshirband, M. Fathi, A. Dehzangi, A. T. Chronopoulos, and H. Alinejad-Rokny. "A review on deep learning approaches in healthcare systems: Taxonomies, challenges, and open issues." *J. Biomed. Inform.*, vol. 113, p. 103627, 2021. doi:10.1016/j.jbi.2020.103627

[35] R. Miotto, F. Wang, S. Wang, X. Jiang, and J. T. Dudley. "Deep learning for healthcare: review, opportunities and challenges." *Brief Bioinform.*, vol. 19, no. 6, pp. 1236–1246, 2018. doi:10.1093/bib/bbx044

[36] Precision Medicine Initiative (NIH). https://nih.gov/precision-medicine-initiative-cohort-program Accessed 12 November 2016.

[37] G. H. Lyman and H. L. Moses. "Biomarker tests for molecularly targeted therapies--The key to unlocking precision medicine." *N. Engl. J. Med.*, vol. 375, no. 1, pp. 4–6, 2016. doi:10.1056/NEJMp1604033

[38] F. S. Collins and H. Varmus. "A new initiative on precision medicine." *N. Engl. J. Med.*, vol. 372, no. 9, pp. 793–795, 2015. doi:10.1056/NEJMp1500523

[39] P. Bede, K. M. Chang, and E. L. Tan. "Machine-learning in motor neuron diseases: Prospects and pitfalls." *Eur J Neurol.*, vol. 29, no. 9, pp. 2555–2556, 2022. doi:10.1111/ene.15443

[40] D. Lopez-Bernal, D. Balderas, P. Ponce, M. Rojas, and A. Molina. "Implications of artificial intelligence algorithms in the diagnosis and treatment of motor neuron diseases—A review." *Life*, 13, no. 4, p. 1031, 2023. https://doi.org/10.3390/life13041031

[41] C. Pancotti, G. Birolo, C. Rollo et al. "Deep learning methods to predict amyotrophic lateral sclerosis disease progression." *Sci. Rep.*, vol. 12, p. 13738, 2022. https://doi.org/10.1038/s41598-022-17805-9

[42] K. Imamura, Y. Yada, Y. Izumi, M. Morita, A. Kawata, T. Arisato, A. Nagahashi, T. Enami, K. Tsukita, H. Kawakami, M. Nakagawa, R. Takahashi, and H. Inoue. "Prediction model of amyotrophic lateral sclerosis by deep learning with patient induced pluripotent stem cells." *Ann Neurol.*, vol. 89, no. 6, pp. 1226–1233, 2021. doi:10.1002/ana.26047

[43] K. Singh and J. Malhotra. Stacked autoencoders based deep learning approach for automatic epileptic seizure detection. Proceedings of the 2018 First International Conference on Secure Cyber Computing and Communication (ICSCCC); Jalandhar, India. 15–17 December 2018; pp. 249–254.

[44] H. A. Glory, C. Vigneswaran, S. S. Jagtap, R. Shruthi, G. Hariharan, and V. S. Sriram. AHW-BGOA-DNN: A novel deep learning model for epileptic seizure detection. *Neural Comput. Appl.*, vol. 33, pp. 6065–6093, 2021.

[45] M. Kołodziej, A. Majkowski, and A. Rysz. "Implementation of machine learning and deep learning techniques for the detection of epileptic seizures using intracranial electroencephalography." *Appl. Sci.*, vol. 13, no. 15, p. 8747, 2023. https://doi.org/10.3390/app13158747

[46] G. Yogarajan, N. Alsubaie, G. Rajasekaran et al. "EEG-based epileptic seizure detection using binary dragonfly algorithm and deep neural network." *Sci. Rep.*, vol. 13, p. 17710, 2023. https://doi.org/10.1038/s41598-023-44318-w

[47] K. Singh and J. Malhotra. "Two-layer LSTM network-based prediction of epileptic seizures using EEG spectral features." *Complex Intell. Syst.*, vol. 8, pp. 2405–2418, 2022. https://doi.org/10.1007/s40747-021-00627-z

[48] Z. Breijyeh and R. Karaman. "Comprehensive review on Alzheimer's disease: Causes and treatment." *Molecules*, vol. 25, no. 24, p. 5789, 2020. doi:10.3390/molecules25245789

[49] A. S. Schachter and K. L. Davis. "Alzheimer's disease." *Dialog. Clin. Neurosci.*, vol. 2. no. 2, pp. 91–100, 2000. doi:10.31887/DCNS.2000.2.2/asschachter

[50] M. G. Alsubaie, S. Luo, and K. Shaukat. "Alzheimer's disease detection using deep learning on neuroimaging: A systematic review." *Mach. Learn. Knowl. Extract.*, vol. 6, no. 1, pp. 464–505, 2024. https://doi.org/10.3390/make6010024

[51] S. Imam and S. Site, "Parkinson's disease diagnosis using modified PCA-KNN classifier", *Int. J. Electr. Electron. Comput. Eng.*, vol. 6, no. 2, pp. 57–63, 2017.

Questions

1. What is the role of artificial intelligence in cardiovascular technology field?
2. Which type of AI system can be used to help patients diagnose and better understand their own illnesses?
3. What is the role of artificial intelligence in diagnosis and treatment of diseases?
4. What is the impact of AI on medical diagnosis and treatment?
5. What are the challenges faced by the researchers while using AI models in several disease diagnoses?
6. How are AI-based techniques helping doctors in diagnosing diseases?
7. Explain in brief the evaluation of supervised learning models in disease diagnosis and prediction.
8. Which deep learning methods are more common in mental disorder data analyses?
9. What is the main application domain of deep learning in mental health disorders?
10. Discuss recent advances in artificial intelligence analyze images and effectively diagnose acute diseases.
11. Explain comprehensive review of the recent development in deep neural networks and medical imaging.
12. What are strengths and weaknesses of deep neural networks in the medical domain?
13. How are AI technologies being utilized in the diagnosis of neurological diseases such as Alzheimer's disease and Parkinson's disease?
14. What role do AI technologies play in predicting the prognosis of cardiovascular diseases like coronary artery disease and heart failure?
15. How can AI technologies aid in predicting survival rates for patients with infectious diseases such as COVID-19 or sepsis?
16. What are the key challenges in implementing AI-based diagnostic tools for neurological, cardiovascular, and infectious diseases?
17. How do AI algorithms analyze medical imaging data to assist in the diagnosis of neurological disorders, cardiovascular conditions, and infectious diseases?
18. What are some examples of AI applications in personalized medicine for patients with neurological, cardiovascular, and infectious diseases?
19. How do AI-driven predictive models contribute to early detection and intervention in neurological, cardiovascular, and infectious diseases?
20. What ethical considerations need to be addressed when deploying AI technologies in disease diagnosis, prognosis, and survival prediction?
21. How do AI-powered decision support systems improve clinical outcomes for patients with neurological, cardiovascular, and infectious diseases?

22. What advancements are needed in AI research to further enhance the accuracy and reliability of diagnostic, prognostic, and survival prediction models for these diseases?
23. How does a deep neural network (DNN) perform segmentation tasks in medical imaging, such as delineating tumor boundaries or identifying anatomical structures?
24. What techniques are employed by DNNs for abnormality detection in medical images, and how do they compare to traditional methods?
25. Can you explain the process by which deep neural networks classify diseases based on medical imaging data, and what are the key challenges in this task?
26. How are DNNs utilized in computer-aided diagnosis systems to assist healthcare professionals in making accurate and timely diagnoses?
27. What role do deep neural networks play in content-based image retrieval systems for medical images, and how do they improve retrieval accuracy compared to conventional methods?
28. What are some common architectures and techniques used in DNNs for medical image segmentation, abnormality detection, disease classification, computer-aided diagnosis, and image retrieval?
29. How do DNN-based approaches handle challenges such as data scarcity, class imbalance, and interpretability in medical image analysis tasks?
30. Can you discuss some real-world applications where DNNs have demonstrated superior performance in medical image analysis compared to traditional machine learning methods?
31. What are the limitations and potential risks associated with deploying deep neural networks in clinical settings for medical image analysis?
32. How can researchers and practitioners ensure the reliability, robustness, and generalizability of DNN-based models in various medical imaging applications?
33. How do deep neural networks contribute to the early diagnosis of neurological diseases such as Alzheimer's disease or Parkinson's disease, and what are the key biomarkers or imaging modalities used in these applications?
34. Can you explain how deep neural networks are utilized in predicting the prognosis of patients with cardiovascular diseases, such as myocardial infarction or heart failure, and what clinical variables are typically considered in these prognostic models?
35. What role do deep neural networks play in predicting the survival outcomes of patients with infectious diseases like COVID-19, and how do they incorporate factors such as demographic information, laboratory test results, and medical imaging findings?
36. How do deep neural networks handle the complexity and heterogeneity of neurological, cardiovascular, and infectious diseases in their diagnostic, prognostic, and survival prediction models?

37. Can you discuss some examples of successful applications of deep neural networks in improving the accuracy and reliability of diagnosis, prognosis, and survival prediction in neurological, cardiovascular, and infectious diseases?
38. What are the challenges and limitations associated with deploying deep neural networks in clinical practice for disease diagnosis, prognosis, and survival prediction, and how can these challenges be addressed?
39. How do deep neural networks compare to traditional statistical models or machine learning algorithms in terms of performance, interpretability, and generalizability in predicting outcomes for neurological, cardiovascular, and infectious diseases?
40. What are some ethical considerations that need to be taken into account when using deep neural networks for disease diagnosis, prognosis, and survival prediction, particularly regarding data privacy, bias, and transparency?
41. Can you discuss the potential impact of deep neural networks on personalized medicine approaches for neurological, cardiovascular, and infectious diseases, and how they can tailor treatment strategies based on individual patient characteristics?
42. How can healthcare providers and researchers collaborate to validate and integrate deep neural network-based diagnostic, prognostic, and survival prediction models into clinical practice, ensuring their accuracy and usability in real-world settings?

Multiple Choice Questions

1. Multiple Choice: What is the primary role of AI technologies in healthcare for neurological, cardiovascular, and infectious diseases?
   a) Diagnosing diseases accurately
   b) Predicting disease prognosis
   c) Estimating patient survival rates
   d) All of the above
2. True or False: AI technologies, such as deep learning models, can only be used for diagnosing neurological diseases.
3. Fill in the Blank: AI technologies can assist in predicting the ________ of patients with cardiovascular diseases based on various clinical factors.
4. Matching: Match the following diseases with their corresponding AI applications: A. Parkinson's disease B. Myocardial infarction C. COVID-19
   1. Disease diagnosis using medical imaging
   2. Prognosis prediction based on clinical variables
   3. Survival rate estimation using demographic data

5. Short Answer: How can AI technologies improve the accuracy of diagnosing infectious diseases compared to traditional methods?
6. Essay: Discuss the potential ethical implications of using AI technologies for predicting survival rates in patients with neurological diseases.
7. Which of the following is NOT a role of AI technologies in healthcare for neurological, cardiovascular, and infectious diseases?
   a) Diagnosing diseases accurately
   b) Predicting disease prognosis
   c) Estimating patient survival rates
   d) Developing new drugs and treatments
8. AI technologies can assist in predicting the prognosis of patients with cardiovascular diseases based on:
   a) Genetic factors b) Imaging data c) Clinical variables d) All of the above
9. Which disease can AI technologies help diagnose using medical imaging?
   a) Parkinson's disease
   b) Influenza
   c) Tuberculosis
   d) All of the above
10. In infectious disease management, AI technologies can be used to:
    a) Track disease outbreaks
    b) Predict the effectiveness of vaccines
    c) Identify drug-resistant strains
    d) All of the above
11. Which AI application is particularly useful for estimating patient survival rates in neurological diseases?
    a) Natural language processing
    b) Computer-aided diagnosis
    c) Deep learning models
    d) Data mining techniques
12. Which of the following tasks can deep neural networks (DNNs) be applied to in medical imaging?
    a) Segmentation
    b) Abnormality detection
    c) Disease classification
    d) Computer-aided diagnosis
    e) All of the above
13. How do deep neural networks contribute to image segmentation in medical imaging?
    a) By identifying and delineating regions of interest
    b) By classifying images into normal and abnormal categories
    c) By predicting the progression of diseases
    d) By recommending appropriate treatments

14. What is the primary objective of abnormality detection using deep neural networks?
    a) To identify healthy regions within medical images
    b) To highlight areas suspected of pathology or abnormalities
    c) To classify diseases based on imaging data
    d) To generate medical reports automatically
15. In disease classification tasks, what role do deep neural networks play?
    a) Identifying key features from medical images
    b) Predicting the likelihood of different diseases based on patient data
    c) Recommending treatment options for specific conditions
    d) Monitoring disease progression over time
16. How do deep neural networks support computer-aided diagnosis (CAD) systems?
    a) By assisting radiologists in interpreting medical images
    b) By automatically generating diagnoses without human input
    c) By predicting the effectiveness of certain treatments
    d) By providing real-time patient monitoring and alerts
17. In what way can deep neural networks aid in medical image retrieval?
    a) By organizing large databases of medical images
    b) By automatically generating medical reports from imaging data
    c) By predicting patient outcomes based on historical data
    d) By recommending relevant images based on similarity to a query image
18. Which of the following diseases can deep neural networks assist in diagnosing?
    a) Neurological diseases
    b) Cardiovascular diseases
    c) Infectious diseases
    d) All of the above
19. How can deep neural networks contribute to the prognosis of neurological diseases?
    a) By predicting disease progression based on patient data
    b) By recommending personalized treatment plans
    c) By identifying biomarkers associated with disease severity
    d) All of the above
20. In cardiovascular disease management, what role can deep neural networks play in predicting survival rates?
    a) By analyzing patient demographics and clinical history
    b) By interpreting medical imaging data for signs of disease progression
    c) By integrating genetic information to assess disease risk
    d) All of the above

21. How do deep neural networks aid in the diagnosis of infectious diseases?
    a) By analyzing patient symptoms and medical history
    b) By detecting patterns in laboratory test results
    c) By identifying specific pathogens in diagnostic samples
    d) All of the above
22. Which of the following statements about the role of deep neural networks in disease diagnosis is true?
    a) They rely solely on medical imaging data for accurate diagnosis.
    b) They can integrate multiple types of data, including imaging, genetic, and clinical information.
    c) They are only effective for diagnosing neurological diseases.
    d) They do not require input from healthcare professionals for accurate diagnosis.
23. What is one advantage of using deep neural networks for disease prognosis?
    a) They can accurately predict disease outcomes without considering patient data.
    b) They provide personalized predictions based on individual patient characteristics.
    c) They require extensive manual feature engineering for accurate predictions.
    d) They are not suitable for predicting long-term disease trajectories.

Chapter 6

Case studies

PIX2PIX GANS FOR BREAST CANCER DETECTION

6.1 INTRODUCTION

In image analysis for digital pathology, generative adversarial networks (GANs) are trending recently. This is because it is critical to acquire rapid and highly precise outcomes without adopting expensive and bulky equipments. The primary reason is that the information being provided for artificial neural network (ANNs) can be incredibly vast, which makes it possible for swift detectors to use it as input and enable minute details and extensive picture analysis. A more recent AI approach to generative modeling that uses deep learning is GANs. GANs are a class of machine learning frameworks designed to generate realistic data by leveraging a competitive process between two neural networks: a generator and a discriminator. GANs are based on unsupervised learning and automatically discover and learn the patterns or regularities of the inputs. Using this technique, the GAN generates new samples that would have been possibly generated using the original dataset. GANs are clever algorithms that performs training of a generative model by making the problem as a supervised learning problem using two submodels one of which is a generator model and the other is a discriminator model. The generator model is the one that is trained to generate new samples, while the discriminator model is the one that performs classification of the samples as either real or generated (fake). Both these models are trained together in an adversarial manner until the discriminator model is fooled. This implies that the generator is generating plausible examples. GANs are exciting and frequently changing algorithms, as they promise generative models with the ability to generate artificial samples that are close to reality, and even humans cannot predict that they are fake.

In nations with advanced economies, lung cancer affects a greater percentage of individuals than any other sort of cancer. At the same time in underdeveloped nations, breast cancer kills far more people than any other type of malignancies. When a breast cancer is so delicate or cryptic that the

DOI: 10.1201/9781003503033-6

radiologist cannot seem to identify it, it is termed as mammographically-occult (M-occult). Retrospective screening is employed for recognizing this type of cancer following preceding mammography that proved negative. Given that the fibrograndular tissue in thick breasts is capable of concealing indications of malignant cells, M-occult cancers are increasingly frequent in females having thick breasts. Bilateral breast tissue differential parameter [1, 2] has been proven to be a successful strategy. In [3], it is demonstrated that a Radon cumulative distribution transform is capable of accurately recognizing M-occult malignancies using the reciprocal breast tissue differential. The identification of M-occult tumors was the subject of only a handful of studies [4]. Magnitude contrast between authentic and mimicked pictures may provide aid in the extraction of additional information regarding the existence of hidden cancer if normal and individualized mammography can be simulated [5]. A conventional mammogram yields four separate views, including the cranial–caudal (CC) and mediolateral–oblique (MLO), which each have left and right views. For obtaining the data necessary for M-occult cancer detection, any one of these viewpoints can be mimicked. The challenging undertaking in this system is to generate healthy, normal images. It is also time-consuming to simulate a personal mammogram. In the last 5 years, machine learning algorithms have become the dominant force in technology. However, efficiency is decreased when artificial intelligence is employed in medical imaging owing to the lack of big databases of medical pictures, which are necessary for deep neural networks to perform well and prevent overfitting. Image augmentation is a newly developed method to expand the current medical dataset. Known image processing techniques for data augmentation include noise insertion, flipping, contrast modulation, and rotation.

6.2 GENERATIVE ADVERSARIAL NETWORKS (GAN) FOR CANCER: THE CASE STUDY

Recent machine learning approaches such as GANs are used to simulate or synthesize images, more commonly referred to as "fake" images [6]. The two main parts of a GAN are a generator and a discriminator. The generator constructs a fake image, and the discriminator evaluates whether the image is a real one derived from the database or a mimicked one produced by the generator. Post undergoing training, the generator proceeds to generate flawless pictures that the differentiator cannot seem to distinguish from real or fake. GANs are not extensively employed in the literature for disease datasets owing to the diversity of their output images. Picture-to-picture conversion is a method that allows one image to be converted into another in a desired profile. A conditional GAN, or CGAN, is the type of GAN that translates images into new images [6, 7]. The distinctive characteristics of the input image are taken advantage of to create the new image. Either right or left mammography fed as input can be used to replicate a contralateral mammogram. The style-Pix2pix, an upgraded version of pix2pix that is designed to perform one-to-many production of pictures, is suggested in [8]. It is based on building the offspring pictures from the input parent picture using style blocks and a mapping affiliation. In [9], skrGAN is proposed. SkrGAN is a method for segmenting blood arteries and microparticles in blood. The technique makes use of fundus pictures and X-ray images. This approach solely relies upon the Sobel edge recognition strategy. Similarly, drawings of pictures are obtained along with pictures from the ultrasonographic procedure in [10]. In [11], pertinent feature masks are used in conjunction with image creation while the surrounding region is kept constant. These pictures were initially extracted from the patient's CT scans. The offerings of this study are as follows: (1) for the inaugural time, we demonstrated the application of Pix2pix GANs for breast malignancy diagnosis along with CNN layers built using U-NET and (2) in relation to transfer learning, which has been carried out on the same database, the preciseness of Pix2pix enriched pictures from the mammogram is higher.

6.3 APPLICATION OF PIX2PIX GAN FOR DETECTION OF BREAST CANCER

A flowchart of the creation of an artificial dataset using GAN is shown in Figure 6.1. The generator is built up of a U-net that assists in converting the input image into a mimicked output image. The differentiator performs the obligation to determine if a specific picture was created via generator. The generator makes adjustments for each image it produces in order to reduce the expected loss. Similar to this, transfer learning is a method for getting around the issue of tiny databases [12–14]. Through transfer learning, primary layers of a CNN or DNN incorporate data out of an affiliation that has previously been trained, while the later levels receive formal training. The production of an output image while employing GAN is dependent on the root picture. The database employed is the Mammographic Image

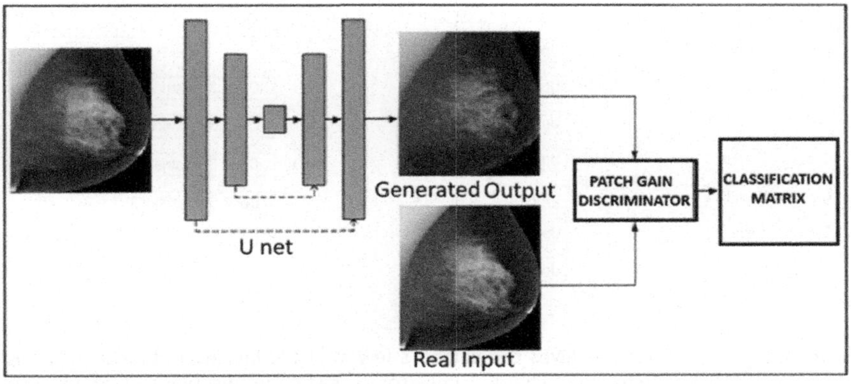

Figure 6.1 Artificial dataset using GAN for cancer image classification.

Analysis Society (MIAS-1.21) dataset, that contains 322 mammography pictures at a resolution of 50 microns and 200 microns, respectively. The images have a 1024 pixel resolution and are in grayscale. The images are resized to 128 × 128 pixels before being sent into the GAN generator and discriminator. The database consists of seven columns; the initial column has the serial number, and the second denotes the type of tissue, such as dense-glandular, fatty glandular, or fatty alone. The classification of the anomaly, such as normal, asymmetric, deformed, hypothesized masses, theorized masses, or cemented, can be seen in the third column. The fourth column categorizes the abnormality's severity as either benign or malignant. The coordinates for the center and diameter of the circles that are sketched to enclose the anomaly are finally described in columns 5, 6, and 7. The supplied picture p may be interpreted as the final picture q using pix2pix GAN. The certified discriminator can spot the bogus images, while the trained generator produces them. The objective of the x and y, which are the supplied and opposing pictures from the mammogram of the exact females, is defined by Equations (6.1) and (6.2) when they are combined.

$$F = E_{x,y}[\log Dis(x,y)] + E_{x,z}[\log(1 - Dis(x, Gen(x,z)))] \tag{6.1}$$

$$Obj = \arg[\min_{Gen} \max_{Dis} (F)] \tag{6.2}$$

Dis is the discriminator function, and Gen is the generator. Now, function F enables the generator to produce believable mammography that is comparable to y by using x (normal) as the supplied mammogram and y (opposite) as the goal mammogram of the exact females also z is latent vector, a latent vector is a set of numerical values that represent compressed,

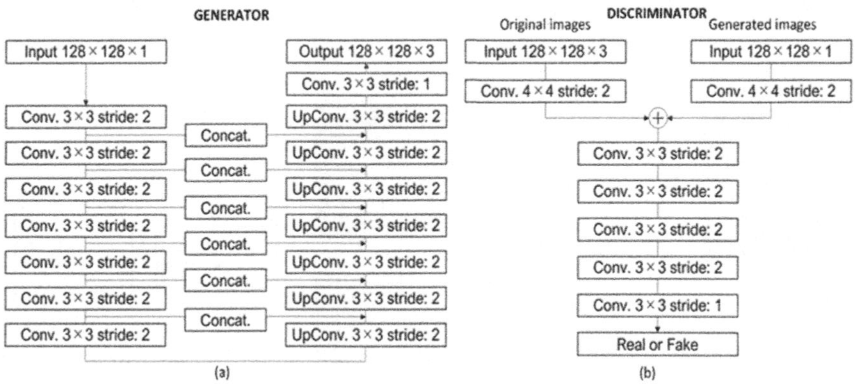

Figure 6.2 (a) Generator receives the dataset's few available images and passing through U-Net structure. (b) The discriminator receives the two types of pictures, real and mimicked, after they are resized to 128 × 128 pixels.

abstract features of data in a lower-dimensional space. The generator seen in Figure 6.2(a) receives the dataset's few available images, which are then sequentially passed through layers of convolutional upsampling and downsampling to create a U-Net structure. Python version 3.0 is the one used for the programming. The database is submitted and provided to the GAN as input. The differentiator, which receives the two types of pictures, real and mimicked, after they are resized to 128 × 128 pixels, is depicted in Figure 6.3. On an NVIDIA server, Google Tensorflow is used to create the suggested GAN. Following the dataset's augmentation with pix2pix and transfer learning, two CNN models, VGG16 [15] and Resnet-50, are used to analyze the final accuracy of the detection. 100 input photos make up the generator design, which has been optimized for RELU in every layer. The number of epochs is assumed to be 350, and the batch size is 10. Faster training is possible with a higher learning rate, while slower training is possible when exploring the details of the database and locating more suitable

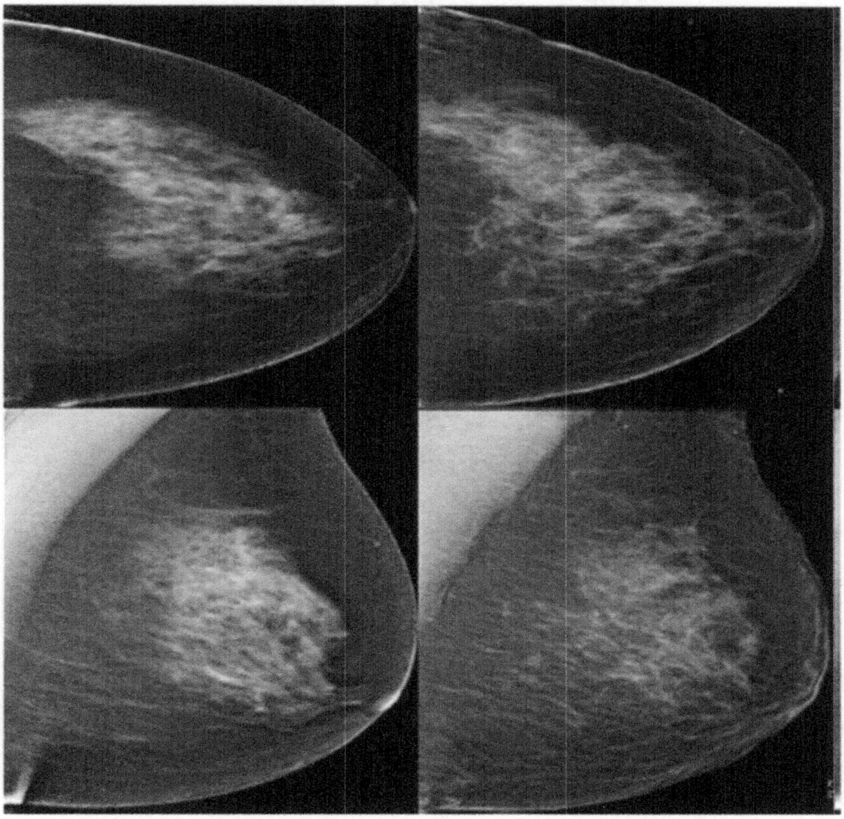

Figure 6.3 Some images of breast created by the proposed algorithm.

characteristics. Owing to which, it is assumed that the rate of getting to know in the suggested algorithm is 0.0001. Figure 6.3 depicts some images of breasts created by the proposed algorithm. Also, Figure 6.4 shows the flow chart of the suggested algorithm for pix2pix breast cancer picture enhancement. Table 6.1 gives a comparison of data augmentation techniques for cancer detection.

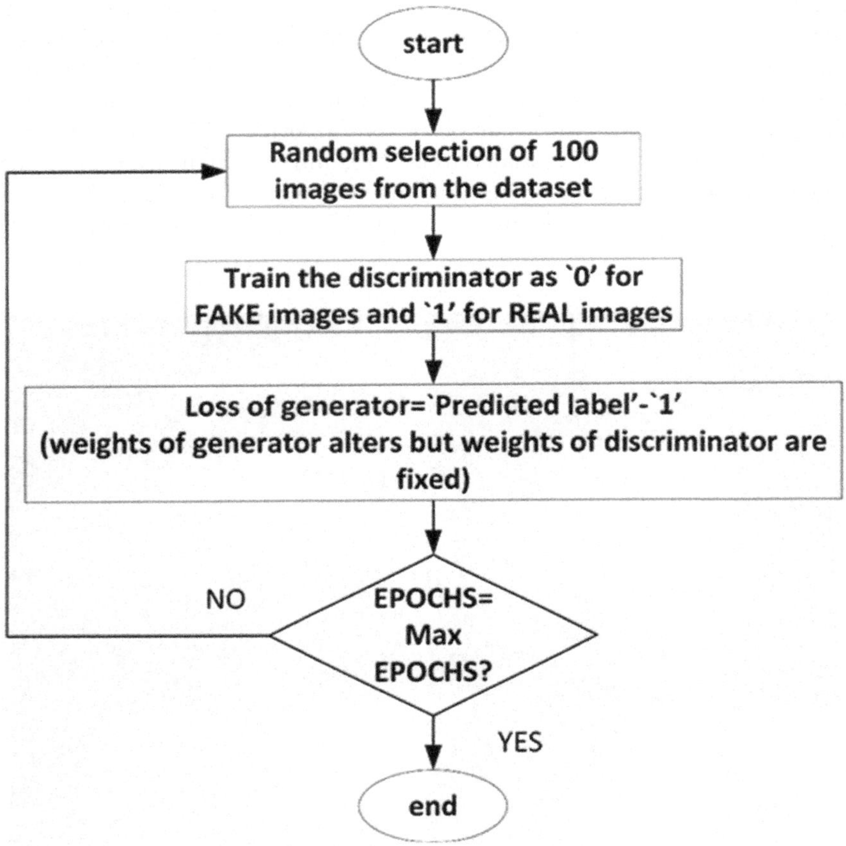

Figure 6.4 The algorithm used for pix2pix Breast Cancer picture enhancement.

Table 6.1 Comparison of data augmentation techniques for cancer detection

Technique	*Precision*	*Recall*	*F-measure*
Pix2pix	0.72	0.78	0.76
Transfer learning	0.70	0.72	0.76

6.4 RESULTS

Results are analyzed in terms of true positive (TP), true negative (TN), false positive (FP), and false negative (FN) receiver operating characteristics. When a picture from mammogram indicates that it is standard and it genuinely is standard, it will be referred to as TP, and if it indicates malignant breast and it genuinely is malignant, it is referred to as TN. If network's result on a standard picture is categorized as malignant, it is designated as FN, and if it is normal, it is designated as FP. Finally, the accuracy, which is the ratio of number of correct assessments and total number of assessments, is given by Equation (6.3).

$$\text{Accuracy} = \frac{\text{TP} + \text{TN}}{\text{TP} + \text{TN} + \text{FP} + \text{FN}} \tag{6.3}$$

The calculation for accuracy is depicted in Equation 6.3. Figure 6.4 shows the algorithm used for pix2pic breast cancer picture enhancement. It can be observed that, Pix2Pix GAN outperforms CNN's transfer learning method for detecting breast cancer in terms of accuracy. Figure 6.6 displays the accuracy values for four models. Two additional criteria are used to evaluate the GANs' output images. The two widely accepted statistics that are typically employed to establish a relation between the picture processing outcomes of whatever methodologies are the peak signal to noise ratio (PSNR) and the structural similarity index (SSIM). The structural resemblance index is used for figuring out how much the mimicked picture differs from the real picture. PSNR is termed as the ratio of the maximum value of the signal to the means square error.

$$\text{PSNR} = 10\log_{10}\frac{\text{max}^2}{\text{mse}} \tag{6.4}$$

where max denotes the highest pixel's potential value, which in this instance is the pixel's brightness. Greater PSNR values are needed to produce output of greater quality, while SSIM values that are closer to 1 are preferable to those that are farther from 1 in terms of quality. As shown in Table 6.2, the images produced by the proposed algorithm perform better than the images produced by styleGAN in [8]. Although the SSIM score of the suggested work is extremely

Table 6.2 PSNR and SSIM of the images generated by the proposed algorithm and styleGAN algorithm [8]

Technique	*PSNR*	*SSIM*
Pix2pix	18.17	0.655
styleGAN [8]	17.98	0.655

similar to [8], the PSNR score of [8] is less than the proposed task. MATLAB software is used for image processing in the calculation of SSIM and PSNR.

THE ROLE OF AI IN REVOLUTIONIZING DENTISTRY

6.5 ABSTRACT

Integration of AI in dental industry is revolutionizing patient care, diagnostics, and operational efficiency. This case study explores practical application of AI in dental management organization (DMO) overseeing manifold dental practices across New York. Outcome of integrating AI tools highlights substantial improvements in patient outcomes and business operations. As acquirer, owner, and operator of DMO, the task was sustaining consistent quality across numerous locations while enhancing patient care. Emphasis lifted to utilizing AI for improved decision-making, operational standards, and diagnostics. Outcomes have been groundbreaking, demonstrating measurable improvements in numerous areas.

6.6 VITAL DISCOVERIES AND BENEFITS OF AI INTEGRATION

Improved Decision-Making at Point of Care: AI's ability to analyze vast datasets enables dentists to make informed decisions quickly. By blending data-driven insights with clinical expertise, AI have the following:

- Amended diagnosis accuracy.
- Augmented case acceptance rates.
- Abridged patient treatment costs.

Standardized Operational Quality: AI has provided scalable tools to ensure consistent standards across numerous locations. These tools not only automate routine tasks but also:

- Augment clinical precision.
- Foster growth by refining patient gratification and retention.

Diagnostic Advancements with AI:
One of the standout contributions of AI was its integration into diagnostic tools, predominantly for X-ray analysis.

Key Features of AI in Diagnostics:

- **Detection of Carious Lesions:** Swiftly identifies decay in real time.
- **Radiographic Bone Levels (RBL):** Measures bone loss to analyze periodontal diseases with precision.

System visually annotates X-rays, aiding dentists in deliberating diagnoses with patients evidently and effectually. Table 6.3 gives types of diagnostic tools in dentistry.

6.7 PERIODONTAL DISEASE MANAGEMENT WITH AI

Diagnosing periodontal disease, exclusively in early stages, can be challenging due to the lack of noticeable symptoms. AI tools abridge this process by evaluating bone levels and annotating severity levels on X-rays utilizing color-coded markers. A seven layer deep neural network was used as a part of this study to detect the periodontal disease. The network used Adam optimizer and learning rate was 0.1. Backpropagation is used in training. The algorithm was trained using 10000 images of patients having periodontal disease. These images were gathered from several clinics as a part of research conducted for oral health. Table 6.4 gives types of markers in the periodontal scan. When the scan on patients teeth is performed, it tries to predict one of the following four important outcomes:

1. No significant bone loss
2. Slight bone loss; early intervention suggested
3. Noticeable bone loss requiring attention
4. Critical bone loss needing immediate care

Figure 6.6 shows this with the help of different markers. It can be observed that the scan successfully detects the areas that needs attention.

Table 6.3 Types of diagnostic tools in dentistry

Diagnostic tool	*Functionality*	*Impact*
Carious lesion detection	Categorizes decay accurately in real time	Quicker diagnosis and amended precision
Radiographic bone level (RBL)	Measures bone levels from cementoenamel junction to alveolar bone. Highlights critical areas	Enhances communication and treatment plans

Table 6.4 Types of markers in the periodontal scan

Marker length	*Severity level*
Small caps	●–●
Large caps	●——●
Small arrows	↔
Large arrows	←——→

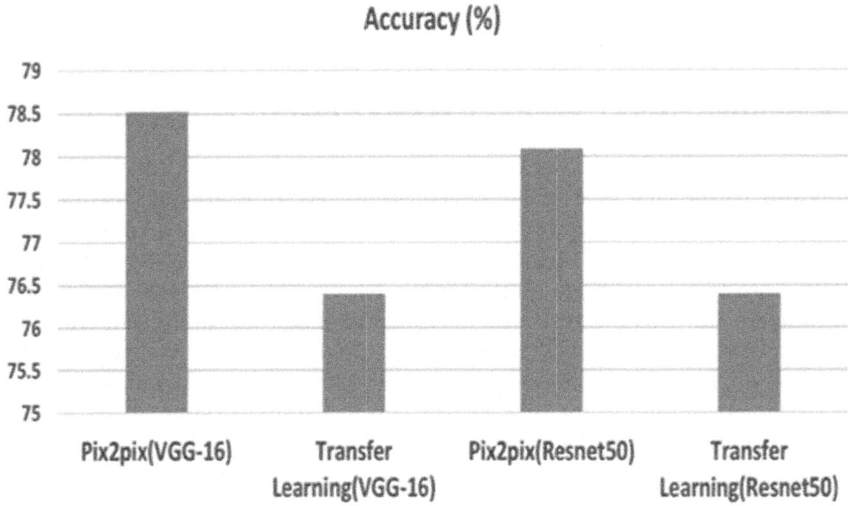

Figure 6.5 Comparison of Pix2pix GANs with transfer learning for image augmentation.

Table 6.5 Types of markers in the periodontal scan and their resultant detection of teeth bone quality

Marker length	*Severity Level*	*Description*
Small caps	Normal	No significant bone loss
Large caps	Mild	Slight bone loss; early intervention suggested
Small stars	Moderate	Noticeable bone loss requiring attention
Large stars	Severe	Critical bone loss needing immediate care

The results are shown in Table 6.5. Figure 6.6 does not show any arrows (small or large) because the patient did not suffer from the conditions that the arrow markers depict. These annotations help in providing dentists with visual aid, enhancing patient understanding and acceptance of treatment plan.

6.8 OPERATIONAL EFFICIENCIES AND PATIENT EXPERIENCE

As shown in Table 6.6, the operational efficiencies of dental procedures with AI have numerous positive outcomes. Broader utilization of AI outspreads beyond clinical diagnostics to overall office management enables:

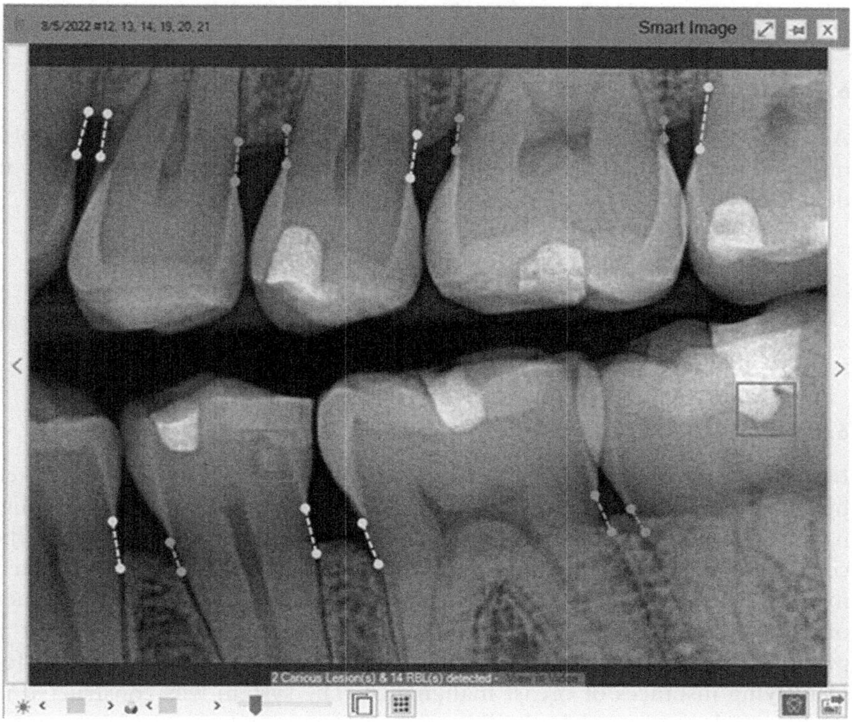

Figure 6.6 Integrating AI into dental practices: DMO's case study.

Table 6.6 Patient experiences from AI-based dental practices

Benefit	*Description*	*Outcome*
Automation of routine tasks	Delegates administrative work to AI	Permits dentists to emphasis on patient care
Predictive analytics	Anticipates patient needs effectively	Upsurges patient retention
Personalized patient care	Tailored treatment plans via AI insights	Augments patient satisfaction and trust

1. **Automation of Routine Tasks**
   - o Appointment scheduling.
   - o Claim processing.
   - o Predictive analytics for patient follow-ups.
2. **Amended Patient Outcomes**
   - o Abridged costs for patients.

- o Advanced case acceptance rates.
- o Personalized care based on data-driven insights.

6.9 BROADER IMPACTS AND FUTURE PROSPECTS

AI's adoption in dentistry addresses oral health disparities and supports underserved populations. Potential of AI to become a standard tool in dental offices within the next decade is substantial, enabling:

- Innovative clinical decision-making.
- Seamless integration of medical and dental care.
- Patient-centered approach that syndicates technology with human expertise.

6.10 CONCLUSION

In this study, a Pix2pix GAN for image enhancement is proposed, suggested by a convolutional neural network for identifying instances of breast malignancy. The simulation was constructed in Python and contrasted along the conventional transfer learning strategy. Accuracy is derived after determining the ROCs and is 78.52% in relation to transfer learning's accuracy of 76.4%. In this research, a Pix2pix GAN for image enhancement is proposed for the first time, afterwards a convolutional neural system for identifying instances of breast malignancy. The system was constructed in Python and contrasted with the conventional transfer learning strategy. Accuracy is derived after determining the ROCs and is 78.52% in relation with the transfer learning's accuracy of 76.4%. Therefore, by improving and creating a better database from a given database containing fewer photos, this approach is employed to obtain more accurate cancer identification processes. This research focuses on GANs, a powerful subset of artificial intelligence that is used to analyze histology image data. GANs have been demonstrated to enhance the performance of detection methods; however, they can also permit more archaic, unworkable applications in this area. Data with morphological changes might occasionally have unclear patterns and be challenging to play with. Cycle GANs are typically more adaptable than less complicated GANs. It is anticipated that due to the recurrent pattern of their implementation, they can be employed in this recognition more effectively because they are capable of handling data with inverted morphology. The lookout for possibilities of various unique methodological techniques, including observed and unobserved machine learning computations, to enhance picture evaluation even more is continually under progress, bearing in mind the current trends and significant advantages of GANs aside. The requirement for greater accuracy of feature extraction could potentially be a significant function in the actual implementation of

ANN-dependent picture evaluation procedures in electronic pathology, even though GANs have the potential to relax and occasionally eliminate the limitations upon the massive volumes of structured information required for perfecting ANN computations.

Moreover, AI has revolutionized various aspects of dental practice, enhancing efficiency, accuracy, and patient outcomes. The case study (b) explores the diverse applications of AI in dentistry and its implications for the future of oral healthcare. The study underscores how AI can harmoniously blend with clinical expertise to elevate dental practices, ensuring excellence in patient care and operational success. By leveraging AI, the DMO can not only improve its operational standards but can also set benchmarks for the future of dental care, ensuring better health outcomes for all.

REFERENCES

[1] J. Lee, R. M. Nishikawa, and G. K. Rohde. "Detecting mammographically occult cancer in women with dense breasts using radon cumulative distribution transform: A preliminary analysis." *Proc. SPIE*, vol. 10575, Feb. 2018, Art. no. 1057508.

[2] J. Lee and R. M. Nishikawa. "Detecting mammographically-occult cancer in women with dense breasts using deep convolutional neural network and radon cumulative distribution transform." *Proc. SPIE*, vol. 10950, Dec. 2019, Art. no. 1095003.

[3] P. Isola, J.-Y. Zhu, T. Zhou, and A. A. Efros. "Image-to-image translation with conditional adversarial networks." In Proceedings IEEE Conf. Comput. Vis. Pattern Recognit. (CVPR), Jul. 2017, pp. 5967–5976.

[4] J. G. Mainprize, O. Alonzo-Proulx, R. A. Jong, and M. J. Yaffe. "Quantifying masking in clinical mammograms via local detectability of simulated lesions." *Med. Phys.*, vol. 43, no. 3, pp. 1249–1258, Mar. 2016.

[5] J. Lee and R. M. Nishikawa. "Identifying women with mammographically-occult breast cancer leveraging GAN-simulated mammograms." *IEEE Trans. Med. Imag.*, vol. 41, no. 1, pp. 225–236, Jan. 2022. doi:10.1109/TMI.2021.3108949

[6] T. Schlegl, P. Seebock, S. M. Waldstein, U. Schmidt-Erfurth, and G. ¨ Langs. "Unsupervised anomaly detection with generative adversarial networks to guide marker discovery." In Information processing in medical imaging, Cham, Switzerland: Springer, 2017, pp. 146–157.

[7] V. Alex, M Safwan K. P., S. S. Chennamsetty, and G. Krishnamurthi. "Generative adversarial networks for brain lesion detection." *Proc. SPIE*, vol. 10133, Feb. 2017, Art. no. 101330G.

[8] R. Toda, A.Teramoto, M. Kondo et al. "Lung cancer CT image generation from a free-form sketch using style-based pix2pix for data augmentation." *Scientif. Rep.*, vol. 12, no. 1, 2022.

[9] T. Zhang, H. Fu, Y. Zhang., et al. "SkrGAN: Sketching-rendering unconditional generative adversarial networks for medical image synthesis." In MICCAI, pp. 777–785, 2019.

[10] J. Liang, X. Yang, H. Li, et al. "Synthesis and edition of ultrasound images via sketch guided progressive growing GANS". In IEEE 17th International Symposium on Biomedical Imaging (ISBI), pp. 1793–1797, 2020.

[11] Q. Wang, Z. Xiaohong, W. Zhang, et al. "Realistic lung nodule synthesis with multi-target co-guided adversarial mechanism." *IEEE Transl. Med. Imag.*, 40, 2343–2353, 2021.

[12] R. K. Samala et al. "Breast cancer diagnosis in digital breast tomosynthesis: Effects of training sample size on multi-stage transfer learning using deep neural nets." *IEEE Trans. Med. Imag.*, vol. 38, no. 3, pp. 686–696, Mar. 2019.

[13] N. Tajbakhsh et al. "Convolutional neural networks for medical image analysis: Full training or fine tuning?" *IEEE Trans. Med. Imag.*, vol. 35, no. 5, pp. 1299–1312, May 2016.

[14] D. Maturana and S. Scherer. "VoxNet: A 3D convolutional neural network for real-time object recognition." In Proc. IEEE/RSJ Int. Conf. Intell. Robots Syst. (IROS), Sep. 2015, pp. 922–928.

[15] K. Simonyan and A. Zisserman. "Very deep convolutional networks for large-scale image recognition." 409.1556, arXiv, 2014.

Subjective Questions

Q1. How does generative adversarial networks contribute to personalized medicine in healthcare?

Q2. Explain how GANs and HPC can be used together to improve cancer detection?

Q3. What are some challenges of GANs in healthcare?

Objective Questions

Q1. A GAN consists of how many individual neural networks?

A) One
B) Two
C) Three
D) Four

Answer: B

Q2. What is the role of discriminator in GAN?

A) Takes random noise as input and generates synthetic data
B) To create data that resembles real data
C) Takes input data (real or generated) and predicts whether it is real or fake
D) Takes input data (real or generated) and creates another data which is different from original data

Answer: C

Q3. How can GANs be used for cancer detection?
   A) By enhancing various aspects of medical imaging, data generation, and analysis
   B) By data analysis
   C) By Segmentation and Localization
   D) By Image-to-Image Translation
   Answer: A, C and D

Q4. Which of the following is true for data augmentation by GANs for cancer detection?
   A) Cancer datasets are often imbalanced, with limited samples of certain cancer types
   B) GANs can generate synthetic medical images (e.g., MRI, CT, histopathological images) that mimic real cancerous and non-cancerous tissue.
   C) Data augmentation increases the dataset's size and diversity, improving the training of machine learning models
   D) Data augmentation cannot do image-to-image translation
   Answer: A, B, and C

Chapter 7

Application of machine learning to gynecological cancers

7.1 INTRODUCTION

Gynecological cancers are the most common cancers among women and thus hold the utmost attention. Due to the lack of knowledge in this field, most women are prone to these cancers and often report at the final stages. Ovarian cancer, cervical cancer (CC), endometrial, and uterine cancer remain the most common cancers. There are a variety of symptoms associated with gynecological cancers. The most common symptom is abnormal bleeding. This can include bleeding between periods, after sex, or after menopause. Other symptoms can include pain in the pelvis, abnormal discharge, and fatigue. Gynecological cancers can be detected through a variety of methods. The most common method is a Pap smear, which can detect CC. Other tests include pelvic exams, ultrasounds, and MRI. Treatment for gynecologic cancers also depends on cancer type and phase of cancer. Most commonly used treatment modalities are radiotherapy, surgery, and chemotherapy. In 2018, ovarian cancer was seen in 295,414 female patients, among which the number of deaths of patients due to cancer in the world was 184,799.

In India, about 74,000 women will be diagnosed with ovarian cancer and about 70,000 women will die from it in the year of 2019. Ovarian cancer is the sixth most common cancer in women worldwide and the fifth most common cause of cancer death in women. In India, ovarian cancer is the eighth most common cancer in women. Carbohydrate antigen 125 (CA125), Carbohydrate antigen 72-4 (CA72-4), and human epididymis protein 4 (HE4) are the promising biomarkers for early detection of ovarian cancer. About 13,000 new cases of CC are discovered each year in the US, and 4,000 women pass away from the disease. The incidence rate of CC is approximately 14.36 per 100,000 women, while the mortality rate is around 7.02 per 100,000 women. The majority of women diagnosed with CC are between the ages of 35 and 44 years. The number of deaths caused by CC in India totals to about 73,831 in 2018. The majority of women who died due to CC (67.5%) were between the ages of 45 and 64 years. CC is a serious health problem in India and a major cause of cancer-related mortality

DOI: 10.1201/9781003503033-7

in Indian women. According to the World Health Organization (WHO), CC is the fourth most common cancer in women in India, with an estimated 96,922 new cases and 73,831 deaths in 2018. CC develops slowly over time. It is most often caused by the human papillomavirus (HPV), which is passed on through sexual contact. Other risk factors include smoking, a weakened immune system, and having multiple sexual partners. The overall rate of ovarian cancer incidence in the US is about 12 per 100,000 women. There are about 21,980 new cases of ovarian cancer diagnosed and about 15,460 ovarian cancer deaths annually. The high mortality rate is attributable to the asymptomatic nature of the disease in its early stages. Patients with early-stage disease are often asymptomatic, and the cancer is discovered only at the time of surgery for an unrelated condition. Patients with advanced disease have a 5-year survival rate of less than 30%. In order to bring down the deathblow because of these gynecological cancers, it is necessary to identify the related risk factors and take prompt measures as early as possible.

Of all the gynecological cancers, CC is the only type which can be diagnosed easily, and thus, the treatment can be effective. Since there are no proper methods to identify gynecological cancers effectively, the need for effective and efficient modern treatment arises. A prolonged duration of intensive medical training is needed for proper disease diagnosis. Even with this training, the diagnostic process is typically challenging and time-consuming. In most regions, the need for specialized knowledge greatly exceeds the available supply. Thus, physicians are under tremendous pressure, which often results in delays in critical patient diagnoses. Recent advances in machine learning (ML), especially in deep learning (DL) algorithms, have greatly enhanced the accuracy and availability of disease diagnosis [1]. Artificial intelligence (AI) is a result of the advancements in computer science during the previous 10 years, and it is now being used in various sectors of science, including medicine. Health healthcare professionals will be better equipped to recognize patients who need extra attention and deliver tailored treatments for each individual with the aid of AI-enabled computer tools. AI can also help to reduce the number of human errors, making it possible to provide patients with more accurate and personalized care. There are many reasons why patients should choose AI-based treatments over traditional ones. For one, AI-based treatments can be administered more quickly and efficiently.

They can also be more accurate, as they do not rely on the human brain to function. AI-based treatments can also be more affordable, as they do not require a lot of equipment or manpower. Because of AI techniques, it has become easy to predict cancer and analyze things one can do to reduce the risks [2]. AI can be used to predict how a person will respond to a certain cancer treatment. The system can also be used to find new cancer treatments. Many women are at a higher risk for gynecologic cancers, and this risk tends to rise with age. It is crucial to be aware of the warning signs, since early detection significantly improves prognosis.

In recent years, prognostication has developed as a major focus in oncology, where decision making is influenced by the predicted probability of future events [3]. Treatment for gynecological cancers varies based on how far the cancer has spread and its specific type. It typically involves options like surgery, chemotherapy, and radiotherapy. Creating oncological prediction algorithms and decision support tools could greatly assist clinicians in selecting the best screening, treatment, and follow-up strategies for their patients. However, challenges arise from the cancers' biological complexity and prognostic variability, alongside the ever-changing clinical, biological, and pathological understanding of these malignancies [4].

Healthcare systems and clinicians currently use several tools to screen, diagnose and treat patients; however, current clinical approaches for many malignancies favor clinical staging and histopathological parameters with multivariate modelling showing limited success [5]. To address these shortcomings, ML approaches have been used to facilitate complex prognostic modelling that may outperform traditional methods [6]. ML methods aim to develop predictive algorithms without requiring complete prior rule definition, a valuable approach in complex clinical settings [6]. Treatment for gynecological cancers varies based on how far the cancer has spread and its specific type. It typically involves options like surgery, chemotherapy, and radiotherapy. Creating oncological prediction algorithms and decision support tools could greatly assist clinicians in selecting the best screening, treatment, and follow-up strategies for their patients. The ML classifiers used to perform the classification tasks include both unsupervised learning, which draws correlations within a dataset without a directed outcome, and supervised learning methods, including support vector machines (SVMs) and artificial neural networks (ANNs), which are goal-directed toward a particular outcome, regression, or classification [6]. In ML workflows, models are initially trained on a dedicated training dataset to learn patterns. During development, a separate validation dataset—which the model hasn't encountered before—helps evaluate its interim performance and guide parameter adjustments. Once finalized, the model is rigorously tested on a completely unseen testing dataset. This final step ensures an objective, unbiased evaluation of how the model might perform in real-world scenarios, as it assesses capabilities without prior exposure to the data.

While these methods have been researched for gynecological cancers, their real-world clinical application remains limited. Current approaches vary widely in both methodology and effectiveness, creating challenges for consistent, successful implementation in patient care. Systematic reviews have previously broadly summarized AI in gynecologic imaging [7], or the application of ML methods broadly to gynecological cancers [8, 9]. To date, no comprehensive synthesis of the literature has thoroughly examined how ML is leveraged to forecast clinical outcomes in gynecological cancers. Our work bridges this critical knowledge gap by pioneering the first systematic appraisal of ML-based prognostic strategies for these malignancies. By scrutinizing the methodological rigor, clinical applicability, and inherent limitations of existing studies, this review aims to clarify the evolving role of ML in enhancing prognostic precision for gynecological oncology. Because of its ability to analyze huge amounts of data, AI has become the best tool to diagnose gynecological cancers effectively and efficiently.

In recent years, machines have almost equaled and also transcended human conduct in many aspects. The influence of modern technology in the medical field is propitious and also may transcend in the upcoming days. The main contributions of this study are identifying the works done till date.

7.1.1 Image processing in medical diagnosis

Image registration, also termed image fusion or matching, is the computational process of spatially aligning two or more images by optimizing their visual or structural similarities. In medical imaging, the core objective of this technique is to identify optimal spatial transformations that precisely align anatomical structures across datasets. Clinically, image registration plays a pivotal role in applications such as surgical guidance, tumor motion monitoring, automated segmentation, radiation dose planning, and longitudinal disease monitoring. Registration methods are broadly classified into four groups based on input image characteristics: multimodal (aligning images from different modalities), unimodal (same modality), intrapatient (same individual over time), and interpatient (across individuals). From a deformation perspective, techniques fall into three categories: rigid (translations/rotations), affine (scaling/shearing), or deformable (non-linear warping). Additionally, approaches can be organized by anatomical regions of interest (ROIs), such as brain, thoracic, or pelvic registrations, each requiring tailored strategies to address organ-specific physiological complexities. According to the dimensions of the image pair, there are three types of registration techniques: 3D to 2D, 3D to 3D, and 2D to 2D/3D [10]. Early cancer detection significantly improves patient survival rates, making timely diagnosis a cornerstone of effective treatment. Traditional diagnostic methods for such malignancies often depend on manual visual inspection of imaging data, which is labor-intensive and inherently subjective. These approaches are susceptible to inconsistencies and human error, particularly when interpreting subtle or complex features in medical scans. To mitigate these challenges, computer-aided diagnosis (CAD) systems emerged in the 1980s [11]. These tools were developed to streamline clinical workflows by offering reproducible, algorithm-driven analyses, thereby enhancing diagnostic accuracy and reducing observer variability. The foundational phase of machine learning-based information system (MLIS) implementation centers on feature extraction design, as this stage determines the integrity of data representation. A systematic approach to selecting attributes directly impacts the reliability of downstream analytical processes, particularly in research contexts where model accuracy hinges on minimizing noise and preserving domain-relevant variables. Methodologically, prioritizing feature engineering frameworks that align with the study's objectives ensures reproducibility and reduces algorithmic bias—a critical consideration for peer-reviewed research. For various cancer types, several feature extraction techniques have been researched [12]. Despite their utility, methodologies reliant on feature extraction are constrained by inherent limitations, including computational overhead, susceptibility to overfitting, and dependency on domain-specific data quality—factors that may compromise generalizability in experimental settings. To address these issues and improve performance, representation learning was proposed by Bengio et al. [13]. A distinct advantage of DL lies in its capacity to autonomously generate hierarchical feature abstractions directly from raw visual data, bypassing labor-intensive manual preprocessing. Furthermore, advancements in graphical processing unit (GPU)-accelerated computing now enable concurrent execution of DL-driven feature extraction and image recognition tasks, optimizing algorithmic performance for real-time or large-scale applications—a critical enhancement in modern computational frameworks. For instance, CNNs have demonstrated promising performance in the detection of cancer [14].

7.2 CANCER DIAGNOSIS USING IMAGE PROCESSING

7.2.1 Preprocessing

Preprocessing constitutes the initial critical stage in image-based detection workflows, aimed at mitigating noise artifacts and enhancing data fidelity to optimize downstream analytical outcomes. In dermatological imaging, for instance, raw inputs often exhibit low contrast between lesions and surrounding tissue, irregular lesion borders, and confounding artifacts such as hair occlusion, epidermal markings, or optical aberrations (e.g., vignetting). These imperfections, if unaddressed, propagate errors into subsequent classification algorithms, risking diagnostic inaccuracies. To counteract these challenges, adaptive filtering techniques—including Wiener, median, and mean filters—are deployed alongside targeted preprocessing operations. These may encompass artifact suppression (e.g., hair removal via inpainting), contrast normalization, color space transformations, and spatial smoothing to homogenize illumination. Such interventions not only reduce signal noise but also standardize inputs for ML pipelines, thereby improving model generalizability. Empirical studies underscore that strategic integration of preprocessing modules, tailored to domain-specific noise profiles, significantly elevates diagnostic precision in applications such as automated melanoma screening. Black frame removal, automated color equalization, hair removal, dull Razor, Karhunen-Loeve transform [15], nonskin masking, Gaussian filter, pseudo-random filter, color space conversion, and contrast enhancement are a few of the preprocessing techniques.

In the case of brain cancer imaging, to modify the contrast, the brain cancer magnetic resonance imaging (MRI) pictures are first converted to greyscale and then subjected to a smoothing procedure [16]. Brain extraction tool (BET) skull stripping is another procedure used on brain MRI scans, along with the removal of brain tissues from different areas of the skull [17]. In clinical workflows, computed tomography (CT) scans acquired for lung cancer diagnosis undergo a standardized preprocessing pipeline. This involves converting raw DICOM images to grayscale, applying intensity normalization to ensure voxel value consistency across scans and implementing noise reduction algorithms (e.g., Gaussian filtering) to enhance anatomical clarity while preserving diagnostically relevant features. These photos are then transformed into binary images, where the undesirable content is subsequently eliminated [18]. In breast cancer imaging workflows, preprocessing mammograms involves three critical steps: (1) tumor segmentation to distinguish malignancies from adjacent healthy tissue, (2) breast parenchyma isolation (e.g., masking non-breast regions), and (3) suppression of pectoral muscle interference to improve diagnostic clarity. However, raw mammographic images often contain artifacts such as adhesive markers, low-intensity annotations, and high-intensity rectangular labels—residual noise from imaging protocols that complicates automated analysis. These artifacts necessitate robust preprocessing pipelines to enhance feature extraction accuracy while preserving clinically relevant anatomical details. As a result, preprocessing is used for mammography labeling, orientation, and segmentation [19]. Transrectal ultrasound (TRUS) pictures, which have poor resolution and intrinsic noise, are used to diagnose prostate cancer. The tree-structured wavelet transform, directional wavelet transform, and tree-structure nonlinear filtering (TSF) are all parts of the preprocessing module that is used to reduce noise and artifacts [20, 21].

Image enhancement techniques can be optimized through dynamic spatial and chromatic adjustments to refine visual output. One approach involves alternating horizontal and vertical rollover components to induce controlled spatial shifts, enabling adaptive pixel repositioning. For brightness modulation, a stochastic framework is applied by selecting random integers within a bounded variation coefficient range, ensuring luminance adjustments remain within thresholds that prevent artifacts like overexposure. Transitioning images to the HSV (Hue, Saturation, Value) color space allows targeted saturation optimization, where the saturation channel is scaled using coefficients sampled from an empirically defined interval to amplify or suppress color intensity while retaining hue fidelity. Similarly, in RGB-based processing, each color channel (red, green, blue) undergoes independent adjustment via distinct randomly selected coefficients, enabling precise spectral balancing without disrupting overall chromatic harmony. These methods emphasize probabilistic parameterization and domain-specific transformations, making them versatile for applications in computational photography, computer vision, and automated image analysis, where adaptive enhancements are critical for improving interpretability and visual quality. Each time, one or more of the four processing techniques is randomly chosen to increase the variety of the picture data [21].

7.2.2 Image segmentation

Image segmentation involves partitioning input data into distinct regions to isolate meaningful information for downstream analysis. In visual processing, this often entails separating ROIs from extraneous background elements. For instance, in medical imaging contexts—particularly when analyzing malignant lesions—segmentation focuses on delineating pathological tissue to extract diagnostically relevant features. Current methodologies are broadly categorized into four frameworks: threshold-based, pixel-based, region-based, and model-based segmentation. Threshold-based techniques leverage algorithms such as Otsu's method, which optimizes class separability, alongside adaptive local/global thresholding and entropy-maximization strategies to define intensity boundaries [22]. Pixel-based approaches employ clustering or statistical models, including fuzzy c-means clustering, Markov random field models, and ANNs to classify individual pixels into semantic groups. Region-based methods prioritize spatial coherence by aggregating pixels with shared attributes, while model-based strategies utilize deformable parametric constructs like level sets to iteratively refine boundaries based on geometric or topological constraints. Each paradigm addresses distinct challenges in feature extraction, balancing computational efficiency with anatomical precision to enhance applications in medical diagnostics and automated image interpretation. There are numerous additional techniques for segmenting images, including gradient flow vector, distributed and localized region identification, adaptive thresholding, histogram thresholding, statistical region growing, and clustering [23], fuzzy-C Mean clustering bootstrap learning, supervised learning, edge detection, active contours probabilistic modeling, sparse coding [24], contextual hypergraph [25], and to increase the system's accuracy, hybrid models of these techniques that combine two or more have been utilized [21].

Accurate identification of cellular and subcellular structures serves as the foundational stage in cytological diagnostics. In CC screening, precise segmentation of nuclear and cytoplasmic morphology is critical, as morphological aberrations in these regions often correlate with pathological anomalies that inform clinical diagnoses. Historically, segmentation algorithms were designed for isolated cells in transparent media, relying on sequential processing pipelines comprising three core stages: background suppression, cell localization, and boundary delineation. Early methodologies predominantly utilized noise-reduction techniques such as mean filtering, followed by basic histogram-based thresholding to isolate cellular regions. These approaches prioritized simplicity and computational efficiency, though they faced limitations in handling overlapping cells or heterogeneous tissue samples. Despite their constraints, such methods laid the groundwork for modern automated screening systems, emphasizing the necessity of robust segmentation to ensure diagnostic reliability in cytopathology. The information retrieved to create the histograms includes optical density information [26], gradient and compactness information [27], and grey level brightness or energy [28]. The most challenging intrinsic problem was determining the ideal threshold [29]. While prior studies demonstrated promising results in controlled experimental settings, their clinical utility for Pap smear diagnostics remained limited. The methods exhibited strong performance on curated datasets but failed to generalize effectively to real-world clinical samples, which often contain heterogeneous cellular morphologies and artifacts that complicate automated analysis. The majority of this section's attention will be on a few strategies that were the subject of further study [30].

7.2.3 Feature extraction

Feature selection and feature extraction represent distinct methodological approaches for deriving optimal feature subsets in ML workflows. While feature selection identifies and retains the most informative variables from the original dataset to enhance model performance and retain interpretability, feature extraction transforms or synthesizes new variables through techniques like principal component analysis to reduce dimensionality while preserving critical patterns in the data. A subset of the initial collection of features is chosen in feature selection as opposed to feature extraction, which retrieves characteristics that could have discriminatory value [31]. Feature selection serves as a critical preprocessing step in ML, aiming to identify a subset of input variables that optimize classification performance. By systematically eliminating features with negligible or redundant predictive value, this process enhances algorithmic efficiency, reduces model complexity, and preserves—or even improves—classification accuracy. In [32], a framework categorizing feature relevance into strong and weak classes is proposed. According to their taxonomy, a feature is deemed strongly relevant if its exclusion from the feature set irreversibly degrades model performance, underscoring its indispensable role in predictive robustness. Conversely, weakly relevant features may contribute marginally to accuracy but lack standalone diagnostic significance. This distinction guides researchers in prioritizing features that are statistically or biologically meaningful, ensuring models remain interpretable and generalizable across datasets. This framework also demonstrates that a characteristic can occasionally improve classification accuracy if it is of weak significance [32]. Feature selection and feature extraction play complementary yet distinct roles in optimizing ML workflows. Feature selection is critical to the predictive modeling pipeline, as classifiers often fail to generalize effectively when trained on suboptimal or redundant features. This underscores the necessity of identifying attributes with high discriminative power, which directly influence model accuracy and interpretability. Existing research highlights several methodological frameworks for feature selection, emphasizing criteria such as statistical significance, correlation with target variables, and domain-specific relevance. These guidelines ensure methodological rigor in distinguishing informative features from noise, thereby enhancing algorithmic robustness and reducing computational overhead. For example, Lippman has mentioned that features need to possess the information demanded to differentiate classes [31]. In character recognition systems, feature extraction represents a critical phase that follows pre-processing. The overarching goal of pattern recognition involves analyzing input samples and accurately assigning them to predefined output categories. This task is accomplished through two interdependent stages: feature selection and classification. Feature extraction serves as the foundational step in designing effective classification frameworks, as it isolates the most discriminative and relevant information that defines each class. These extracted features are compiled into feature vectors, which classifiers subsequently use to map input data to corresponding output labels. By reducing data dimensionality and emphasizing class-specific attributes, feature extraction simplifies the classifier's task of delineating boundaries between distinct classes. In essence, this process distills meaningful patterns from raw data by identifying variables that uniquely and precisely describe the structural or visual properties of characters or objects. Such precision ensures robustness in recognition tasks, particularly in scenarios involving variability in input quality or style. Feature vectors extracted in this process play as identities of the associated objects or characters [33]. The feature extraction's primary goal is to construct a similar feature set for several instances of the same symbol and extract a collection of features that maximizes the rate of recognition with the minimum number of components [34]. Contemporary methodologies in the field emphasize the application of diverse feature extraction approaches to enhance data representation and analytical accuracy in computational models. Contour profiles, geometric moment invariants, Graph description, zoning, Zernike moments, projection histograms, spline curve approximation, Gabor features, gradient features, and Fourier descriptors are a few of the frequently used techniques [35, 36].

7.3 IMPORTANCE OF FEATURE EXTRACTION IN IMAGE PROCESSING

Following the completion of preprocessing and the successful segmentation of data into relevant units—whether symbols, words, lines, or characters—various feature extraction techniques are employed to derive pertinent features from these segments. This critical step precedes the application of classification and postprocessing algorithms. The feature extraction stage is of particular importance as its design significantly influences the recognition system's overall performance. Indeed, within feature extraction, the task of feature selection stands out as the most vital component for achieving high levels of recognition accuracy. The goal of feature extraction is to transform raw data into a set of features that are optimally informative for classification. This involves identifying and isolating information that effectively distinguishes between different classes, while minimizing variations within the same class. Therefore, the careful selection of a feature extraction method, tailored to the specific nature of the input data, is paramount. With all of these things taken into account, it becomes crucial to evaluate the numerous feature extraction approaches that are several feature extraction methods available in a given domain that cover a large variety of conceivable circumstances [37]. In image classification systems, localized visual features within a digital image play a critical role in discriminating between distinct visual categories, enabling accurate categorization and analysis. These characteristics are categorized based on several essential picture data elements, including color intensity, the boundaries of the objects in the image, and texture [35]. The efficacy of feature extraction methodologies serves as a critical determinant in enhancing downstream image processing tasks. These extracted attributes are integral to applications such as image matching, pattern recognition, and content-based retrieval systems. To achieve robust accuracy, such systems rely on discriminative and relevant feature representations, as raw input images often inherently contain redundant or extraneous data that complicates computational analysis. Using this data to decrease a collection of features (or feature vectors) is a technique known as feature selection [38]. Image analysis involves the systematic extraction and quantitative evaluation of visual features from digital imagery to derive actionable insights for downstream applications. Unlike related techniques such as computational enhancement, data compression, or noise reduction, its primary focus lies in feature interpretation rather than visual optimization or structural preservation of the image itself. Techniques for detection, segmentation, extraction, and classification are used in image analysis [39]. Feature extraction methodologies are employed to derive pertinent characteristics from extensive visual datasets, with the goal of maximizing information retention. In contemporary research, the efficient and effective selection and extraction of features present a considerable challenge.

Medical imaging stands out as a highly valuable source of diagnostic information; however, its reliance on human interpretation and the increasing strain on resources pose ongoing difficulties. Particularly in low and developing countries, the demand for and availability of diagnostic pictures is outpacing the abilities of the professionals who are now available [13]. This issue could be solved by automated diagnosis using medical imaging using AI, particularly in the field of DL [14, 15]. While DL models demonstrating diagnostic capabilities on par with, or even exceeding, human performance have generated considerable excitement, it is crucial to temper this enthusiasm with rigorous evaluation. Within the field, concerns have been raised regarding potential biases in favor of novel technologies within certain proposed studies. Key questions persist, including the generalizability of research findings, the context of study execution (clinical versus controlled environments), and consequently, the real-world applicability of reported outcomes. The US Food and Drug Administration has now given its approval to more than AI algorithms [16]. As AI diagnostic tools approach clinical implementation, it becomes critical to systematically evaluate the existing evidence validating their use in medical imaging. This study conducts a rigorous comparative analysis of DL algorithms and healthcare professionals in diagnostic imaging interpretation, while critically examining reporting quality, clinical relevance, and methodological robustness within the global research landscape. By addressing gaps in transparency, practical utility, and experimental design, this work seeks to clarify the readiness of AI-driven systems for integration into real-world clinical workflows. They also carried out a meta-analysis to evaluate the diagnostic performance accuracy of DL algorithms in comparison to health care professionals [40].

DL is proving quite versatile, finding uses in many areas, but especially standing out for its potential to improve medical diagnostics. This encompasses but is not limited to biomedicine, magnetic resonance image analysis, and health informatics [40]. DL is being applied to a range of specialized tasks within medical imaging, including classification, diagnosis, prediction, segmentation, and the identification of specific anatomical areas of interest (ROI). A key advantage of DL over traditional ML lies in its architecture: with multiple hidden layers, DL can learn directly from raw data. This capability allows DL models to grasp complex concepts directly from the input data itself [41]. Indeed, DL models have demonstrated a remarkable ability to quickly and accurately identify and classify objects. Consequently, DL has driven significant advancements across core medical image processing tasks like segmentation, classification, diagnosis, and recording. The layered neural network approach inherent in DL enables the extraction of more abstract features from images. This inherent capacity is anticipated to offer solutions to long-standing challenges associated with traditional CAD systems in medicine. Automated systems have the potential to enable less experienced technicians, physicians, and other health care staff to prepare an equivalent assessment to those of specialists [5]. The purpose of these systems is to provide a diagnosis with acceptable accuracy, in the shortest possible time, with the least human intervention [24]. Furthermore, DL uses several intermediate layers located between the input and output layers that help to discover complex structures in a large set of data [42]. This capacity for learning hierarchical representations allows DL models to achieve exceptional precision and efficiency in object identification, classification, and segmentation tasks. In medical imaging, DL has demonstrated transformative potential by enhancing core processes such as lesion detection, anatomical segmentation, diagnostic decision-making, and automated reporting. Its multilayer neural network architecture facilitates the extraction of increasingly abstract image features, which may resolve longstanding limitations of traditional CAD systems, including reliance on handcrafted features and susceptibility to variability in image quality. Recently, Litjens et al. [43] achieved a very thorough analysis of the same topic by Shen et al. Both give a comprehensive image of the prevalence and applicability of DL techniques in the community [44]. The subsequent section offers a concise overview of contemporary research focused on several of these established tasks.

Specifically, challenges in medical image classification are structured to assist in the identification of irregularities within images obtained through medical diagnostic procedures. Numerous neural network architectures have been applied for this purpose over the past few years, including restricted Boltzmann machines applied to discriminative learning techniques and lung CT analysis, combining reproductive (van Tulder and de Bruijne), and stacked auto-encoders were used to identify moderate cognitive impairment and Alzheimer's disease by utilizing the latent nonlinear intricate linkages among different characteristics [45, 46]. Convolutional neural networks (CNNs) are rapidly being used for classification and detection tasks in recent years [47–51].

7.4 GYNECOLOGICAL CANCERS DETECTION APPROACHES

7.4.1 Cervical cancer

Histopathological assessment of cervical biopsy specimens is fundamental to establishing a diagnosis. For individuals presenting with symptoms suggestive of CC, a comprehensive diagnostic approach necessitates cervical cytology, a pelvic examination, and evaluation of the transparency of the vaginal mucosa and cervix. Visual examination of the cervix and vaginal mucosa, facilitated by speculum insertion, is crucial. It is important to note that in cases of microinvasive disease or when malignancy is confined to the endocervical canal, the cervix may exhibit a normal macroscopic appearance. CC is characterized by its potential for lymphatic dissemination, enabling metastasis to regional lymph nodes, including pelvic, inguinal, mediastinal, para-aortic, and supraclavicular lymph node groups. In advanced illness, enlarged, indurated inguinal, and supraclavicular lymph nodes may be visible [4]. When infection is clinically suspected, yet definitive lesions are not immediately visible upon initial examination, the diagnostic protocol should include colposcopy followed by biopsy for definitive assessment. If cancer is supposed clinically or by cervical cytology but is not proven through histopathologic analysis of cervical samples, a cone biopsy is required [52]. Sustained activation of the immune response, driven by persistent HPV infection, disrupts the regulated cellular division within the cervical epithelium, primarily affecting squamous cells. This dysregulation leads to the development of a precancerous condition known as cervical intraepithelial neoplasia (CIN), previously termed dysplasia. CIN lesions are stratified into CIN1, CIN2, and CIN3 based on the severity of the pathological changes and the extent of involvement within the squamous epithelial layer [53]. The World Health Organization (WHO) further refines the classification of precancerous cervical lesions: CIN1 is also designated as low-grade CIN, indicative of mild dysplasia where dysplastic characteristics are evident in approximately one-third of the epithelial thickness. Progression of a precancerous lesion to encompass two-thirds of the epithelium, resulting from uncontrolled cell proliferation, is classified as moderate dysplasia, or CIN2. CIN3 is diagnosed when dysplasia extends beyond two-thirds of the epithelial layer and is associated with a significant decrease in epithelial thickness. Collectively, CIN2 and CIN3 are categorized as high-grade CIN. According to the WHO research, there are four common ways to diagnose CC [54]: conventional cytology (Pap smear), liquid-based cytology, human papillomavirus deoxyribonucleic acid (HPV DNA) test, visual inspection with acetic acid (VIA) using a manual colposcope and digital colposcope [55]. This research has prioritized the evaluation of DL methodologies in the development of automated systems for CC detection. Among medical imaging modalities, MRI has emerged as the preferred imaging technique for training such algorithms due to its high-resolution soft tissue characterization [46]. A critical analysis of task-specific implementations reveals that image segmentation—a process enabling precise delineation of tumor boundaries and anatomical structures—dominates current methodological frameworks. To enhance the generalizability and clinical viability of these systems, researchers emphasize the integration of diverse datasets from multiple sources, including multimodal imaging and heterogeneous patient demographics. This approach not only mitigates overfitting during model training but also addresses variability in real-world clinical settings, thereby improving diagnostic reliability. Furthermore, the incorporation of cross-institutional data has been shown to bolster algorithmic robustness, a prerequisite for scalable deployment in global healthcare systems. For expert-level assessment, MRIs, fundus photography, computerized tomography scan images, and other procedures of data can be used [41]. Early CAD systems for medical imaging relied heavily on manual feature extraction, requiring domain experts to identify and annotate clinically relevant patterns in visual data. However, advancements in CNNs have transformed this paradigm, enabling automated learning of hierarchical feature representations directly from raw pixel data. By leveraging supervised training on annotated datasets, CNNs autonomously derive complex nonlinear relationships between input images and diagnostic outcomes, eliminating the need for handcrafted feature engineering. Empirical studies consistently demonstrate that DL models achieve diagnostic accuracy comparable to—and in some cases exceeding—human performance across tasks such as lesion detection and classification. A landmark example of this progress occurred in 2015, when a DL architecture surpassed human-level accuracy in the ImageNet Large-Scale Visual Recognition Challenge, a benchmark competition for image classification. This breakthrough underscored the potential of data-driven approaches to replicate and augment human perceptual capabilities in visual analysis. In clinical contexts, such advancements are particularly transformative, as they reduce subjectivity in image interpretation while scaling diagnostic workflows. Since then, DL-based models and algorithms in the field of computer vision have advanced in a variety of tasks, including object identification and segmentation, in addition to image classification [56].

7.4.2 Ovarian cancer

As per the reports, 85%–91% of malignancies of ovaries are epithelial carcinomas which are further classified as serous carcinomas (52%), clear cell carcinomas (6%), mucinous carcinomas (6%) and endometrioid carcinomas (10%). According to 2020's statistics (3,13,959) women are in the spotlight of incidence of ovarian cancer and (2,07,252) have lost their lives due to this cancer. Histopathological images play a vital role in prognosis of ovarian cancer and recently prognosis through computer-aided design has been used for cancers. To diagnose ovarian cancer, healthcare professionals utilize a combination of procedures including a pelvic exam to physically assess pelvic organs, imaging tests like ultrasound or CT scans to visualize the ovaries' size and structure, blood tests to evaluate overall health and organ function, and potentially surgery for definitive diagnosis and staging. Genetic testing may also be recommended to identify inherited gene mutations that increase ovarian cancer risk, which can inform treatment decisions.

7.4.3 Endometrial cancer

Endometrial cancer can be categorized as Type 1 and Type 2 cancer. Type 1 cancer has an easy prognosis and is a low grade cancer, in which abnormal cells do not grow abruptly and about 80% of the endometrial cancer are type 1 whereas the identification of type 2 cancer is not facile. About 20% of the endometrial cancers are of this type.

Endometrioid cancer is a kind of adenocarcinoma and is the most occurring cancer among all types of endometrial cancer, whereas, uterine carcinosarcoma happens in less than 5% of the women, but is extremely detrimental and rapidly spreading cancer. Endometrial cancer too has the survival rate, the localized endometrial cancer has no chance to spread the cancer out of the uterus, and according to the studies, it has a 5-year survival rate of 96%. Regional endometrial cancer can spread to the lymph nodes, and it has a 5-year survival rate of 76%. Distant endometrial cancer can spread to distant organs like the liver, lungs, or other, and it has a survival rate of around 20%. During the past decade, the role of classification algorithms in various medicinal specialities like cancers is on a stepping scale. Implementing models which have the use of AI is the key to introduction of brisk and accurate results. As the complexities of tumors are growing day by day, the prognosis of cancer has reached a complex stage and needs to be intervened by ML and DL algorithms.

7.5 PUBLICLY AVAILABLE DATASET

Dataset used for training the prediction models play a major role in giving accurate and precise results. So, it is very much important to have a good dataset. SIPaKMeD, CC (risk factors), Mendely, Herlev, histopathological image dataset for EC diagnosis, and histopathological whole slides image dataset are the few datasets available which are used to predict cervical, uterine, and ovarian cancer summarize the publicly available datasets used in the gynecological cancer's prediction.

7.5.1 SIPaKMeD

The SIPaKMeD database comprises 4,049 high-resolution cellular images obtained through a standardized imaging protocol using a charge-coupled device camera mounted on a light microscope. These images were derived from 966 multicellular clusters isolated from conventional Pap smear slides, with individual cells meticulously annotated and segmented by clinical experts to ensure diagnostic accuracy. This curated collection serves as a critical resource for advancing computational pathology research, particularly in developing ML models for automated cervical cytology analysis and early cancer detection. The dataset's methodological rigor—combining optical microscopy, expert validation, and digital preservation—supports reproducible studies in cellular morphology and diagnostic algorithm development. These cells are classified into five different classes, i.e., normal (superficial intermediate, parabasal), abnormal (koilocytotic, dyskeratotic) and benign (metaplastic) cells. In each image, both the region of the nucleus and the cytoplasm of each cell 26 concerning features are calculated. Cell features are divided into nuclei and cytoplasm features. These features are employed for the classification of the cells using SVM and standard multilayer perceptrons. The trained VGG-19 convolution neural network is employed as a feature extractor by feeding an input cell image and employing the preactivations of the intermediate layer to form a feature vector. Image features are obtained by employing the preactivations of the last convolutional layer (layer conv5). These features are added up by sum-pooling to form a feature vector of size 512 to represent each cell image. For each cell, there are three types of features: raw features 512 size, compressed features 256 size, and compressed features 32 size. Deep features are obtained by employing the preactivations of the first fully connected layer (layer fc6). These features are of size equal to the number of neurons in the corresponding layer, i.e. 4096. For each cell, there are three types of features: raw features 4096 size, compressed features 256 size, compressed features 32 size. In the preprocessing stage, two phases of data augmentation task are executed; first is to employ some geometric manipulation, e.g. affine transformations, addition of noises (Gaussian, Laplace), canny filter, edge detection, color filter, change of brightness, and contrast to enhance the training samples. Second is to employ the in-place data augmentation technique using the Keras "Image- Data Generator" API, where the images are reconstructed randomly during the training time. SIPakMeD dataset is employed to measure the performance of the CC detection proposed model by calculating accuracy, precision, recall, and F1 score. Some of the classification systems found in the SIPaKMeD database are validated in the hope of checking their efficiency in discrimination of the various cell types. Several experiments have been performed for the classification of these images, which include feature and image-based classification schemes. Various DL and ML classifiers like K-nearest neighbor, stochastic gradient descent, SVMs, random forest, AlexNet, ResNet, and K Means clustering are applied on this dataset to classify the cervical cells. Both supervised and unsupervised techniques, that is, SVMs and fuzzy logic, were applied. The dataset can be also used for evaluation of image segmentation methods for isolated cells (cropped images) or overlapping cells (cell clusters). The SIPaKMeD database provides new challenges, and it constitutes a solid basis for competitive evaluations for the cell image analysis community. Figure 7.1 gives SIPaKMeD dataset of cells.

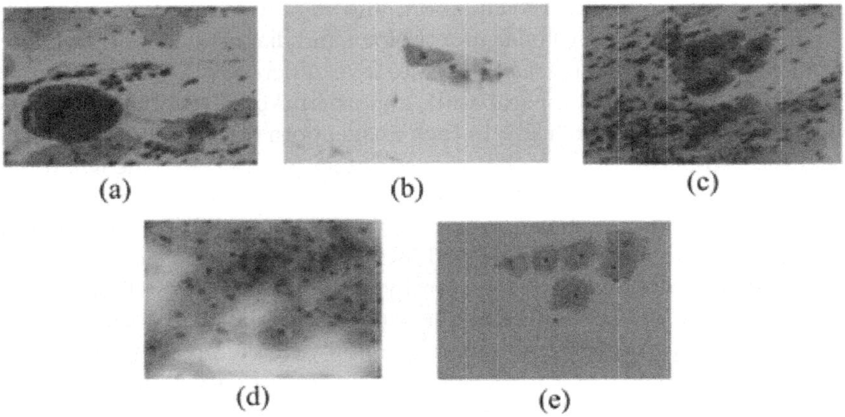

Figure 7.1 SIPaKMeD dataset (a) dyskeratotic, (b) koilocytotic, (c) metaplastic, (d) parabasal, and (e) superficial intermediate.

7.5.2 UCI risk factors

The data were collected at 'Hospital Universitario de Caracas' in Caracas, Venezuela. This is a dataset for CC cases. This dataset is classified with classifiers like Naive Bayes, Random Forest, Decision Tree, K-nearest neighbor and SVM to classify the risk factor of CC. The dataset includes demographic information, habits, and medical history of 858 patients. The dataset consists of 835 instances, 36 attributes, and also missing values. Many people restrained themselves from giving information because of privacy concerns. These data include 3,622 missing values out of 27,456 observations, which forms 13.2% of the data. These data consist of missing values and imbalanced data. Missing values in the data must be treated with techniques like sample mean data imputation technique for numerical data and mode imputation technique for categorical value attributes. We can see that 13% of total questions were not answered i.e., missed. STDs: time since first diagnosis and STDs: time since last diagnosis had enormous missing data so they have been excluded from the dataset and classifications made based on remaining 34 attributes. These two attributes have missing values rate around 92%, and the missing values rates above 15% may severely impact the interpretation. To address the imbalanced data techniques like oversampling, under sampling and both together are used. Data is said to be unbalanced when one class has a small number of examples whereas the other has a large number of examples, which gives rise to the class imbalance problem.

From the raw data, first the null values are removed and then the dataset is normalized. Feature selection methods are then applied to find the main risk factors of CC. The CC risk classification dataset is utilized as a preparation set to assess and look at the execution of various classifiers in terms of accuracy and other evaluation measures. Research has been done on evaluating performance of various ensemble-based classification models. Classifiers like linear regression, decision tree, Naive Bayes, SVM, random forest, K-nearest neighbor also have been evaluated to check their performance.

7.5.3 Mendeley data

Images of the dataset are gathered from the liquid-based cytology test of medical diagnostic centers of NER regions, India i.e. Babina Diagnostic Pvt. Ltd, Imphal, Gauhati Medical College and Hospital, Guwahati and Dr. B. Barooah Cancer Institute, Guwahati. This dataset can be utilized for the comparative study of the work carried out using other similar datasets like SIPaKMeD database for the CC prediction. This data has been utilized by several researchers for the feature selection, feature extraction, and image segmentation algorithms in the classification process (both multi as well as binary classification). For binary classification, negative for intraepithelial malignancy (NL) is taken as normal, and high squamous intraepithelial lesion (HSIL), low squamous intraepithelial lesion (LSIL), and squamous cell

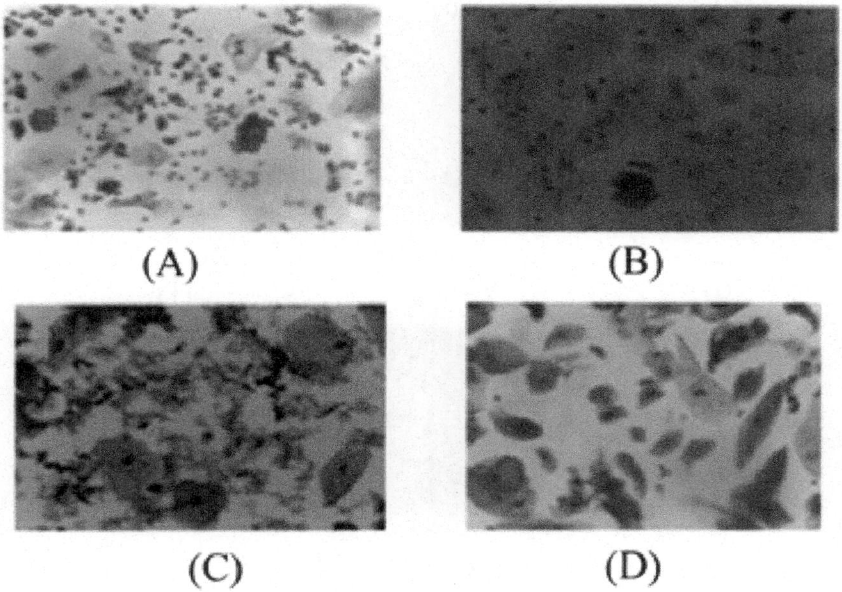

Figure 7.2 Mendeley dataset (a) High squamous intraepithelial lesion, (b) low squamous intraepithelial lesion, (c) Negative for intraepithelial malignancy, and (d) squamous cell carcinoma.

carcinoma (SCC) are taken as abnormal. Mendeley dataset comprises 993 pap smear images at 400× magnification from pap smear slides out of which 613 images are negative for intraepithelial malignancy i.e. normal category, and the remaining 350 images are HSIL, LSIL and SCC i.e., abnormal category as illustrated in Figure 7.2. The 400× magnification gives a clearer view of a smear level image per slide than 100× and 200× with clear cellular features as per the concerned categories.

7.5.4 Herlev dataset

The publicly available Herlev Pap smear dataset is used for the training and testing purpose. It includes 917 photos of single cervical cells that have been classified and segmented using ground truth. There are seven different

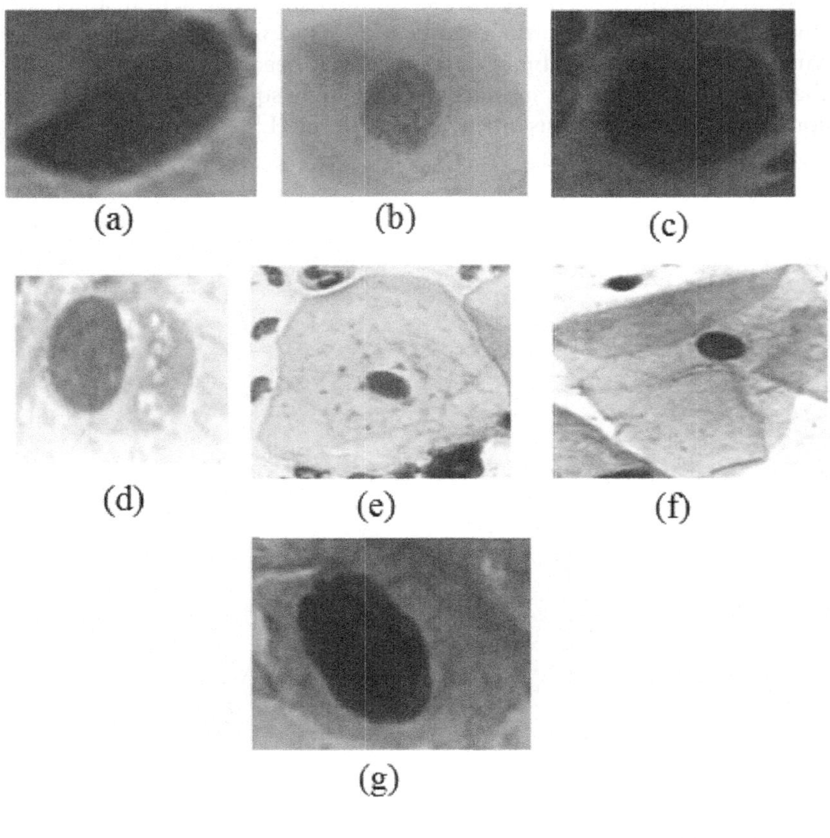

Figure 7.3 Herlev dataset (a) carcinoma in situ (b) light dysplastic (c) moderate dysplastic (d) normal columnar (e) normal intermediate (f) normal superficial, and (g) severe dysplastic.

classes into which the cells are divided. To improve the accuracy of the diagnosis, cytologists and clinicians diagnose these seven classes. Additionally, these seven types can be divided roughly into two groups: malignant and benign. First through third grade are considered normal or benign, whereas fourth through seventh grade are considered aberrant or cancerous. It is evident that the nucleus of abnormal or cancerous cells is larger than that of normal cells. The challenging challenge from the perspective of classification is that the chromatin distribution and nucleus size of normal columnar cells are identical. Figure 7.3 gives Herlev dataset images.

7.5.5 Histopathological image dataset for EC diagnosis

Histopathological image dataset of endometrium is developed to decrease the ML and DL methods nonsuccess in diagnosing endometrial cancer

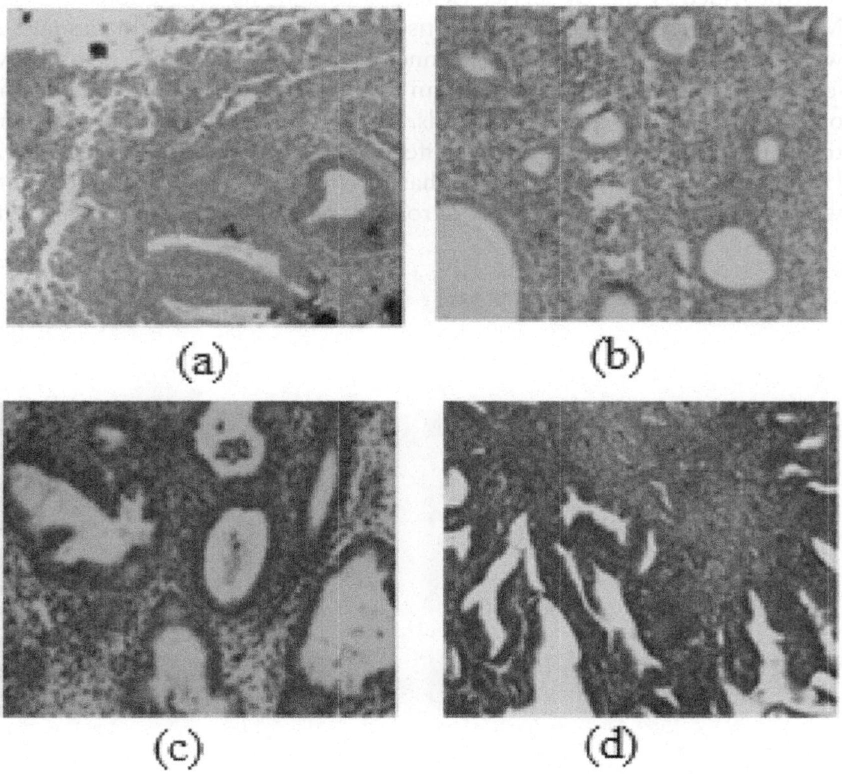

Figure 7.4 Histopathological image dataset for EC diagnosis. (a) Endometrial hyperplasia complex, (b) endometrial hyperplasia simple, and (c) endometrial adenocarcinoma.

efficiently. The aforementioned dataset contains 3,302 pathologically confirmed joint photographic experts' group (JPEG) images from around 500 endometrial specimens which are stained with hematoxylin and eosin (H&E). Normal endometrium (NE), endometrial polyp (EP), endometrial hyperplasia (EH), and endometrioid adenocarcinoma (EA) are the four mainstream endometrial tissues this dataset contains. NE consists of three data subtypes which are defined by the menstrual cycle phases, that is the luteal phase, menstrual phase, and follicular phase. Figure 7.4 shows Histopathological image dataset for EC diagnosis.

7.5.6 Histopathological whole slide images dataset for ovarian cancer

The data set consists of 288 whole slides stained with hematoxylin and eosin (HE) that are deidentified and contain clinical data for 78 patients. The slides were provided by the Tri-Service General Hospital and the National Defense Medical Center in Taipei, Taiwan's tissue bank. Whole slide images (WSIs) were taken with a digital slide scanner (Leica AT2) with a 20× objective lens. The average size of the ovarian cancer slides is 27.34 × 20.66 mm, or 54342 × 41048 pixels in pixels. In the data sets, the bevacizumab treatment is effective in 126 and ineffective in 162. The Tri-Service General Hospital research ethics committee has provided its clearance, and the data were deidentified and used for a retrospective analysis without having any

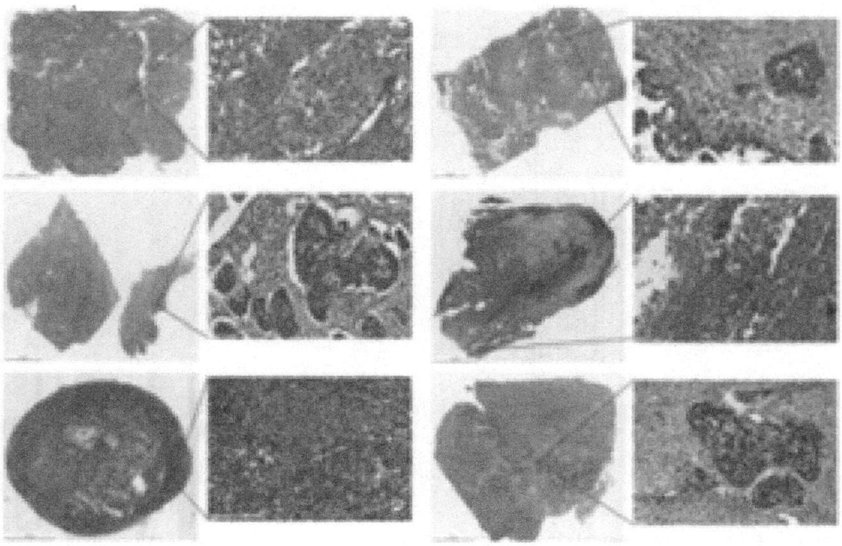

Figure 7.5 Histopathological whole slide images dataset for ovarian cancer.

Table 7.1 Summary of publicly available dataset for research in gynaecology oncology

S. No	*Cancer type*	*Dataset*	*General class*	*Sub type*	*Number of instances*
1	Cervical	SIPaKMeD (Pap smear images)	NA	Superficial Intermediate cells	126 images,831 cells
				Parabasal cells	108 images,787 cells
				Koilocytotic cells	238 images,825 cells
				Metaplastic cells	271 images,793 cells
				Dyskeratotic cells	223 images,813 cells
2	Cervical	UCI risk factors (integers, real)	NA	NA	835 instances, 36 attributes
3	Cervical	Mendeley (Pap smear images)	NA	High squamous intraepithelial lesion	350
				Low squamous intraepithelial lesion	
				Squamous cell carcinoma	
				Negative for intra epithelial malignancy	613
4	Cervical	Herlev (cervical cell images)	Normal	Superficial squamous epithelial	74
				Intermediate squamous epithelial	70
				Columnar epithelial	98
			Abnormal	Mild squamous nonkeratinizing dysplasia	182
				Moderate squamous nonkeratinizing dysplasia	146
				Serve squamous nonkeratinizing dysplasia	197
				Squamous cell carcinoma in situ intermediate	150
5	Endometrial	Histopathological image dataset for ET (histopathological images)	Benign	Luteal phase, menstrual phase	600, 21
				NA	636
				Simple	516
				Complex	282
			Malignant	NA	535
6	Ovarian	Histopathological image dataset for ovarian cancer Histopathological images	Hematoxylin and eosin (H&E)	NA	288

influence on patient treatment. The data managers of the Gynaecologic Oncology Center documented the clinicopathologic features of the patients. Age, serum CA-125 before and after treatment, histologic subtype, recurrence, and survival status were all documented. Figure 7.5 shows histopathological WSIs dataset for ovarian cancer.

7.6 CONCLUSION

For the purpose of this systematic review, we have searched Science direct, IEEE, springer, PubMed databases, Google Scholar, and forward and backward citations from 2005 to 2022. We have searched all the articles on gynecological cancer prediction using DL and ML techniques which were not date or country limited. We studied papers by various authors to obtain statistics of the modern treatment in gynecology oncology. We did individual meta-analyses for cervical, uterine, and ovarian gynecological cancers. Sixty studies were identified in which SIPaKMeD, Herlev, Mendeley, UCI risk factors, histopathological image dataset for EC diagnosis, and histopathological WSIs dataset for ovarian cancer has been used in 12, 15, 4, 7, 1, 2 papers, respectively. Other 24 papers from the conducted review have worked on some private datasets. It has been observed that DL and ML techniques work efficiently in predicting gynecological cancers. Figure 7.1 gives an overview of the flow of the work done in classifying, predicting the cancers. Firstly, the required model needs to be trained with an efficient dataset. In order to bring down the time and other complexities of the program, the datasets are brought down into machine readable forms using the segmentation techniques in the preprocessing stage. Datasets are divided into training and testing sets to train the model efficiently. Data augmentation techniques are used to increase the dataset size because larger datasets yield good results. In order to extract important features from the raw images of the dataset, segmentation of images is done. After the dataset is converted into a presentable form, various classification models are implemented for predicting or detecting cancer lesions from the dataset. The proposed models are evaluated using statistical analysis, i.e., calculating accuracy, precision, recall, sensitivity, specificity, and area under the curve. Table 7.1 gives a summary of publicly available datasets.

REFERENCES

[1] K. Adem, S. Kiliçarslan, and O. Cömert. "Classification and diagnosis of cervical cancer with softmax classification with stacked autoencoder." *Expert Syst. Appl.*, vol. 115, pp. 557–564, 2019. https://doi.org/10.1016/j.eswa.2018.08.050

[2] M. Ahmed, M. M. Jahangir Kabir, M. Kabir, and M. M. Hasan. Identification of the risk factors of cervical cancer applying feature selection approaches. In 3rd International Conference on Electrical, *Computer and Telecommunication Engineering, ICECTE* 2019, pp. 201–204, 2019. https://doi.org/10.1109/ICECTE48615.2019.9303554

[3] S. Kim et al. "Cancer survival classification using integrated data sets and intermediate information." *Artif. Intell. Med.*, vol. 62, no. 1, pp. 23–31, 2014.

[4] H.M. Zolbanin et al. "Predicting overall survivability in comorbidity of cancers: A data mining approach." *Decis. Supp. Syst.*, vol. 74, pp. 150–161, 2015.

[5] K. Matsuo. "A pilot study in using deep learning to predict limited life expectancy in women with recurrent cervical cancer." *Am. J. Obstet. Gynaecol.,* vol. 217, no. 6, pp. 703–705, 2017.

[6] A. B. Shinagare. "High-grade serous ovarian cancer: use of machine learning to predict abdominopelvic recurrence on CT on the basis of serial cancer antigen 125 levels." *J. Am. Coll. Radiol.*, vol. 15, no. 8, pp. 1133-1138, **2018**.

[7] K. Matsuo. "Survival outcome prediction in cervical cancer: cox models vs deep-learning model." *Am. J. Obstet. Gynaecol.,* vol. 220, no. 4, pp. 381.e1–381.e14, 2019.

[8] J. Ruan. A novel algorithm for network-based prediction of cancer recurrence *Genomics*, vol. 111, no. 1, pp. 17–23, 2019.

[9] Q. Wang. "Prognostic potential of alternative splicing markers in endometrial cancer." *Mol. Ther. Nucleic Acids*, vol. 18, pp. 1039–1048, 2019.

[10] Y. Fu, Y. Lei, T. Wang, W. J. Curran, T. Liu, and X. Yang, "Deep learning in medical image registration: A review," *Phys. Med. Biol.*, vol. 65, no. 20, Oct. 2020, Art. no. 20TR01.

[11] K. Doi, "Computer-aided diagnosis in medical imaging: Historical review, current status and future potential," *Comput. Med. Imag. Graph.*, vol. 31, pp. 198–211, Jun. 2007. doi:10.1016/j.compmedimag.2007.02.002

[12] G. M. T. Brake, N. Karssemeijer, and J. H. C. L. Hendriks. "An automatic method to discriminate malignant masses from normal tissue in digital mammograms." *Phys. Med. Biol.*, vol. 45, no. 10, pp. 2843–2857, Sep. 2000, doi:10.1088/0031-9155/45/10/308

[13] Y. Bengio, A. Courville, and P. Vincent. "Representation learning: A review and new perspectives." *IEEE Trans. Pattern Anal. Mach. Intell.*, vol. 35, no. 8, pp. 1798–1828, Aug. 2013. doi:10.1109/TPAMI. 2013.50

[14] Y. LeCun, Y. Bengio, and G. Hinton. "Deep learning." *Nature*, vol. 521, no. 7553, pp. 436–444, Sep. 2015. doi:10.1038/nature14539

[15] M. Messadi, A. Bessaid, and A. Taleb-Ahmed. "Extraction of specific parameters for skin tumour classification." *J. Med. Eng. Technol.*, vol. 33, no. 4, pp. 288–295, Jul. 2009, doi:10.1080/03091900802451315

[16] B. V. Reddy, P. B. Reddy, P. S. Kumar, and S. Reddy. "Developing an approach to brain MRI image preprocessing for tumor detection." *Int. J. Res.*, vol. 1, pp. 725–731, Jul. 2014.

[17] E. I. Zacharaki, S. Wang, S. Chawla, D. S. Yoo, R. Wolf, E. R. Melhem, and C. Davatzikos. "Classification of brain tumor type and grade using MRI texture and shape in a machine learning scheme." *Magn. Reson. Med.*, vol. 62, no. 6, pp. 1609–1618, Dec. 2009.

[18] M. B. A. Miah and M. A. Yousuf. "Detection of lung cancer from CT image using image processing and neural network." In Proc. 2nd Int. *Conf. Electr. Eng. Inf. Commun. Technol.*, May 2015, pp. 1–6, doi:10.1109/ICEEICT.2015.7307530

[19] D. N. Ponraj, M. E. Jenifer, P. Poongodi, and J. S. Manoharan. "A survey on the preprocessing techniques of mammogram for the detection of breast cancer." *J. Emerg. Trends Comput. Inf. Sci.*, vol. 2, no. 12, pp. 656–664, 2011.

[20] Y. Zhang, R. Sankar, and W. Qian. "Boundary delineation in transrectal ultrasound image for prostate cancer." *Comput. Biol. Med.*, vol. 37, no. 11, pp. 1591–1599, Nov. 2007. doi:10.1016/j.compbiomed.2007.02.008

[21] K. Munir, H. Elahi, A. Ayub, F. Frezza, and A. Rizzi. "Cancer diagnosis using deep learning: A bibliographic review." *Cancers*, vol. 11, no. 9, pp. 1–36, 2019. doi:10.3390/cancers11091235

[22] X. Tan, K. Li, J. Zhang, W. Wang, B. Wu, J. Wu, X. Li, and X. Huang. "Automatic model for cervical cancer screening based on convolutional neural network: A retrospective, multicohort, multicenter study." *Cancer Cell Int.*, vol. 21, no. 1, pp. 1–10, Dec. 2021. doi:10.1186/s12935-020- 01742-6

[23] M. E. Celebi, H. A. Kingravi, H. Iyatomi, Y. A. Aslandogan, W. V. Stoecker, R. H. Moss, J. M. Malters, J. M. Grichnik, A. A. Marghoob, H. S. Rabinovitz, and S. W. Menzies. "Border detection in dermoscopy images using statistical region merging." *Skin Res. Technol.*, vol. 14, no. 3, pp. 347–353, Aug. 2008.

[24] B. Bozorgtabar. "Sparse coding based skin lesion segmentation using dynamic rule-based refinement." In *Proceedings of 13th international workshop on machine learning in medical imaging*, 2016, pp. 254–261.

[25] X. Li, Y. Li, C. Shen, A. Dick, and A. V. D. Hengel. "Contextual hypergraph modeling for salient object detection." In *Proceedings of IEEE International Conference on Computer Vision*, Dec. 2013, pp. 3328–3335.

[26] A. Kale and S. Aksoy. "Segmentation of cervical cell images." In Proceedings of 20th International Conference on Pattern Recognition, Aug. 2010, pp. 2399–2402, doi:10.1109/ICPR.2010.587

[27] H. Borst, W. Abmayr, and P. Gais. "A thresholding method for automatic cell image segmentation." *J. Histochem. Cytochem.*, vol. 27, no. 1, pp. 180–187, Jan. 1979, doi:10.1177/27.1.374573

[28] C.-W. Chang, M.-Y. Lin, H.-J. Harn, Y.-C. Harn, C.-H. Chen, K.-H. Tsai, and C.-H. Hwang. "Automatic segmentation of abnormal cell nuclei from microscopic image analysis for cervical cancer screening." In *Proceedings of IEEE 3rd International Conference on Nano/Molecular Medicine and Engineering*, Oct. 2009, pp. 77–80, doi:10.1109/NANOMED.2009.5559114

[29] K.-B. Kim, D. H. Song, and Y. W. Woo. "Nucleus segmentation and recognition of uterine cervical pap-smears." In Proceedings of 11th International *Conference on Rough Sets, Fuzzy Sets, Data Mining Granular Computing*, 2009, pp. 153–160. doi:10.1007/978-3-540-72530-5_18

[30] T. Conceicao, C. Braga, and L. Rosado. "A review of computational methods for cervical cells segmentation and abnormality classification." *Int. J. Mol. Sci.*, vol. 20, no. 20, p. 5114, 2019, doi:10.3390/ijms20205114

[31] G. Kumar and P. K. Bhatia. "A detailed review of feature extraction in image processing systems." In Proceedings of 4th International *Conference on Advanced Computer and Communication Technologies,* Feb. 2014, pp. 5–12, doi:10.1109/ACCT.2014.74

[32] M. Mohamad, H. Hassan, D. Nasien, and H. Haron. "A review on feature extraction and feature selection for handwritten character recognition." *Int. J. Adv. Comput. Sci. Appl.*, vol. 6, no. 2, pp. 204–212, 2015. doi:10.14569/ijacsa.2015.060230

[33] X. Li, C. Li, M. M. Rahaman, H. Sun, X. Li, J. Wu, Y. Yao, and M. Grzegorzek. "A comprehensive review of computer-aided whole slide image analysis: From datasets to feature extraction, segmentation, classification and detection approaches." *Artif. Intell. Rev.*, vol. 55, pp. 4809–4878, Jan. 2022.

[34] B. Ghojogh, M. N. Samad, S. A. Mashhadi, T. Kapoor, W. Ali, F. Karray, and M. Crowley. "Feature selection and feature extraction in pattern analysis: A literature review." 2019, arXiv:1905.02845

[35] D. P. Tian. "A review on image feature extraction and representation techniques." *Int. J. Multimed. Ubiquitous Eng.*, vol. 8, no. 4, pp. 385–395, Jul. 2013.

[36] M. A. Joshi and M. H. Chavan. "Techniques of feature extraction based on," *Image*, vol. 1, p. 3, Jan. 2017.

[37] T. C. Asogwa, E. Fidelis, C. Obodoeze, and I. N. Obiokafor. "A review of feature extraction techniques for image analysis." *Int. J. Adv. Res. Comput. Commun. Eng.*, vol. 3297, pp. 153–155, Feb. 2017. doi:10.17148/IJARCCE

[38] S. Gharsellaoui, M. Mansouri, S. S. Refaat, H. Abu-Rub, and H. Messaoud. "Multivariate features extraction and effective decision making using machine learning approaches." *Energies*, vol. 13, no. 3, p. 609, Jan. 2020.

[39] R. Revathi and M. Hemalatha. "An emerging trend of feature extraction method in video processing." *Cs-Cscp,* pp. 69–80, May 2012.

[40] X. Liu, L. Faes, A. U. Kale, S. K. Wagner, D. J. Fu, A. Bruynseels, T. Mahendiran, G. Moraes, M. Shamdas, C. Kern, and J. R. Ledsam. "Articles a comparison of deep learning performance against health care professionals in detecting diseases from medical imaging: A systematic review and meta-analysis." *Lancet Digit. Heal.*, vol. 1, no. 6, pp. 271–297, 2019. doi:10.1016/S2589-7500(19)30123-2

[41] M. Bakator and D. Radosav. "Deep learning and medical diagnosis: A review of literature." *Multimodal Technol. Interact.*, vol. 2, no. 3, p. 47, Aug. 2018. doi:10.3390/mti2030047

[42] G. Van Tulder and M. De Bruijne. "Combining generative and discriminative representation learning for lung CT analysis with convolutional restricted Boltzmann machines." *IEEE Trans. Med. Imag.*, vol. 35, no. 5, pp. 1262–1272, May 2016.

[43] G. Litjens, T. Kooi, B. E. Bejnordi, A. A. A. Setio, F. Ciompi, M. Ghafoorian, J. A. Van Der Laak, B. Van Ginneken, and C. I. Sanchez. "A survey on deep learning in medical image analysis." *Med. Image Anal.*, vol. 42, pp. 60–88, Dec. 2017.

[44] H. P. Chan, R. K. Samala, L. M. Hadjiiski, and C. Zhou. "Deep learning in medical image analysis." *Adv. Exp. Med. Biol.*, vol. 1213, pp. 3–21, Jun. 2017. doi:10.1007/978-3-030-33128-3_1

[45] H.-I. Suk, S.-W. Lee, and D. Shen. "Latent feature representation with stacked auto-encoder for AD/MCI diagnosis." *Brain Struct. Funct.*, vol. 220, no. 2, pp. 841–859, 2015.
[46] T. Brosch, R. Tam, for the Alzheimer's Disease Neuroimaging Initiative. (2013). Manifold learning of brain MRIs by deep learning. In: Mori, K., Sakuma, I., Sato, Y., Barillot, C., Navab, N. (eds), *Medical Image Computing and Computer-Assisted Intervention – MICCAI 2013*. MICCAI 2013. Lecture Notes in Computer Science, vol. 8150. Springer, Berlin, Heidelberg. https://doi.org/10.1007/978-3-642-40763-5_78..
[47] M. Talo, O. Yildirim, U. B. Baloglu, G. Aydin, and U. R. Acharya. "Convolutional neural networks for multi-class brain disease detection using MRI images." *Comput. Med. Imag. Graph.*, vol. 78, Dec. 2019, Art. no. 101673. doi:10.1016/j.compmedimag.2019.101673
[48] M. Talo, U. B. Baloglu, Ö. Yildirim, and U. R. Acharya. "Application of deep transfer learning for automated brain abnormality classification using MR images." *Cogn. Syst. Res.*, vol. 54, pp. 176–188, May 2019. doi:10.1016/j.cogsys.2018.12.007
[49] O. Yildirim, T. R. San, and U. R. Acharya. "An efficient compression of ECG signals using deep convolutional autoencoders." *Cognit. Syst. Res.*, vol. 52, pp. 198–211, Dec. 2018.
[50] O. Yildirim, M. Talo, B. Ay, U. B. Baloglu, G. Aydin, and U. R. Acharya. "Automated detection of diabetic subject using pretrained 2D-CNN models with frequency spectrum images extracted from heart rate signals." *Comput. Biol. Med.*, vol. 113, Oct. 2019, Art. no. 103387.
[51] U. Raghavendra, H. Fujita, S. V. Bhandary, A. Gudigar, J. H. Tan, and U. R. Acharya. "Deep convolution neural network for accurate diagnosis of glaucoma using digital fundus images." *Inf. Sci.*, vol. 441, pp. 41–49, May 2018.
[52] WHO. (2020). Cervical cancer. Accessed 14 June 2020. [Online]. Available at www.who.int/health-topics/cervical-cancer
[53] S. D. Balasubramaniam, V. Balakrishnan, C. E. Oon, and G. Kaur. "Key molecular events in cervical cancer development." *Medicina*, vol. 55, no. 7, p. 384, Jul. 2019.
[54] WHO. (2019). Guidelines for screening and treatment of precancerous lesions for cervical cancer prevention. [Online]. Available: www.who.int
[55] T. A. Berman and J. T. Schiller. "Human papillomavirus in cervical cancer and oropharyngeal cancer: One cause, two diseases." *Cancer*, vol. 123, no. 12, pp. 2219–2229, 2017. doi:10.1002/cncr.30588
[56] M. V. Enriquez, "A deep learning approach for pneumonia detection in chest X-ray," Univ. Vigo, Pontevedra, Spain, Tech. Rep., 2019.

Chapter 8

Wearable healthcare devices

8.1 INTRODUCTION

Different wearables and applications for smartphones are developed recently which provide many healthcare facilities. Research in this area is ongoing [1]. Healthcare facilities provided by wearable devices are not restricted by the location of individuals' as it provides remote support. For senior citizens who have limited mobility and for patients who lack access to medical care, wearables are becoming a better choice. Healthcare institutions and insurance companies are preferring wearable technology, as monitoring and virtual care of the patient are the key features of wearables, which helps in cost savings. The demand for wearable devices has risen in the last few years because of the unleashing capability like patients' health data collection. Wearables provide ecological momentary evaluations by capturing long-term data in research participants' naturalistic surroundings [2].

Based on the research conducted by Radin et al. [3], COVID-19 outbreak probability was calculated with the data obtained from wearables, which included physical activity, sleep, and weather data. Forecasting of the number of COVID-19 infections for the next 4 days was done based on the obtained data. Wearable medical devices facilitate health improvement, fitness goal tracking, and early detection of health concerns. Figure 8.1 shows the features of wearable devices. They are beneficial for diverse age groups and health conditions and with ongoing advancements and research in this field. Many more possibilities are upcoming.

With advancements in technology, wearables are becoming smaller in size with less power requirements. The data-driven by wearable technology by any device has reached 2.3 trillion (GB) per day in 2020 and 847 zettabytes (ZB) in 2021 up from 218 ZB in 2016 per year [4]. The market for wearable medical technology has expanded globally, at an annual growth rate of 30%, from 2.5 billion dollars in 2015 to 12 billion dollars in 2020. The global wearable healthcare devices market was valued at USD 14.3 billion in 2022, and it is anticipated to grow up to USD 45.8 billion by 2032, at

DOI: 10.1201/9781003503033-8

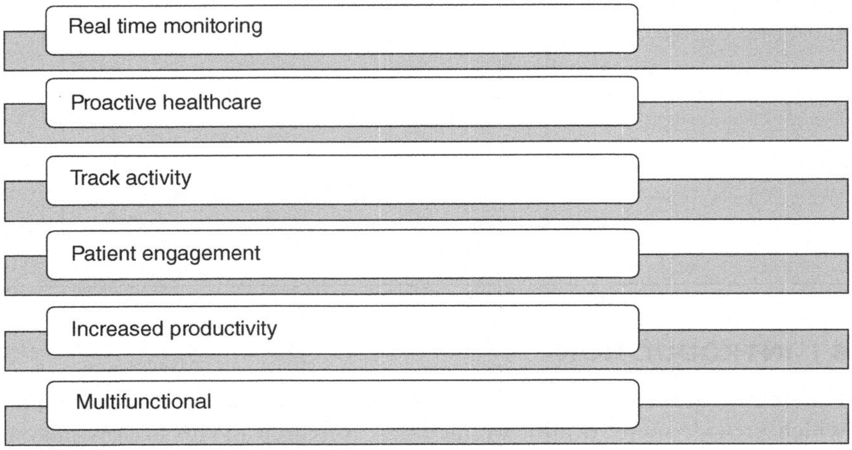

Figure 8.1 Features of wearable devices.

a CAGR of 12.4% during the forecast period, according to global insight services.

8.2 THE MEDICAL FIELD AND WEARABLE TECHNOLOGY

The applications of wearable technology have skyrocketed with the rise in the use of mobile phone technology, Internet of things, and smart sensing [5–7]. In the healthcare industry, for instance, IBM provides a broad range of mobile services via its Mobile Wireless Health Solutions, while GE Healthcare created Vscan (a general purpose diagnostic ultrasound imaging equipment) to deliver quicker and more precise healthcare services that are location- and time-independent [8, 9]. Wearable fitness trackers, smart health watches, blood pressure monitors, ECG monitors, and biosensors are just a few examples of the many types of wearable technology used in healthcare. Numerous healthcare services have been made possible by the development of smartphone applications, and this trend is anticipated to continue in the future. Fitbit's Versa 2, Xiaomi's Mi Band 4, Samsung Electronics' Galaxy Watch Active 2, and Apple's Watch 5 are all excellent examples [10, 11].

The five primary characteristics of wearable technology as a standard health care intervention are (1) wireless mobility; (2) interactivity and intelligence; (3) sustainability and durability; (4) easy operation and downsizing; and (5) wearability and portability [12]. The 4P medical paradigm, which is defined by preventative, predictive, personalized, and participatory medicine, is the framework that modern medicine uses to use wearable technology in the medical area [13]. Wearable technologies have the potential to significantly advance precision medicine by facilitating the assessment of clinically relevant indicators that indicate an individual's health condition [14]. However, in [15], it is also suggested that wearable medical devices are a significant enabler and catalyst for the development of linked health care.

The use of several wearable technologies, including sensor technology, medical chip technology, wireless communication technology, power management technology, display technology, and information feedback technology, is necessary for the operation and deployment of these devices. The internet receives real-time medical data from these devices for additional analysis or input from a healthcare professional.

There is a lot of room for development when it comes to wearables in the healthcare sector. Figure 8.2 lists some desirable features of wearable

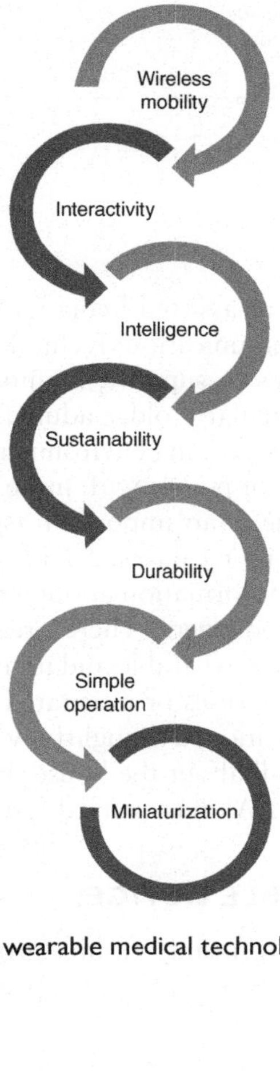

Figure 8.2 Desirable features of wearable medical technology.

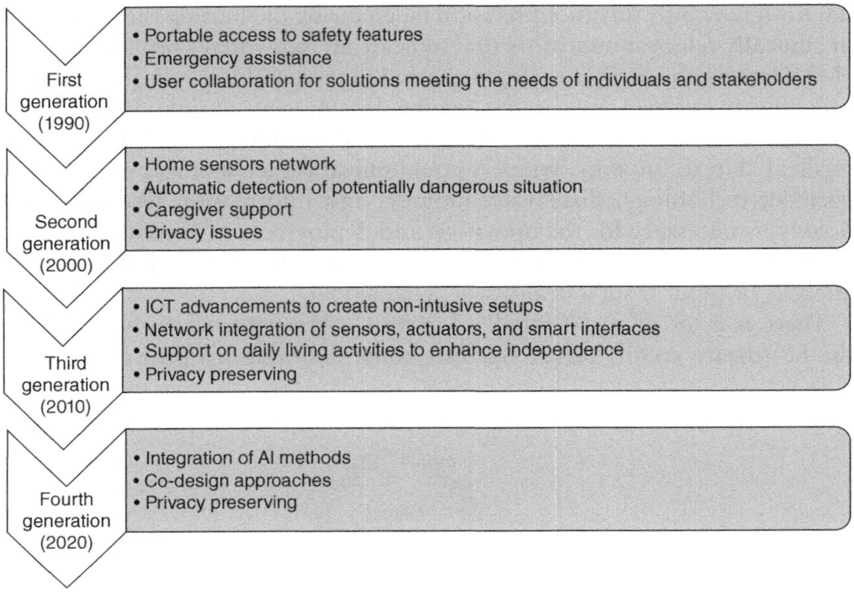

Figure 8.3 AAL timeline.

medical technology. Ambient-assisted living (AAL) refers to a concept that uses Information and Communication Technologies, assistive devices, and sensor network technologies to support, monitor, and enhance the quality of life for individuals, particularly older adults, or people with disabilities, within their daily living and working environment. It provides technological solutions into surroundings of people with more self-sufficiency, liberty, and security. Subject monitoring is an important aspect of AAL, which makes use of various sensors in order to access data, giving caretakers and medical experts important new information about a patient's everyday activities, health issues, and possible dangers. There are two primary categories of sensors from which to choose: wearable and nonwearable. The first one may be worn by the user as accessories or integrated into garments. Conversely, nonwearable sensors are positioned thoughtfully on doors, walls, appliances, furniture, and other items all about the house. Figure 8.3 shows AAL timeline, which represents how AAL has evolved form 1990's to the present day.

8.3 TYPES OF WEARABLE DEVICES

Wearable devices have promising future growth. The demand for it has increased significantly in recent years specially for features like data generation for cutting-edge health research. Wearables as medical devices are used in various forms [16]. Initially, wearable health gadgets may be wristwatches or other accessories. Well-being and fitness are the most commonly used functions of wristwatches. Syncing with apps on smartphones, storage and management of information like the user's psychological status, sleep patterns, tracking calories burned and consumed; and recording distance travelled are some key functions of such wearables. Second, wearable health devices can be in the form of clothing. Electrical signals and data are exchanged using chips that measures variations in blood flow, biological rhythm, respiration, and the health of its users and data collecting, or connects with a smartphone using certain materials to perform a variety of tasks. Third, it is possible to affix wearable medical technology to the body. Patients with glaucoma wear a contact lens-like medical device made by the Swiss company Sensimed, which measures their intraocular pressure continuously. The most crucial component in the diagnosis of glaucoma is changes in intraocular pressure, which can be continuously monitored to slow down the disease's progression. These contact lenses assess the wearer's intraocular pressure using sensors and antennae inside the lens. The data are then transmitted and recorded in real time to a smart device and stored on the physician's computer via Bluetooth. Biologic wearables are the fourth category. The most cutting-edge wearables can be ingested by users or implanted within them. These kinds of technologies currently include ingestible sensors on prescription drugs that detect whether the drug is being taken in real time by the patient, as well as technology that enables a wireless sensor to be inserted beneath the skin to detect changes in blood sugar levels in real time for individuals who require continuous monitoring, such as diabetics. The aging population's increasing need for healthcare services is driving the acceptance and application of digital health in the treatment and care of the aged.

8.4 BENEFITS OF WEARABLE TECHNOLOGY

Wearables can empower patients in several ways [16]. Firstly, health care of patients is possible without disturbing their daily routine. Table 8.1 discusses various locations on human body on which wearable devices can be used. Wearables greatly reduce the patients' requirement to allocate time spent in scheduling appointments with medical specialists, changing their daily routine because of these appointments, or spend money and time on travel linked to appointments. The use of wearables has shown reduction in the need for certain in-person appointments. Secondly, data collected by wearables if taken frequently provides a richer dataset as compared to the examining documents acquired when visiting a medical facility. Data may be gathered at the comfort level of the participants while doing normal daily activities. Multiple readings can be taken by patients' themselves like

Table 8.1 Application of wearables devices on the human body

Wearable device type	*Position*	*Application*
Helmet	Head	GPS monitoring and microphone
Camera	Headband	Sporting video
Glasses	Eyes	Information display
Throat tattoo	Neck	Inbuilt microphone for communication
Earphones	Ears	Fitness tracking, communication
Lenses	Eyes	Monitor glucose level
Sports clothing	Body	Heart rate, step count, GPS tracking
Watch	Wrist	voice activation, and activity monitoring are measured.
Jewellery	Neck, finger, ears	Monitoring
Gloves	Hands	Capturing and safeguarding
Shoes	Feet	Foot ailments, blood pressure, steps counting

checking sugar levels daily over the course of months. This increases the richness of the data set and improves the chances of better diagnosis and treatment. Patients' privacy and dignity are preserved using wearables as healthcare monitoring devices. For example, taking off clothes to reveal the patient's chest, which is required in some traditional medical tests, but it is not required with wearables. Wearables also provide immediate warning whenever any drastic change in data is observed. Moreover, behavioral changes are possible in individuals using wearables, as motivation and challenges are given to individuals like daily step challenge, goal setting. This has positive health effects and aids in the fight against the obesity crisis that health systems are dealing with and that the COVID-19 pandemic has made worse. Remote patient monitoring decreases the number of patient consultations as a result of the healthcare industry's emphasis on patient care and wearables' adaptability to meet a variety of objectives, from managing chronic ailments to serving as a preventive tool for fitness promotion. Figure 8.4 shows common tasks performed by wearables.

8.5 BARRIERS TO USE WEARABLE TECHNOLOGY

Wearable gadgets are lightweight instruments and a person can always have on their body [16]. To transfer data, these devices are linked with other devices. All the data that are collected daily or minute-by-minute basis, such as heart rate, heart rhythm, caloric burned, and length of sleep, create an excellent user database. They are becoming popular and many people have started using them but its cost is a barrier. Apart from the cost, wearable medical device applications face numerous technical obstacles. Some of them are demonstrated in Figure 8.5.

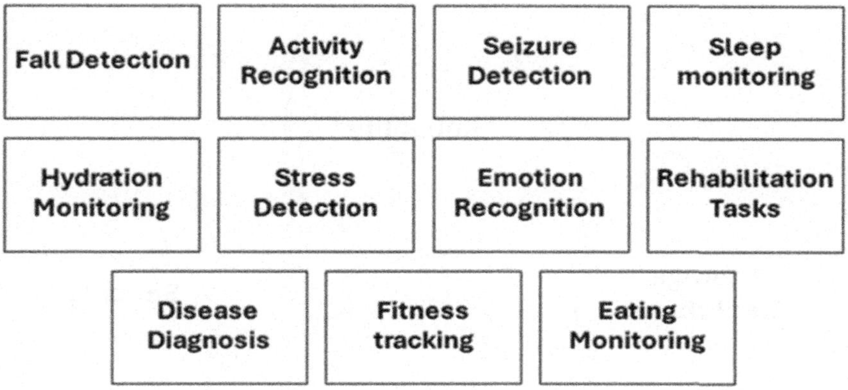

Figure 8.4 Common tasks performed by wearables.

Data Accuracy: Use of wearables is highly dependent upon its accuracy. If the data set is not reliable, then its significance is reduced. Only tested and accurate devices are beneficial, so regulatory standards are set to ensure the reliability. Sensor while taking reading detects nonclinical signals which leads to incorrect diagnosis and needless testing and contributes to the patient's anxiety. Sometimes, due to the sensor's limited sensitivity, pathological clinically significant values are overlooked, delaying therapy and making a diagnosis impossible.

Single Function: Wearable gadget compatibility is not very good. Several tasks are performed by only few wearable devices. The primary focus of the functions is health monitoring, with clinical therapy progressing slowly. Moreover, unfamiliarity with or lack of tech savvy makes wearables complicated for users specially for older adults as connecting wearables to smartphones is required. In fact, not having a smartphone, which is a must to connect to wearables, limits interest in tracking activities altogether.

Poor Battery Life: Battery and power consumption are one of the key-performing parameters of wearables. Wearables with a large energy storage capacity and low power consumption are required. The primary obstacle to the further advancement of sensors for continuous monitoring is their constant power need, necessitating battery changes or recharge under all circumstances. Numerous studies have been conducted on energy harvesting for sensors through the use of motion or body heat.

Equipment Safety: Sometimes false alarms by the wearables are generated, which causes annoyance to the user and reduces user alertness and results in noncompliance of the user from the feedback provided. Medical equipment must prioritize safety and security. Thus, effective methods

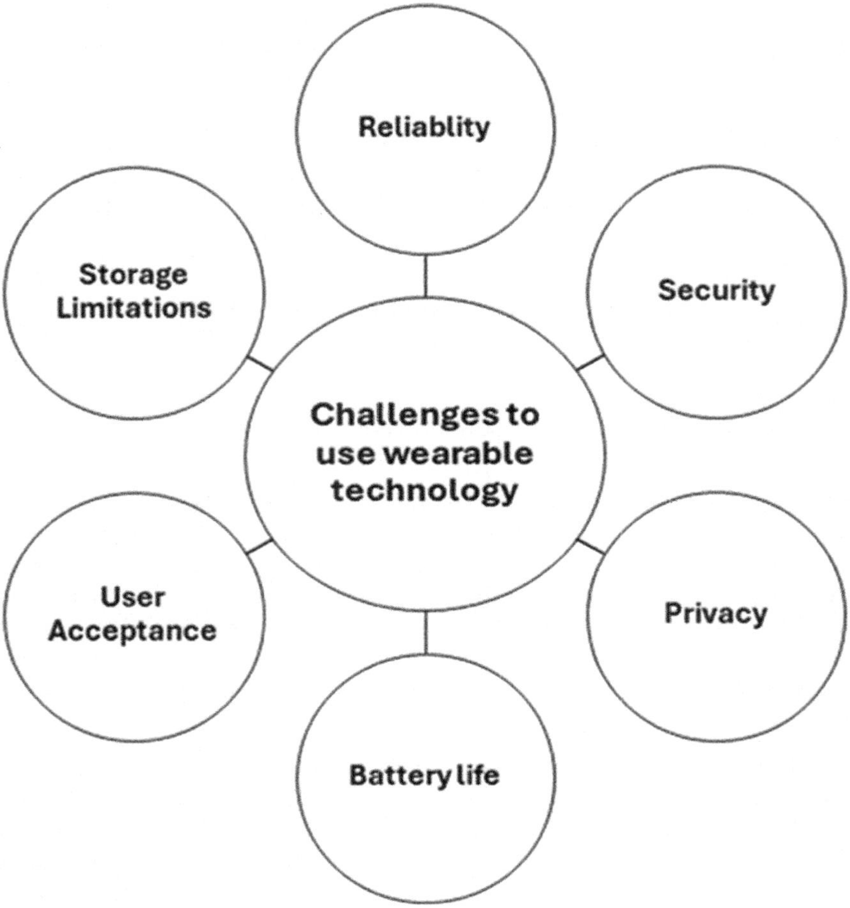

Figure 8.5 Common barriers faced while using wearables.

must be in place to identify and address any anomalies in the data that is being collected.

Security and Privacy: Information on health, location, and lifestyle are all collected by wearables in the form of data, which raises security and privacy concerns. The risk of leakage and tampering increases because these data are available in various formats, large scale, and numerous mobile links. To guarantee the data's security and the privacy of individuals, some strategies are required.

Absence of Industry Regulations and Standards: Industry standards and regulations are required to be set-up, as it is challenging to integrate resources since corporations aim to create their own standards and rules based on their core products, as there is no such standard. Therefore, it is necessary to establish and implement new regulatory standards. Despite people's apparent eagerness to utilize wearables, usage seems to be uneven. A study reported that more than 90% of the participants suspended use. Further improvements are required for other difficulties like cost, inefficient data collecting and processing, unreliable human–computer interfaces, and unfinished big data health cloud building. Another among the obstacles to use that were noted were hospitalization, forgetting to apply, losing interest, and momentary misplacing of the wearable device. Feelings of fatigue stemming from the use of technology, loss of interest, and malfunctioning of the devices that require replacement by the manufacturer are also some factors, which contribute as a barrier to the use of wearables.

8.6 WEARABLE MEDICAL DEVICES USING FPGA

Wearable medical devices are becoming more and more popular for continuous patient monitoring and surveillance [17]. Field programmable gate arrays (FPGAs), which provide high-performance computing and power-saving features, enhance these devices. Examples comprise the following:

ECG Monitors: FPGAs allow ECG signals to be processed in real time, identifying anomalies and giving patients and medical professionals instant feedback.

Blood Glucose Monitors: FPGAs help patients manage their diabetes more successfully by assisting with quick data analysis and precise glucose level monitoring.

Wearable Health Trackers: FPGAs are used to process sensor data, measure movement, keep an eye on vital signs, and analyze sleep patterns for health and fitness applications.

8.6.1 RNS-based FPGA accelerators for high-quality 3D medical image

Medical image processing includes the utilization and investigation of 3D picture datasets of the human body. There are various types of medical data sets like ultrasound images, Computed tomography (CT) scan, X-ray, magnetic resonance imaging (MRI) images, optical and radionuclide etc. are used to analyze pathologies and diagnosis purposes for public healthcare [18]. Figure 8.6 represents the basic steps involved in image processing. Several visual data processing issues are present in modern medical imaging systems. Since 2D and 3D images are not containing enough information to identify abnormalities in the image and further diagnosis of patient, images taken from multiple angles of an organ and combining them to analyze the

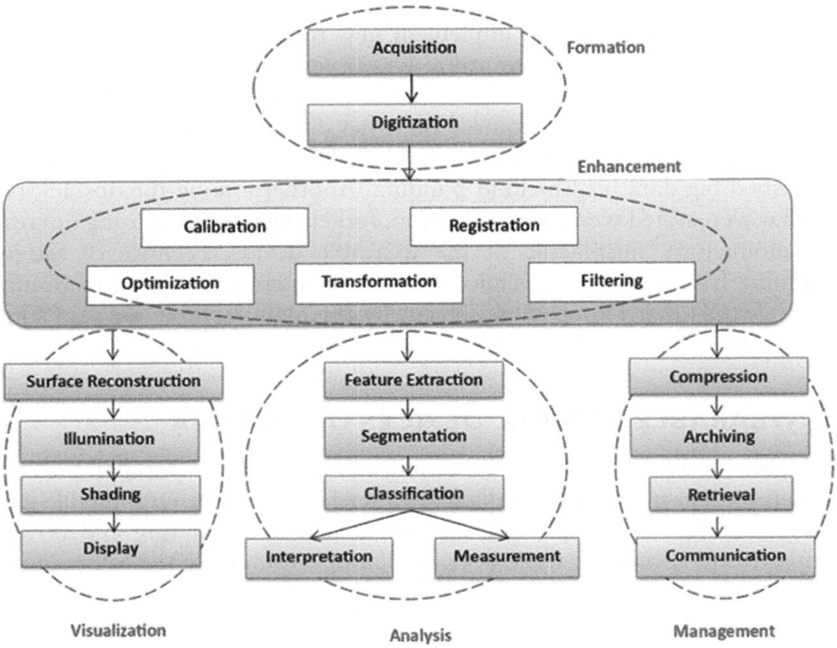

Figure 8.6 Steps involved in Image processing [21].

action of the organ cells are one of the ways to overcome this problem [19]. Also, this will give a comprehensive picture of the behavior of the organs and their anatomical structure.

Another major problem for many imaging techniques is medical image denoising. Images can contain noise, which skews information and makes it difficult to diagnose and cure diseases. Low-resolution images from ultrasound imaging are typically deteriorated by speckle noise, necessitating the use of imaging techniques to enhance image quality and facilitate accurate medical diagnosis [20].

Scanning technologies are constantly improving, leading to medical imaging systems producing more accurate images with higher spatial resolutions and color bit-depth. This increases the amount of information needed for storage, processing, and transmission, particularly for 3D scanning technology. Medical imaging sets can be large, requiring large amounts of data to be processed and transmitted. The rapid data generation and storage of such data require enormous computing resources, space, and high throughput. Therefore, effective 3D image compression is an urgent issue for modern medical imaging systems [22].

8.6.2 Hardware accelerator for medical image processing

Applications for medical imaging have high system requirements. Higher picture resolutions and the merging of many modalities have been fueled by earlier prediction and treatment, necessitating the use of complex software and hardware systems for medical image registration, storage, analysis, and processing. The evolution of technology demands complex computations and real-time processing of large amounts of imaging data. This is crucial for improving patient experience and reducing clinical costs. Lowering equipment prices, developing and implementing them, and increasing their lifespan is essential for more affordable and accessible healthcare. Under these conditions, working with imaging technologies and real-time image processing in healthcare applications has made developing and applying innovative hardware architectures imperative [23].

Using hardware description languages, FPGAs are integrated circuits that enable hardware functionality and postfabrication modification. They are made up of logic blocks coupled by input/output ports and programmable interconnects, which enable high performance and unique hardware design, often with real-time processing, while avoiding the complexity of ASIC design [24]. Because of their numerous configurable logic blocks, FPGAs are well renowned for their huge parallelism, programmability, and configurability, making them very popular as hardware accelerators.

The authors of ref. [25] present a high-level synthesis programming design flow for hardware acceleration. Also, parallel algorithm for maximum likelihood expectation maximization tomographic image reconstruction is discussed. For medical image processing, a highly integrated general-purpose hardware accelerator that can efficiently boost 2D labeling algorithms' computational efficiency and lower FPGA devices' power consumption is proposed in [26]. With the use of parallel computing and data reuse, the design combines image denoising, edge detection, and image segmentation algorithms into a hardware IP core built on a deep pipelining framework. This effectively increases the speed of the 2D labeling method during heavy medical image processing. The FPGA-based 2D labeling accelerator offers a considerable advantage over CPU and GPU accelerators in terms of processing speed and power consumption, according to experimental results, and the labeling results are highly accurate.

Ref [27] presents the tradeoff dilemma between data accuracy and storage and transmission resources by proposing an INR-based approach for parametrizing 3D medical images. A dedicated hardware accelerator for the INR-based reconstruction algorithm is discussed by optimizing computation flow and memory access. On the basis of it, an identical hardware design is also suggested, which receives the coordinate of the spot where three scans (3D medical image) overlap and outputs all of the voxel intensities.

The author of ref. [28] introduces an l Fourier-domain optical coherence tomography (FDOCT) imaging processor for portable OCT applications, which is capable of all OCT image generation operations. The design uses a "1RHC" CFFT-based RFFT(complex-valued FFT-based real-valued fast Fourier transform) unit, reducing power consumption and enabling calibration awareness with minimal area overhead. A test chip was designed, with lower power consumption than without CFFT-based optimization. The FPGA platform was used for design verification, achieving A-line scanning and OCT image display at 30 fps. An ultrasound transceiver application-specific integrated circuit (ASIC) for 3D ultrasonic imaging of the carotid artery is described in [29]. The ASIC interfaces a piezo-electric transducer array with an imaging system using only 24 transmit and receive channels. The ASIC is implemented in a 0.18 μm high-voltage bipolar CMOS DMOS (BCD) process and has been successfully tested in electrical and acoustic experiments.

Residue Number Systems: A residue number system (RNS) is a numeral system that represents integers by their values modulo several coprime integers, known as moduli. This representation is enabled by the Chinese remainder theorem, which states that if M is the product of the moduli, there is exactly one integer with any given modular values in an interval of length M. Multimodular arithmetic is widely used for large integer computation, polynomial greatest common divisor, Gröbner basis computation, and cryptography [30].

The product of the moduli, M = m1. m2. m3... mj, determines the dynamic range M in an RNS that uses the mutually prime numbers m1, m2, m3,....,mj as moduli. The residues can be used to uniquely represent the numbers between 0 and M – 1. As an alternative, numbers can be expressed between—M/2 and ((M/2) – 1) for even values of M and—((M – 1)/2) and (M – 1)/2 for odd value of M. As a result, when a large number is divided by a set of moduli, it can be represented by a number of smaller numbers called residues. Thus, we can conduct several tiny word length operations on these residues in place of large word length operations. Thus, it is possible to carry out modulo addition, modulo subtraction, and modulo multiplication operations rather effectively.

A nonweighted number system is the RNS. As a result, it differs greatly from weighted number systems like binary or decimal. Arithmetic operations with residue, such as multiplication, subtraction, and addition, are intrinsically carry-free, meaning that every resultant digit is a function of just one digit independent of all other digits, from each operand. This function aids in significant improvement in processing speed, the primary requirement in DSP software [31].

A collection of independent moduli is provided in the RNS. Each modulus's residue serves as an integer's representation, and arithmetic operations are predicated on each residue separately. The RNS arithmetic operations can be carried out independently on different moduli to avoid the carry in addition, subtraction, and multiplication, which is often lengthy.

8.7 RNS-BASED HARDWARE ACCELERATORS

Many applications that require speed and great performance use digital image processing. However, the high speed and functional demands of these applications result in higher power consumption. Therefore, it is crucial to find a solution to the power-performance problems. The authors of ref. [32] describe the use of the RNS and the static voltage scaling (SVS) strategy to improve the power performance of a two-dimensional (2D) discrete wavelet transform (DWT) image processor. Examining how the RNS and SVS schemes affect the suggested image processor is the goal of this work. The low-complexity hardware architecture of the RNS-based filter banks, optimized transposition units, and taking advantage of the SVS scheme to lower power consumption are some of the unique features of the suggested design. In order to reduce hardware complexity, the RNS-based filter banks' multiplierless scheme and binary-coded number format are employed. Also, for boosting system performance, modular arithmetics and 6-bit dyadic fraction filter coefficients are used. The images are compressed using the bi-orthogonal DWT because of its multiresolution characteristics and capacity to locate limited signals.

As an alternative to the traditional binary number representation, an efficient convolutional neural network (CNN) accelerator design called RNSiM is described in [33], which is based on the RNS. Unlike traditional arithmetic implementation, which is inevitably plagued by a long carry propagation chain, RNSiM is new in that all data including computation and communication are carried out within the RNS domain. This includes stored weights. Power and delay are greatly decreased because RNS arithmetic is inherently parallel. Additionally, to reduce the overhead caused by nonmodular operations, an improved integrated intermodulo operation core is built. By creating effective processing-in-memory (PIM) designs that utilize a variety of volatile CMOS and nonvolatile post-CMOS technologies to speed up RNS-based multiplication-and-accumulations (MACs), systems' performance efficiency can be further increased.

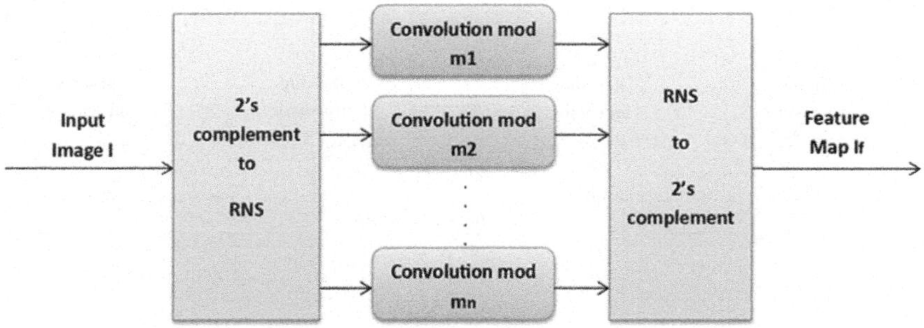

Figure 8.7 Convolution operation in RNS [34].

The technique for implementing the CNN on hardware for pattern recognition utilizing RNS computations is presented in [34]. Figure 8.7 shows the steps involved in the convolution operation. The CNN's reduced configuration consists of a classifier that is structured like a conventional multilayer perceptron, a max pooling layer, and a convolutional layer. The convolution layer's hardware implementation demonstrates that using RNS can save hardware expenses by 7.86%–37.78% when compared to the two's complement. The average time for image recognition is lowered by 41.17% when the suggested heterogeneous solution is used. The findings of the study can be used to develop efficient video surveillance systems that can identify people, objects, handwriting, and terrain. Figure 8.8 shows the front-end design of an RNS-based processor.

A fundamental component of many applications that may be dealt with on embedded devices is modular arithmetic. One method to increase the efficiency of modular arithmetic is to find algorithmic changes that would improve the target arithmetic's parallelization and allow it to make use of parallel architectures and hardware. Data-level parallelism is made possible by the RNS. This allows parallelization of algorithms based on modular arithmetic that have multiple data dependencies. However, it might be difficult to transfer generic algorithms to fully RNS-based implementations, and appropriate hardware designs that can scale and react to various demands must be used. In this study, a scalable architecture that fully utilizes the RNS for the concurrent implementation of algorithms based on modular arithmetic is proposed and discussed. A logical mapping between the architecture and

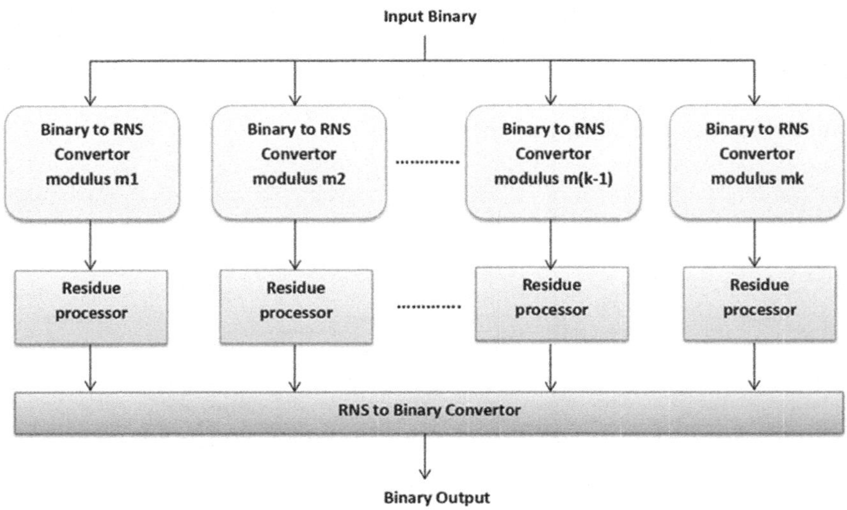

Figure 8.8 RNS-based processor.

a general modular arithmetic algorithm is demonstrated. For an application-specific integrated circuit (ASIC) or FPGA design flow that targets modular arithmetic algorithms, it can be used as a high-level synthesis phase.

8.8 FPGA DESIGN CONSIDERATIONS FOR MEDICAL IMAGING

Applications like image processing, static, and real-time analysis are prominent in medical imaging with a broad range of hardware and software design considerations. We will discuss some important factors for an effective FPGA design.

8.8.1 Selection of development tools

FPGA development tools provide efficient development, testing, and debugging of designs. They are an important factor in the design and implementation of applications on a field programmable gate arrays. For applications like medical imaging, these development tools/platforms determine capability to process data and resources and the viability for jobs involving medical imaging. Xilinx and Altera are two tools. Table 8.2 lists the key features of these tools.

8.8.2 FPGA programming languages

Programming languages offer a way to explain how FPGA circuits operate and behave. VHDL and Verilog are commonly used hardware description languages for the design of applications on FPGAs. For FPGA development, specific IDEs, simulators, and synthesis tools are available in addition to these languages and tools. With the help of these tools, engineers can

Table 8.2 The key features of FPGA tools

FPGA development tools	*Key features*
Xilinx Vivado	With Xilinx Vivado's user-friendly interface, developers can easily write and edit code in multiple programming languages, including Verilog and VHDL, for FPGA development. For complex designs Vivado provides built-in libraries and modules for common functions so that every-time those commonly used functions are selected making programming easier. It also provides inclusive development environment which offers advanced synthesis, placement and routing capabilities
Altera Quartus	To design Intel FPGA devices Quartus is used which is an effective instrument for creating Intel FPGA devices. It has a graphical interface with a library to provide sophisticated tools for synthesis and verification

Table 8.3 The key features of FPGA languages

FPGA languages	*Key features*
Verilog	Hardware description language (HDL) is used for modelling and designing digital systems. It enables circuit behavior and structure to be described at different abstraction levels by designers. Hardware description languages (HDLs) like Verilog and VHDL can be used to program and configure FPGAs. With HDLs, the user can use a high-level language to explain how the digital circuit behaves. The tool finds the best place for the logic gates and interconnect routing on the FPGA in order to satisfy the design timing and hardware requirements
VHDL	Another HDL for FPGA development is VHDL, which supports both sequential and concurrent programming styles and has a robust type system
System Verilog	System Verilog is an extension for Verilog that adds more features for assertions, verification, and test-bench development
Python	Python's simplicity and versatility make it a popular choice for automating FPGA workflows and generating hardware designs

create and improve FPGA designs more quickly, which eventually results in improved performance and a shorter time to market. New versions, updates, improvements, and continuous evolution of FPGA development tools and languages is in progress. Table 8.3 demonstrates the key features of FPGA languages.

8.8.3 Resource management and optimization

Resource Utilization: For medical image processing, resource allocation of logic gates, memory, and DSP blocks must be done efficiently for optimal usage of resources. For efficient resource utilization, pipelining and parallelization are two strategies that are used.

Power Efficiency: FPGA designs aim at efficient power consumption, as power consumption is a critical concern. Particularly in high-frequency applications or resource-demanding designs, FPGAs utilize a lot of power. In portable medical devices, power consumption is an issue. To reduce power consumption, strategies like clock gating, dynamic scaling of frequency and voltage, and power design methodologies are preferred.

8.8.4 Safety and reliability concerns

Redundancy and Fault Tolerance: In applications that involve medical imaging, designers should make a reliable system. For smooth operations in monitoring and diagnosis systems redundancy check, fault-tolerance mechanism must be adopted. These fault-tolerant techniques help in the proper functioning of medical imaging systems in real time.

Testing and Verification: In imaging systems based on FPGA simulation, verification and testing is required. These steps are necessary for identification and rectification of the design.

8.8.5 Compliance with regulatory standards

Medical Device Regulations: For patient safety and data security medical imaging devices must follow safety regulation guideline. FPGA-based systems must strictly follow safety standards and FDA guidelines.

Data Security and Privacy: Medical data needs to be protected from unauthorized access and security threats, as patient information is confidential. Strong access control, data handling protocols and encryption protocols must be adopted.

8.9 CONCLUSION

Healthcare facilities have received a great support by the application of wearable medical devices. Wearable technology is not only getting popular but also enhancing the quality of healthcare. Much research and development are ongoing in this field as there are some limitations of wearable technology which is discussed in this chapter. Technology must be developed for data transfer, preservation, sharing, gathering, and legal infrastructure, which will improve the efficiency of the whole system and better healthcare for the patient. The autonomy of the patient should be maintained while using wearable health devices so that the patient takes active participation in their own care. Similarly, cases like when using wearable devices, it is best to avoid misdiagnosis, missed diagnosis, and false alarms caused by faulty or delayed data. In this chapter, we have discussed how wearable technology is contributing to health care. We have discussed about different types of wearables and how sensors are used for collecting information. Benefits and challenges related to wearables are also discussed.

Wearable gadgets have become a big component of the lifestyle and fitness industry, but the growth of wearable sensors in the health care sector has been relatively modest. However, as wearable sensor technology advances, there are a ton of prospects for its application in the medical field, particularly in precision medicine and connected health care, where wearables can evaluate a person's health in real time and with high quality. In conclusion, wearable technology will unavoidably play a bigger part in the field of health care and become more seamlessly incorporated into our daily lives as science and technology advance and personalized health concepts gain popularity. To investigate further wearable gadget uses in the medical field, more research is necessary.

REFERENCES

[1] T. O'Donovan, J. O'Donoghue, C. Sreenan, D. Sammon, P. O'Reilly, and K. O'Connor. "A context aware wireless body area network (BAN)." In 3rd International Conference on IEEE *Pervasive Computing Technologies for Healthcare*, 2009.

[2] S. Shiffman, A. A. Stone, and M. R. Hufford. "Ecological momentary assessment." *Annu. Rev. Clin. Psychol.*, vol. 4, pp. 1–32, 2008. doi:10.1146/annurev.clinpsy.3.022806.091415

[3] J. M. Radin, N. E. Wineinger, E. J. Topol, and S. R. Steinhubl. "Harnessing wearable device data to improve state-level real-time surveillance of influenza-like illness in the USA: a population-based study." *Lancet Digit Health*, vol.2, no. 2, p. e85–93, 2020. doi:10.1016/S2589-7500(19)30222-5

[4] M. Jiang, P. Maass, and T. Page. "Regularizing properties of the mumford-shah functional for imaging applications." *Inverse Problems*, 2014.

[5] P. Rubel, J. Fayn, L. Simon-Chautemps, H. Atoui, M. Ohlsson, D. Telisson, S. Adami, S. Arod, M. C. Forlini, C. Malossi, J. Placide, G. L. Ziliani, D. Assanelli, and P. Chevalier. New Paradigms in Telemedicine: Ambient Intelligence, Wearable, Pervasive and Personalized. In A. Lymberis, & D. de Rossi (Eds.), *Wearable eHealth Systems for Personalised Health Management: State of the Art and Future Challenges* (Vol. 108, pp. 123–132, 2004). IOS Press. http://iospress.metapress.com/link.asp?id=gmfhkj0yqdd61kwb]

[6] R. Qian and Y. Long. "Wearable chemosensors: a review of recent progress." *Chemistry Open.*, vol. 7, no. 2, pp. 118–130, 2018. doi:10.1002/open.201700159 [PMC free article] [PubMed] [CrossRef] [CrossRef] [Google Scholar]

[7] K. Guk, G. Han, J. Lim, K. Jeong, T. Kang, E. Lim, et al. "Evolution of wearable devices with real-time disease monitoring for personalized health care." *Nanomaterials (Basel)*, vol. 9, no. 6, 2019. [Medline:31146479]

[8] M. Zhang, R. Saeed, S. Saeed, S. Stankovski, and Z. Xiaoshuan. Wearable technology and applications: A systematic review. 5–16.

[9] F. John Dian, R. Vahidnia, and A. Rahmati. "Wearables and the internet of things (IoT), applications, opportunities, and challenges: A survey." *IEEE Access*, vol. 8, pp. 69200–69211, 2020. doi:10.1109/ACCESS.2020.2986329

[10] K. Tehrani and M. Andrew. "Wearable technology and wearable devices: Everything you need to know." *Wearable Devices Magazine*. 2014 [Online]. Available at WearableDevices.com

[11] V. Sharma, Vineeta, S. Som, and S. K. Khatri. "Future of wearable devices using IoT synergy in AI." In Proc. 3rd Int. Conf. Electron. Commun. Aerosp. Technol. ICECA 2019, pp. 138–142, 2019. doi:10.1109/ICECA.2019.8821915

[12] D. R. Witt, R. A. Kellogg, M. P. Snyder, and J. Dunn. "Windows into human health through wearables data analytics." *Curr. Opin. Biomed. Eng.*, vol. 9, pp. 28–46, 2019. doi:10.1016/j.cobme.2019.01.001

[13] R. S. Spaho. Wearable devices in palliative care for people 65 years and older: A scoping review, 2023. doi:10.1177/20552076231181212
[14] A. Chatterjee, A. Aceves, R. Dungca, H. Flores, and K. Giddens. "Classification of wearable computing: A survey of electronic assistive technology and future design." In Proceedings of 2016 2nd IEEE International Conference on Research in *Computational Intelligence and Communication Networks*, ICRCICN 2016, pp. 22–27, 2017. doi:10.1109/ICRCICN.2016.7813545
[15] M. Mardonova and Y. Choi. "Review of wearable device technology and its applications to the mining industry." *Energies*, vol. 11, no. 3, 2018. doi:10.3390/en11030547
[16] S. Canali, V. Schiaffonati, A. Aliverti. Challenges and recommendations for wearable devices in digital health: Data quality, interoperability, health equity, fairness. *PLOS Digit Health*, vol. 1, no. 10, p. e0000104, 2022. doi:10.1371/journal.pdig.0000104
[17] M. Vaithianathan, S. Udkar, M. Reddy, D. Roy, and S. Rajasekaran. FPGA-based smart health monitoring systems for wearable devices. 2024. doi:10.13140/RG.2.2.33185.62567
[18] Z. Yan, X. Xu, Y. Wang, T. Li, B. Ma, L. Yang, Y. Lu, and Q. Li. "Application of ultrasonic Doppler technology based on wavelet threshold denoising algorithm in fetal heart rate and central nervous system malformation detection." *World Neurosurg.*, vol. 149, pp. 380–387, May 2021. doi:10.1016/j.wneu.2020.10
[19] B. M. G. Rosa and G. Z. Yang. "Bladder volume monitoring using electrical impedance tomography with simultaneous multi-tone tissue stimulation and DFT-based impedance calculation inside an FPGA." *IEEE Trans. Biomed. Circuits Syst.*, vol. 14, no. 4, pp. 775–786, Aug. 2020, doi:10.1109/TBCAS.2020.30088
[20] T. Deserno. "Medical image processing." In Optipedia, SPIE Press, Bellingham, WA, 2009.
[21] N. N. Nagornov, P. A. Lyakhov, M. V. Valueva and M. V. Bergerman. "RNS-based FPGA accelerators for high-quality 3D medical image wavelet processing using scaled filter coefficients." *IEEE Access*, vol. 10, pp. 19215–19231, 2022, doi:10.1109/ACCESS.2022.3151361
[22] E. Alcaín, P. R. Fernández, R. Nieto, A. S. Montemayor, J. Vilas, A. Galiana-Bordera, P. M. Martinez-Girones, C. Prieto-de-la-Lastra, B. Rodriguez-Vila, M. Bonet et al. "Hardware architectures for real-time medical imaging." *Electronics*, vol. 10, no. 24, p. 3118, 2021. https://doi.org/10.3390/electronics10243118
[23] V. K. Tiwari et al. "A high-speed ANN-based data acquisition hardware accelerator targeting electrical impedance tomography." *IEEE Trans. Circuits Syst.*, vol. 71, no. 9, pp. 4078–4091, 2024.
[24] M. Ravi, A. Sewa, T. G. Shasidhar, and S. S. S. Sanagapati. "FPGA as a hardware accelerator for computation intensive maximum likelihood expectation maximization medical image reconstruction algorithm." *IEEE Access*, vol. 7, pp. 111727–111735, 2019. doi:10.1109/ACCESS.2019.2932647
[25] X. Xu, W. Su, B. Li, Y. Wei, D. Kong, H. Zeng, and X. Zhang. "An FPGA-based hardware accelerator for 2D labeling." In Proceedings of the 6th International Conference on Biomedical Signal and Image Processing

(ICBIP '21). Association for Computing Machinery, New York, NY, USA, pp. 72–78, 2021. https://doi.org/10.1145/3484424.3484436

[26] C. Rao, Q. Wu, P. Zhou, J. Yu, Y. Zhang, and X. Lou. "An energy-efficient accelerator for medical image reconstruction from implicit neural representation." *IEEE Trans. Circuit Syst. I*, vol. 70, no. 4, pp. 1625–1638, Apr. 2023, doi:10.1109/TCSI.2022.3231863

[27] S.-N. Tang and F.-C. Jan. "Energy-efficient and calibration-aware Fourier-domain OCT imaging processor." *IEEE Trans. Very Large Scale Integr. Syst.*, vol. 27, no. 6, pp. 1390–1403, Jun. 2019. https://doi.org/10.1109/TVLSI.2019.2894751

[28] E. Kang et al. "A reconfigurable ultrasound transceiver ASIC With 24×40 Elements for 3-D Carotid Artery Imaging." *IEEE J. Solid-State Cir.*, vol. 53, no. 7, pp. 2065–2075, Jul. 2018, doi:10.1109/JSSC.2018.2820156

[29] A. O. Sharoun. "Residue number system (RNS)." *Poznan Univ. Technol. Acad. J. Electr. Eng.*, vol. 76, pp. 265–270, 2013.

[30] P. V. A. Mohan. Residue number systems. Cham: Springer International Publishing, 2016. doi:10.1007/978-3-319-41385-3

[31] A. Safari, C. V. Niras, and Y. Kong. "Power-performance enhancement of two-dimensional RNS-based Dwt image processor using static voltage scaling." *Integration*, vol. 53, pp. 145–156, 2016.

[32] A. Roohi, M. Taheri, S. Angizi and D. Fan. "RNSiM: Efficient deep neural network accelerator using residue number systems." In 2021 IEEE/ACM International Conference On Computer Aided Design (ICCAD), Munich, Germany, 2021, pp. 1–9, doi:10.1109/ICCAD51958.2021.9643531

[33] M. V. Valueva, N. N. Nagornov, P. A. Lyakhov, G. V. Valuev, and N. I. Chervyakov. "Application of the residue number system to reduce hardware costs of the convolutional neural network implementation." *Math. Comput. Simul.*, vol. 177, pp. 232–243, 2020. https://doi.org/10.1016/j.matcom.2020.04.031

[34] S. Antão and L. Sousa. "A flexible architecture for modular arithmetic hardware accelerators based on RNS." *J. Sign. Process Syst.*, vol. 76, pp. 249–259, 2014. https://doi.org/10.1007/s11265-014-0879-y

QUESTIONS

Q1. What is an FPGA, and how does it differ from other types of hardware?
Q2. What are the benefits of using an FPGA in a design?
Q3. What are the key features of an FPGA?
Q4. What is the design flow for an FPGA, and what are the challenges in designing an FPGA?
Q5. How do you verify the design of an FPGA, and what tools do you use for debugging and troubleshooting?
Q6. FPGA architecture consists of?
Q7. What is the use of programmable interconnects in FPGA?
Q8. How FPGA performs better than ASIC and in which applications?

Q9. What are the challenges in FPGA design process?
Q10. Define HDL?
Q11. What are the differences between Verilog and VHDL?
Q12. What are the benefits of using an FPGA?
Q13. What are the key features of an FPGA?
Q14. How does an FPGA work?
Q15. What are the applications of an FPGA?
Q16. What is the design flow for an FPGA?
Q17. How do FPGAs differ from microprocessors in terms of functionality?
Q18. What are the differences between FPGA and CPLD?
Q19. What is the significance of FPGAs in modern day electronics?
Q20. Why is programmability so important in designing chips
Q21. What does "field-programmable" mean?
Q22. How FPGAs contribute in the field of healthcare?
Q23. What does EMS stand for?
Q24. How FPGA is used in EMS?
Q25. What is digital watermarking, and what is its significance in medical sector?
Q26. How FPGA is used in digital watermarking?
Q27. What is real-time processing capability?
Q28. What is design complexity, and how it is a limitation of FPGA?
Q29. List some applications of FPGA in medical diagnostic?
Q30. What is the usage of FPGAs in medical imaging?
Q31. How does a medical imaging system works?
Q32. List some development tools for FPGA?
Q33. List some programming languages for FPGA?
Q34. What are the imitations of FPGA?
Q35. Why data security is important with regards to the usage of FPGA in medical imaging?
Q36. What are wearable devices?
Q37. How are wearables contributing to healthcare?
Q38. List some features of wearables?
Q39. What does AAL stands for?
Q40. What is the use of sensors in wearables? What are the benefits of wearable technology?
Q41. What are nonwearable sensors, how do they work?
Q42. How patient's privacy is maintained in doing diagnosis using wearable devices?
Q43. What are misdiagnosis, how it contributes to the anxiety of patient?
Q44. How data accuracy becomes a drawback of wearables?
Q45. How big is the Wearable Healthcare Device market?
Q46. Are wearables power-efficient devices?
Q47. According to research, what is the most common reason for people who suspend the use of wearables?

Q48. What types of problem faced by today's medical imaging system?
Q49. What are moduli in residue number systems?
Q50. Residue number system is ....? (weighted/nonweighted)
Q51. What are the advantages of using RNS-based systems?
Q52. What is the advantage of using RNS-based hardware accelerator?

Chapter 9

High-performance computing systems for healthcare

9.1 INTRODUCTION TO HIGH-PERFORMANCE COMPUTING IN HEALTHCARE

High-performance computing (HPC) systems provide a number of significant benefits when connecting hospital and lab data centers. More precise diagnoses and well-informed research are made possible by HPC systems' ability to integrate data from various institutions, which offers a unified view of clinical results, research data, and patient records. Accelerated research discoveries and timely interventions are made possible by the rapid data processing capabilities of HPC systems. The development of new medications, therapies, and technologies is accelerated by pooling resources and data, which improves collaborative research. Faster and more accurate treatment decisions are made when vital information is available in real time, and infrastructure costs are decreased and performance is maximized through effective resource use. For better forecasting of disease outbreaks and patient outcomes, advanced predictive analytics is utilized in conjunction with centralized data management to ensure regulatory compliance and security. Comprehensive data analysis strengthens the case for precision medicine and makes customized treatments possible. Better patient care practices and creative solutions are also produced by the connectivity, which encourages cooperation and knowledge exchange between researchers and healthcare professionals. In general, the long-term advantages of HPC infrastructure include reduced costs and improved research and patient care efficiencies, despite the fact that the initial investments can be substantial.

The significant influence of HPC in healthcare is exemplified by several recent instances as shown below:

1. Czech Republic Medical Image Processing: Using HPC, deep learning algorithms for segmenting tissue in medical images can be developed, leading to better abnormality detection. With verified data, this automated system continuously improves its accuracy, showcasing how HPC has the potential to completely transform medical diagnostics.

DOI: 10.1201/9781003503033-9

2. Nutritional Support (Belgium): By measuring intragastric pressure and analyzing stomach motility, VIPUN Medical [1] uses HPC to combat malnutrition in critically ill patients. HPC contributes to the development of tailored nutritional support, enhancing patient outcomes by reducing risks associated with malnutrition.
3. Pharmaceutical Research (Belgium): Molecular dynamics simulations, which offer comprehensive insights into protein drug targets, are a key tool used by HPC to propel pharmaceutical innovation. The role of HPC in personalized medicine is highlighted by these simulations, which speed up drug discovery and make it possible to develop more potent treatments.
4. Swiss Aortic Valve Prosthesis Design: By modeling the turbulence of blood flow surrounding the valves, HPC aids in the improvement of aortic valve prosthesis design. By making minor design adjustments based on these simulations, durability and biocompatibility can be increased, leading to better surgical results.
5. Child Radiation Dosimetry (Greece): The PediDose [2] intimate tool, created with HPC, calculates the harmful radiation doses that organs of children will absorb.
6. Utilizing HPC for Cloud-Based Pulmonary Shunting Guidance (Italy): In Italy, HPC is employed to provide assistance for systemic pulmonary shunting operations through a cloud-based platform. This platform delivers pre-determined results for vascular shunt implantation, enabling surgeons to scrutinize patient-specific conditions using a Medical Digital Twin (MDT), thereby improving the accuracy of surgical decisions.

Figure 9.1 demonstrates the principle of HPC.

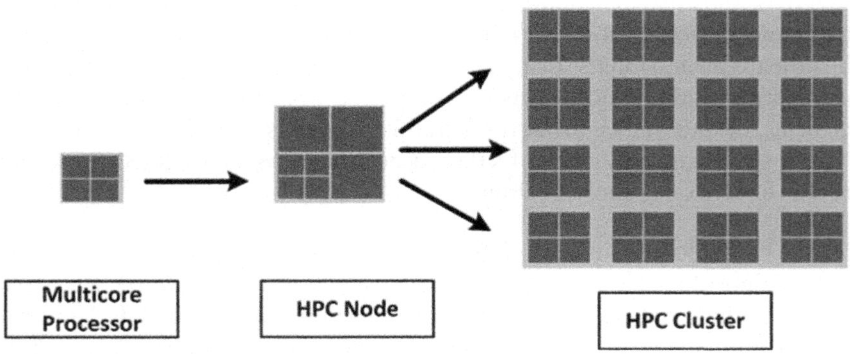

Figure 9.1 Principle of high-performance computing (HPC).

9.2 MEDICAL EQUIPMENT USING HIGH-PERFORMANCE COMPUTING WITH LOW-POWER PROCESSORS: CUTTING-EDGE COMMERCIAL DESIGN ENVIRONMENTS

In the last 20 years, the IT sector has moved from physical servers to virtualized environments and then to Kubernetes and OpenShift-managed container-based solutions. Unfortunately, the difficulties in implementing these platforms have prevented HPC environments from embracing containerization as quickly. Because they are flexible, modular, and have lower overhead, containers are a good choice for jobs that require a lot of bandwidth and latency. Although containers have benefits, they are difficult to use and frequently require complicated command-line processes. Another method involves creating an architecture that combines seamless hardware with an intuitive user interface. This architecture features dynamic workload placement that is based on scheduling that is machine learning-based and real-time performance analysis. This methodology targets problems with Kubernetes [3], like improper workload distribution, and concentrates on enhancing energy efficiency, a critical issue in HPC. The suggested solution consists of an application that installs Kubernetes automatically on a variety of hardware platforms, showing promise in workload scheduling speed and placement accuracy as well as increased energy efficiency. This design holds significance for enhancing low-power processor performance in medical equipment, especially in commercial design settings and health care processor prototyping boards.

Modern IT increasingly needs to move away from static data center designs and toward more dynamic and efficient models, especially in HPC. Conventional data centers frequently use fixed resource allocation and design patterns, which make it difficult to accommodate the changing needs of modern workloads. HPC environments are now investigating the advantages of container orchestration platforms like Kubernetes, having previously relied on specialized hardware and software to attain maximum performance. Recent research has shown that CPU hardware-assisted hypervisor features have a major performance impact. For example, virtual machines (VMs) provide advantages like live migration, which enables the seamless transfer of running VMs between hosts. Using physical servers or containers is not possible for this capability. Research on scheduling multiple VM live migrations to maximize efficiency has demonstrated the benefits of VMs in specific scenarios. Moreover, ideas like VMware Distributed Resource Scheduler (DRS) can improve VM scheduling. Resource allocation is automated by DRS, which has shown improvements in efficiency and environmental awareness over time when compared favorably to human experts. This is especially true of advanced features like predictive DRS.

Notwithstanding these benefits, studies comparing the performance overhead of containers versus hypervisors show that containers are typically more efficient. Because of their reduced overhead and capacity to manage bandwidth- and latency-sensitive tasks, containers, a more flexible and lightweight version of traditional hypervisors have become increasingly popular. Docker containers [4] provide scalable, high-performance solutions when they are used on virtual or bare metal servers. Further improving their usability and efficiency is the integration of containers with Kubernetes and DevOps workflows. While designs, deployments, and lifecycle management are more complicated with containers, they are still a good substitute for hypervisors in large-scale environments due to their practical advantages.

The overheads of virtualization and containerization have been studied in the past. In terms of I/O operations, for instance, KVM (Kernel-based VM) adds overhead that influences overall performance based on the size of the I/O. Generally speaking, however, containers are better at handling I/O-intensive workloads. Comparing Kubernetes to Docker and Podman [5], studies show that Kubernetes performs significantly better, making it a powerful tool for managing large-scale containerized applications. Although they provide more security and flexibility, containers such as Podman, which enable rootless operation, are not as suitable for HPC workloads.

Docker and Podmanto have been found to be useful solutions in studies on the use of containerization in machine learning and scientific computation scenarios. It has been discovered that HPC applications require finer-grained scheduling in order to ensure effective resource management, as the default Kubernetes scheduler is insufficient. This difficulty has prompted more research into Kubernetes optimization for HPC environments, including the application of Quality of Service (QoS) guidelines for pod auto-scaling. There is a need for specific methods to package HPC applications, and auto-scaling with QoS awareness can help to ensure consistent performance. Kubernetes still lacks native hardware monitoring solutions, despite its advancements. In this regard, machine learning techniques for identifying cluster anomalies can be useful in proactive system management. Efficiency gains in operations and sustainability can be achieved through dynamic workload placement that is informed by real-time metrics, resource availability, and energy efficiency. Better resource use, a smaller carbon footprint, and alignment with contemporary business requirements are all promised by such strategies.

An important development in HPC environment optimization is the emphasis on adaptable and dynamic infrastructure in data centers. Organizations can effectively manage energy consumption and expenses while maintaining optimal performance by utilizing containerization and orchestration technologies to better meet the changing needs of modern workloads. Core technologies that improve IT scalability and efficiency include virtualization, orchestrators, containers, and HPC. While orchestrators like Kubernetes automate management, virtualization and containers optimize resource usage and application consistency. Through parallel processing, HPC promotes scientific research. They are the foundation of the contemporary digital ecosystem when combined. Listed below are a few of the techniques.

1. Multiple VMs, each running a different operating system, are created by vitalizing physical hardware. VMs are managed via hypervisors. Type 1 (bare metal) is more efficient than Type 2 (hosted). Although it has a larger overhead than containerization, key benefits include strong isolation, live migration, and dynamic resource allocation.
2. Containerization leverages technologies such as Docker, Linux Containers (LXC), and Podman to provide lightweight, portable, and consistent environments for application deployment. In terms of resource consumption, startup times, density, and consistency across environments, containers outperform VMs. Containerization makes managing dependencies easier and enables safe, isolated testing; it started with BSD jails. Modern scalable applications benefit greatly from containers because they maximize hardware utilization and minimize overhead by sharing the host system's kernel.
3. With FreeBSD 4.0, BSD jails were added, enabling the partitioning of a FreeBSD system into separate mini-systems that share the host kernel. Because of this, virtualization is safe and effective, which makes it perfect for environments used for testing and development that require fewer resources.
4. Docker, which packages applications and dependencies into lightweight containers that share the host OS kernel and require less overhead than traditional VMs, completely changed the way applications are deployed. It provides quick startup times, great efficiency, and cross-environment consistency. Docker's capabilities are enhanced through its integration with orchestration tools such as Kubernetes, which makes it a crucial technology in contemporary DevOps practices. Docker became the industry standard for application packaging even though it did not create containerization; rather, it popularized the idea.
5. An open-source platform called Kubernetes makes it easier to deploy, scale, and manage containerized applications. It has a primary worker architecture, groups apps into Pods, and allows for load balancing, service discovery, and horizontal scaling. While orchestration tools like Kubernetes and Open Shift improve application resilience, fault tolerance, and high availability, declarative configuration in Kubernetes makes management easier. Kubernetes, which started out in big IT companies, is now a necessity in contemporary

cloud native environments because it increases the effectiveness and scalability of container management.

Historically, HPC workloads have been dependent on physical and VMs because of their sophisticated hardware features, which containers frequently do not offer, like PCIe pass through and SR-IOV. HPC workloads need close-to-hardware execution for best performance; however, containerizing these workloads presents difficulties, such as re-packaging, deploying Kubernetes, and ineffective scheduling for real-time applications. The issue of hardware-software co-design, particularly in HPC settings, emphasizes the necessity of better integration and context-aware scheduling algorithms to improve scalability, energy efficiency, and performance in contemporary data centers. Optimizing HPC workloads based on Kubernetes requires addressing these problems.

9.3 RECONFIGURABLE INTEGRATED CIRCUITS IN HEALTHCARE

In healthcare sector, field programmable gate array (FPGAs) are in high demand as they enhance the performance, flexibility, and utility of various medical instruments. Their usage has transformed the healthcare system as they can be reprogrammed and customized for specific tasks. Emergency medical service (EMS) is a system that aims at providing emergency medical care. One of the most useful and emerging EMS system is made by using FPGA. An FPGA-based medical system, as shown in Figure 9.2, is proposed in [6] which is applicable for outside and inside of hospitals. This FPGA-based integrated system has strengthened the concept of EMS system.

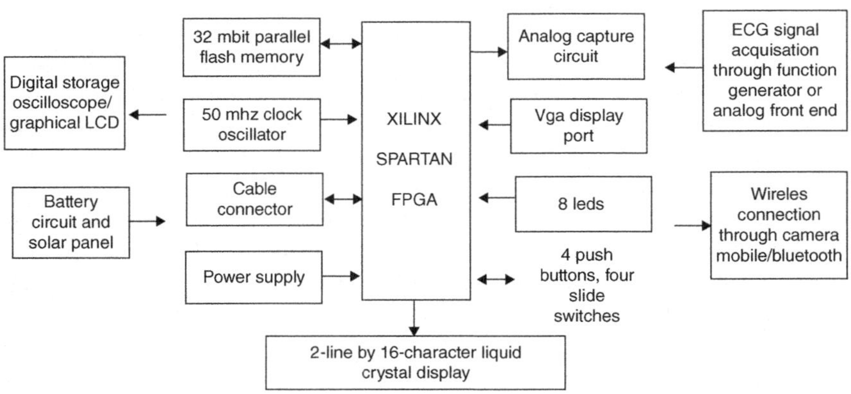

Figure 9.2 Block diagram of an FPGA-based EMS system.

Especially in rural areas in countries like India are far behind in health care facilities. So, the proposed system which is discussed here aims at providing quick diagnosis of life-threatening clinical syndromes. This system is cost-effective also, so it is affordable. This system is used to display electrocardiogram (ECG) waveforms to diagnose the diseases. It is robust, simple, and a portable system. It can be used in places where there is a shortage of electricity. There is a lot of research going on in "FPGA based digital image watermarking" [7, 8]. Transmission and reception of biomedical information like patients' reports, encryption, and decryption are done using FPGA. The technique of digital image watermarking is used to conceal a hidden information so that copyright is protected for multimedia contentor to demonstrate that the information is true, up-to-date, and has not been altered. Protective digital information is encoded and decoded, and the recipient authenticates the received information. Digital image watermarking using FPGAs is discussed in [9, 10].

Extensively used in the biomedical industry, this technique is efficiently implemented by FPGAs. It is used in ultrasound images, disease image authentication, and other types of biomedical images. These images become part of their diagnosis and treatment and radiologists and surgeons watermark these images to make sure that the title does not disappear or change hands without proper authorization. One method of doing digital image watermarking is discrete cosine transform (DCT) [11]. It transforms real signals into frequency domain values and operates on the real portion of complex signal, and the image is represented as a group of sinusoids with different frequencies and magnitudes. FPGA-based Zynq edge processing system is used, and the design flow is shown in Figure 9.3.

The first stage determines the specifications and requirements of the system. Tasks are partitioned programmable logic (PL) or processing system (PS) during the design. Then, the hardware and software components are developed and tested. Finally, the design process is completed when system integration and testing are done. Block diagram of DCT general architecture which is shown in Figure 9.4 consists of a hardware accelerator implemented by XilinxVivado, and it uses DCT technique.

9.4 COMPARATIVE ANALYSIS OF FPGA WITH OTHER ICS

Computing system that uses FPGA offer performance, parallelism, and flexibility, so they are preferred for many applications. Whereas, the general purpose or digital signal processing architecture has limited memory bandwidth and fewer arithmetic logic units. Moreover, FPGA system can be implemented for special applications, such as 3D real-time medical applications. As they contain enough logic cells and function units, FPGA chips can be customized into a circuit architecture like an application-specific integrated circuit (ASIC). Customized digital circuits are made and

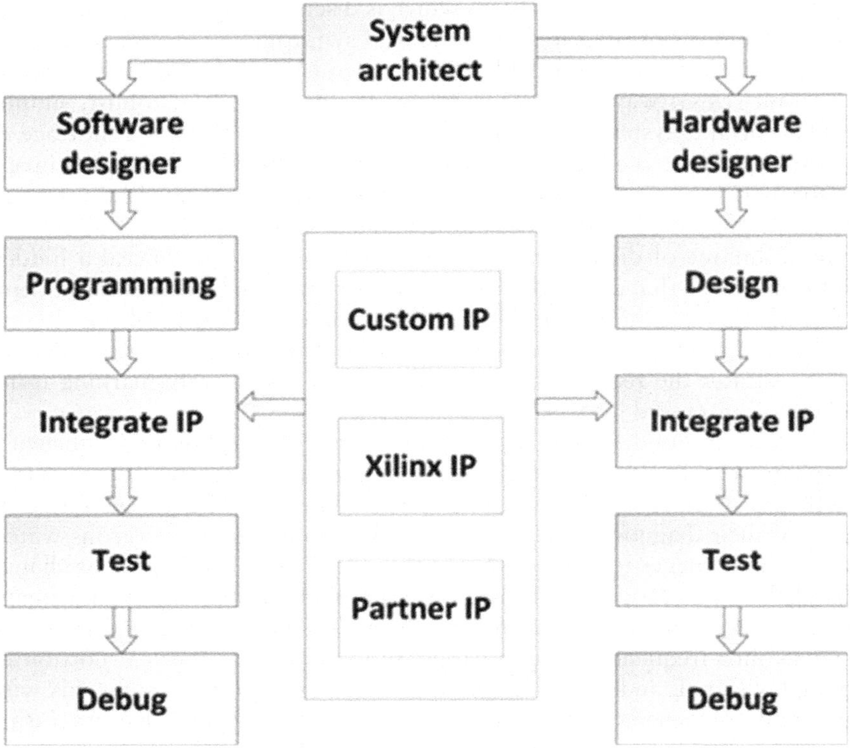

Figure 9.3 Hardware software co-design flow for digital watermarking.

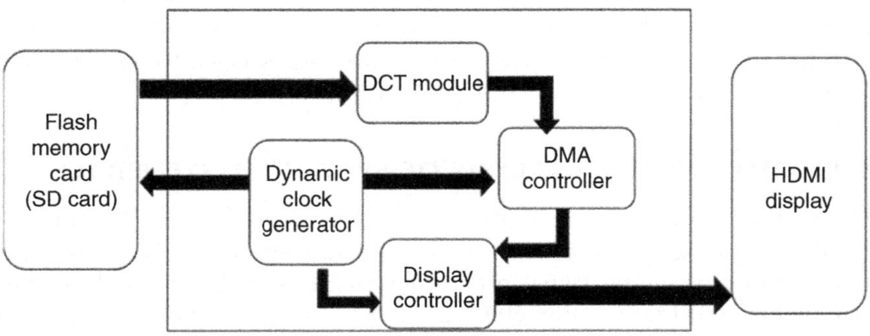

Figure 9.4 Block diagram of DCT hardware accelerator.

reconfigured by SRAM-based FPGA systems. This reconfigurability feature optimizes algorithm design and validation. Software algorithm can be conveniently ported to hardware implementation with the help of design tools available in FPGA programming language library. For example, using high level algorithm description Altera's DSP Builder is capable of generating netlist [12].

Small, wireless handy devices are available for mobile monitoring of patient's health such as heart pacing, blood pressure, and glucose tracking. These devices are made-up of discrete components and a CPU. Implementation of such devices is time-consuming and requires more resources. If custom blocks are made instead of standard blocks, then it will be efficient. One of the unique features of FPGA is that Application-specific Standard Product (ASSP) devices are integrated with it, and the processor is made into a single chip. All the application-specific features and other benefits can be integrated into a single chip and standard intellectual property blocks with platform designer. This feature provides many benefits like reusing previous internal engineering IP development efforts, leveraging additional FPGA and partner IP blocks, and separating application-specific analog input/output and sensor circuits onto modular daughter cards. Figure 9.5 shows an FPGA implementation on a programmable chip solution using a processor and custom logic. It includes user interface, application-specific analog functionality, and network connectivity.

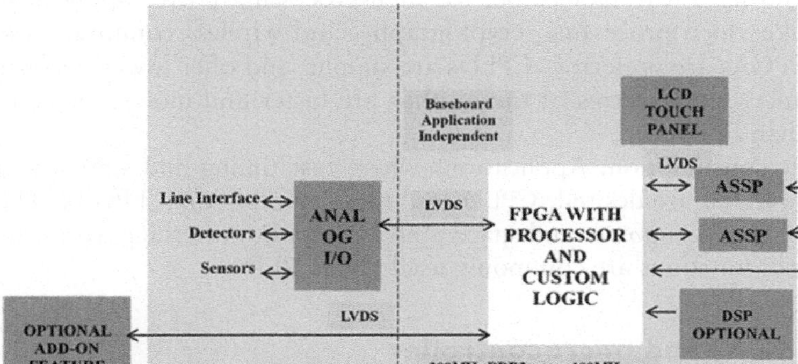

Figure 9.5 An FPGA implementation on a programmable chip solution using a processor and custom logic.

9.4.1 FPGAs and ASICs

Flexibility: FPGAs when deployed can be reconfigured and modified without changing the hardware. ASICs are fixed circuits that cannot be modified.

Development Time: Applications where quick implementation with new designs is required. FPGAs are better option, as ASICs development is a time-consuming process.

Power Efficiency: For battery-operated devices and power-constrained applications, ASICs becomes energy-efficient and consumes lesser power compared to FPGA.

Performance: ASICs are opted for a specific task and are capable of providing higher performance levels in comparison to general purpose processors or FPGAs.

9.4.2 FPGAs and CPLD

Architecture: FPGA architecture includes a matrix of configurable logic blocks (CLBs), interconnects, and input/output (I/O) blocks that perform complex tasks. Programmable switches interconnect several logic blocks in complex programmable logic device (CPLDs).

Flexibility: Any digital logic function can be performed by highly flexible FPGA. CPLDs are good for medium-sized logic circuits as they are smaller and less flexible than FPGAs.

Performance: FPGAs have better performance than CPLDs because they are more complex. They include logic resources, extended memory, and hardware blocks. So, for high-processing power applications like video processing, cryptography, and wireless communication FPGAs are preferred. CPLDs are simpler and offer lower performance, but in terms of timing they are faster and more predictable than FPGAs.

Power consumption: Applications where fast timing and simple logic function are desired, CPLDs are more suitable than FPGAs. They require less power and space than FPGAs. Bus interfacing and control functions are commonly used with CPLDs.

9.4.3 FPGAs and microcontroller

Flexibility and Reprogrammability: For applications which require frequent modifications, FPGAs are preferred. Whereas microcontroller is less flexible and less suitable for such applications.

Parallel Processing Capabilities: FPGAs are preferred for the execution of complex algorithms or tasks that require significant processing power, as they perform parallel processing. For high-speed data processing applications like signal processing and real-time data analysis, FPGAs are the best choice. Compared to FPGAs, microcontrollers usually have lower computational capabilities and limited memory.

High-Speed Performance: Quicker execution time is possible in FPGAs as hardware is customizable. So, FPGAs are preferred when a quick response is required.

Higher Cost and Complexity: FPGAs are less suitable for applications with budget constraints as skilled programmers are required. There are affordable prices for microcontrollers.

Higher Power Consumption: FPGA are high-power consuming devices because of features like parallel processing capabilities and the presence of numerous logic blocks. Microcontroller consumes less power. Table 9.1 shows a comparison of FPGA with other ICs.

9.5 ADVANTAGES OF USING FPGAS IN HEALTHCARE

Power Efficient and Portable: FPGA-based systems provide improved battery life and lower consumption as optimization for specific tasks is possible. It greatly reduces the power consumption compared to

Table 9.1 Comparison of FPGA with other ICs

	FPGA	*CPLD*	*ASIC*	*Microcontroller*
Architecture	Configurable logic blocks (CLBs)	Complex programmable logic devices (CPLDs)	Fixed and nonreprogrammed	Fixed hardware and execute instructions sequentially. They integrate RAM, ROM, I/O ports, and other peripherals
Power consumption	Moderate to high	Low	Lower power consumption	Use less power than FPGAs
Flexibility	Highly flexible	Less flexible	Fixed	They are designed for specific tasks which makes it less flexible
Cost	High	Low	Cost-effective for large-scale production	Cost-effective option for simple applications
Processing power	High-speed parallel processing capabilities	Low	High	Lower processing power compared to FPGAs

other processors performing the same task. For portable or battery-operated medical devices, this feature is crucial.

Flexibility and Customizability: FPGAs provide flexibility as new algorithms/protocols are easily upgraded. Unlike ASICs, which cannot be customized or reprogrammed, FPGAs save time and resources when changes or enhancements are required.

High Performance: FPGAs are ideal for computationally intensive tasks and real-time applications because of parallel processing, which helps to execute intricate algorithms and deliver timely outcomes.

Real-time Processing Capabilities: Real-time signal processing provides quick outcomes in FPGAs so that quicker diagnosis and prompt actions are possible. In medical applications, real-time processing is essential for patient monitoring and diagnosis.

9.6 LIMITATIONS OF USING FPGAS IN HEALTHCARE

Complexity in Design: Designing an FPGA-based healthcare system requires trained professional, and it is a time-consuming process. In healthcare, skilled engineers with medical domain knowledge are required.

Verification and Validation: Verification and validation techniques are required to find and correct faults and errors in the design. The development timeline might need to be further extended as a result of this requirement.

Standards for Safety and Regulatory Compliance: FPGA-based medical devices need to adhere to strict safety regulations and standards in order to ensure patient safety and data privacy. It can be difficult to obtain regulatory approval, particularly when using innovative FPGA-based technology.

Cost: Although FPGAs can be customized and reconfigured, compared to pre-made fixed hardware solutions, they are more costly.

Resource Utilization: Underutilization or excessive resource consumption in FPGAs will negatively impact the overall system performance. Resources must be properly used in order to get better results.

9.7 FPGA APPLICATIONS IN MEDICAL DIAGNOSTICS

To analyze and interpret patient data, FPGAs are used. Features of FPGAs like parallel processing, real-time signal analysis, and hardware acceleration have made it the best choice for medical diagnosis. Some examples of areas where FPGA is being used in diagnostic imaging, as shown in Figure 9.6.

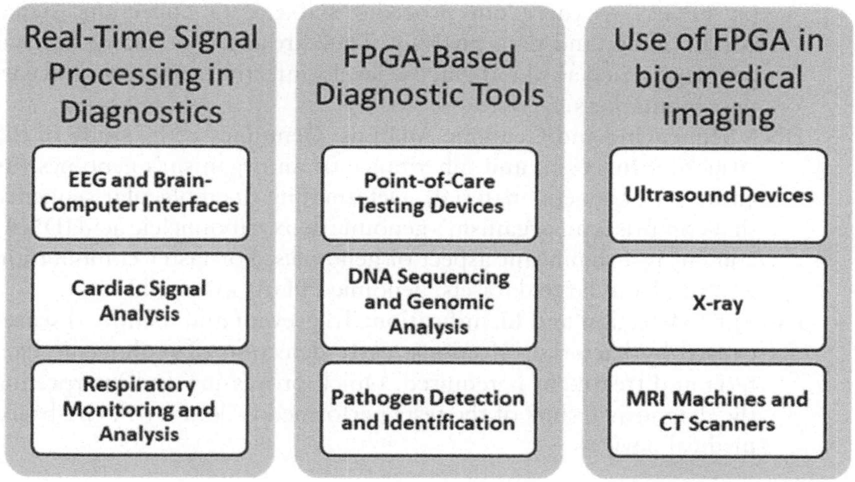

Figure 9.6 FPGA applications in medical diagnostics.

9.7.1 Real-time signal processing in diagnostics

Electroencephalogram (EEG) and Brain–Computer Interfaces (BCIs): Brain–computer interfaces (BCIs) are used to study electroencephalogram (EEG) signals. It provides information and control signals for the treatment of patients with disabilities like amyotrophic lateral sclerosis, spinal cord injuries, stroke, and muscular dystrophies. Real-time EEG signal processing is made possible by FPGA, which reduces noise, identifies aberrant patterns, and filters out background noise to aid in the diagnosis of diseases.

Cardiac Signal Analysis: In an emergency, prompt identification of potentially fatal heart conditions and abnormal cardiac rhythms is required. FPGAs provide real-time signal processing of ECG signals so that diagnosis is possible.

Respiratory Monitoring and Analysis: To monitor breathing patterns and lung infection, diagnostic devices are used, which process data from FPGA-based sensor. These sensors provide real-time analysis for early detection of any respiratory issue in patient.

9.7.2 Diagnostic tools using FPGA

Devices for Point-of-Care Testing: Point-of-Care Testing (POCT) is a testing method which is conducted close to the patient. It provides quick results so that appropriate treatment can be implemented. It can be performed by various healthcare professionals and, in some cases, even by patients themselves. These devices are based on FPGAs to carry out procedures like data collection, signal conditioning, and data analysis. They are used for many medical problems, such as blood glucose levels, infectious diseases, and cardiac biomarkers.

DNA Sequencing and Genomic Analysis: Genomics is the study of the structure, function, and inheritance of an organism's genomes (its entire set of genetic material). Determining the molecular sequence that comprises an organism's genomic deoxyribonucleic acid (DNA) content is a significant aspect of genomics. For faster computation and results in large datasets, genomic FPGAs are used [13].

Pathogen Detection and Identification: To prevent and identify diseases caused by bacterial infections, early detection of pathogenic bacteria and treatment is required. Quick processing and interpreting the diagnosis results of the tests performed is done by FPGA-based medical devices.

9.7.3 Use of FPGA in biomedical imaging

Medical imaging allows the visualization and investigation of the interior organs and bodily processes. FPGAs provide the ability to process data swiftly and optimize image quality, which helps in accurate diagnoses and better therapy. Imaging system uses FPGA in order to process real-time images and recreate it. Some examples are

a. **Ultrasound Devices:** With the use of FPGAs, ultrasound equipment can perform real-time beamforming and image processing, producing sharper, more detailed images that aid in diagnosis. The use of FPGAs is making modern ultrasound devices powerful tools for healthcare professionals.
b. **X-ray:** FPGAs provide better image quality and lower radiation doses for patients as it use advanced image filtering and noise reduction techniques.
c. **MRI Machines and CT Scanners:** FPGAs enable speedy image reconstruction for magnetic resonance imaging (MRI) and computed tomography (CT). So, the scan time is greatly reduced. While maintaining image quality, it also enables faster image acquisition and reconstruction.

Regarding medical imaging, the commonly used medical diagnostic method is image fusion. Previous studies [13–15] have shown that in image fusion, the time between patient diagnosis and therapy is shortened. The image integration is a useful technique for gathering data from the sensors, which helps in quick decision-making. The precise diagnosis of cancer stage and tumor response to radiation exposure is aided by the combination of various imaging modalities. These multimodality imaging systems have been the subject of the most important studies. Figure 9.7 describes the methodology, which is used to achieve the medical image fusion of two clinical figures. To perform image processing relevant to medical diagnostics, two medical images of the brain, such as a CT and MRI scan, are imported into the Matlab tool. By using the commands in the Matlab tool, both the images are converted into grayscale which every pixel in the digital representation carries data about the brightness of the light. In these kinds of photos, the contrast between the lightest white and the darkest black is usually all that is visible. To put differently, there are only three colors in the image: black, white, and gray, which is available in a range of shades. To process the pixels as binary values, these grayscale images are transformed into binary images. An image that has just two possible colors for each pixel—typically

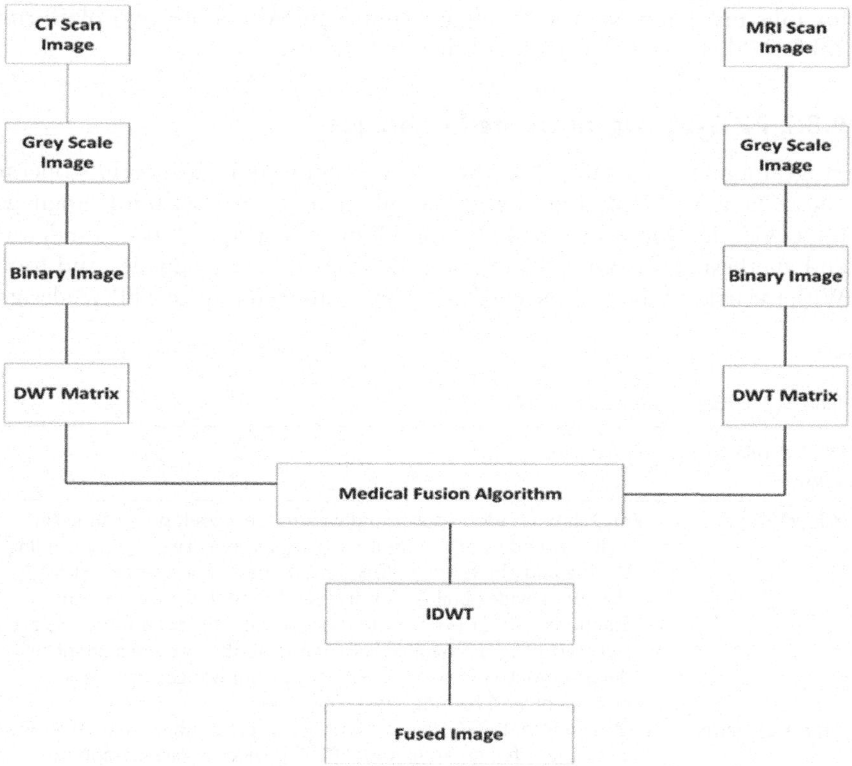

Figure 9.7 Flowchart of medical image fusion using MATLAB tool.

black and white—is called a binary image. When two colors are used in pixel art, it is sometimes called 1-Bit or 1bit.

9.8 FPGA DESIGN CONSIDERATIONS FOR MEDICAL IMAGING

In medical imaging systems for applications like image processing and real-time analysis, a broad range of hardware and software design considerations are required. We will discuss some important factors for an effective FPGA design.

9.8.1 Selection of development tools

FPGA development tools provide efficient development, testing, and debugging of designs. They are an important factor in the design and implementation of FPGAs. For applications like medical imaging, these development tools/platforms determine the processing capability, resources, and suitability for jobs involving medical imaging. Xilinx and Altera are two platforms. Table 9.2 lists the key features of these platforms.

9.8.2 FPGA programming languages

Programming languages offer a way to explain how FPGA circuits operate and behave. VHDL and Verilog are popular hardware description languages for FPGA development. For FPGA development, specific IDEs, simulators, and synthesis tools are available in addition to these languages and tools. With the help of these tools, engineers can create and improve FPGA designs

Table 9.2 FPGA development tools

FPGA development tools	*Key features*
Xilinx Vivado	With Xilinx Vivado's user-friendly interface, developers can easily write and edit code in multiple programming languages, including Verilog and VHDL, for FPGA development. For complex designs, Vivado provides built-in libraries and modules for common functions so that every time those commonly used functions are selected, programming is made easier. It also provides an inclusive development environment, which offers advanced synthesis, placement, and routing capabilities
Altera Quartus	To design Intel FPGA devices, Quartus is used, which is an effective instrument for creating Intel FPGA devices. It has a graphical interface with a library to provide sophisticated tools for synthesis and verification

Table 9.3 Languages for FPGA development

FPGA languages	*Key features*
Verilog	Hardware description language (HDL) is used for modelling and designing digital systems. It enables circuit behavior and structure to be described at different abstraction levels by designers. Hardware description languages (HDLs) like Verilog and VHDL can be used to program and configure FPGAs. With HDLs, the user can use a high-level language to explain how the digital circuit behaves. A netlist, or list of logic gates and interconnects that implement the circuit, is created by synthesizing the HDL code. The place-and-route tool is then used to map the netlist onto the FPGA architecture. The tool finds the best place for the logic gates and interconnects on the FPGA in order to satisfy the design's timing and resource requirements
VHDL	Another HDL for FPGA development is VHDL, which supports both sequential and concurrent programming styles and has a robust type system
System Verilog	System Verilog is an extension for Verilog that adds more features for assertions, verification, and test-bench development
Python	Python's simplicity and versatility make it a popular choice for automating FPGA workflows and generating hardware designs

more quickly, which eventually results in improved performance and a shorter time to market. New versions, updates, improvements, and continuous evolution of FPGA development tools and languages are in progress. Table 9.3 gives languages developed for FPGA.

9.8.3 Resource management and optimization

Resource Utilization: For medical image processing, resource allocation of logic gates, memory, and DSP blocks must be done efficiently for optimal usage of resources. For efficient resource utilization, pipelining and parallelization are two strategies that are used.

Power Efficiency: FPGA designs aim at efficient power consumption, as power consumption is a critical concern. Particularly in high-frequency applications or resource-demanding designs, FPGAs utilize a lot of power. In portable medical devices, power consumption is an issue. To reduce power consumption, strategies like clock gating, dynamic scaling of frequency and voltage, and power design methodologies are preferred.

9.8.4 Safety and reliability concerns

Redundancy and Fault Tolerance: In medical imaging applications, designers should make a reliable system. For smooth operations in monitoring and diagnosis systems, redundancy check, and fault-tolerance mechanism must be adopted. These fault-tolerant techniques help in the proper functioning of medical imaging systems in real time.

Testing and Verification: In imaging systems based on FPGA simulation, verification and testing are required. These steps are necessary for identification and rectification of the design.

9.8.5 Compliance with regulatory standards

Medical Device Regulations: For patient safety and data security, medical imaging devices must follow safety regulation guidelines. FPGA-based systems must strictly follow safety standards and FDA guidelines.

Data Security and Privacy: Medical data needs to be protected from unauthorized access and security threats, as patient information is confidential. Strong access control, data handling protocols, and encryption protocols must be adopted.

9.8.6 Challenges and ethical considerations

While FPGAs offer significant advantages in the field of medical imaging, they also present various challenges and raise ethical considerations that must be addressed to ensure their responsible and effective use.

Privacy and security issues in medical imaging

Data Security: Medical picture transmission and storage must be protected from unauthorized access and potential breaches since they frequently contain sensitive patient data. Real-time data processing using FPGAs calls for strong access control and encryption protocols.

Cybersecurity: FPGAs are vulnerable to cybersecurity threats, including malware and hardware attacks. Ensuring the security of FPGA-based medical imaging systems is paramount to prevent data tampering or system compromise.

Ethical use of medical data

Informed Consent: Strict informed consent guidelines must be followed when collecting and using medical imaging data for study or diagnosis. Patients should be fully informed about how and why their data will be utilized.

Data Ownership: Determining the ownership of medical imaging data, especially when it is used for research or training AI models, can be a complex issue. Ethical frameworks need to address who has the right to use and benefit from such data.

Regulatory and legal framework

Compliance: FPGAs used in medical imaging must adhere to legal requirements by the Health Insurance Portability and Accountability Act (HIPAA) in the United States or the General Data Protection Regulation (GDPR) in the European Union. To prevent legal repercussions, compliance with these requirements must be guaranteed.

Liability: Liability issues arise from the usage of FPGAs in medical imaging in the event of mistakes or malfunctions. For patient safety and legal remedies, defining precise legal obligations and accountability for FPGA-based systems is essential.

Ethical considerations in AI integration

Bias and Fairness: When FPGAs are integrated with AI algorithms for image analysis, ethical concerns related to bias and fairness in AI models become pertinent. Efforts must be made to reduce bias and ensure equitable healthcare outcomes.

Transparency: Ensuring transparency in AI decision-making processes is crucial. Healthcare practitioners should be able to understand and interpret AI-driven diagnostic recommendations to maintain the human touch in patient care

9.9 CONCLUSION

From aerospace to healthcare, from the use in blockchain technology to telecommunication networks, FPGAs are providing immense potential for innovative and advancement in technology. FPGAs can be optimized for power efficiency because of their flexibility, which makes them appropriate for battery-powered devices where energy consumption is critical. In this chapter, we have discussed how high processing power, reprogrammability, configurability, flexible nature, and real-time operations are becoming the key factors for high demand of FPGAs. The chapter presents how FPGAs have revolutionized medical imaging systems and healthcare industry. Image processing using FPGA provides powerful and affective results is also discussed in this chapter. FPGA accelerates, provides real-time results, and enables advanced functionalities image processing applications. Real-time applications such as medical imaging, surveillance, autonomous vehicles, and quality control have greatly benefited from FPGA-based image processing. Future advancements in FPGA hardware, integration of AI and machine learning algorithms, and addressing scalability and flexibility challenges will shape the future of FPGA-based image processing systems. In conclusion, FPGA-based image processing provides a robust and efficient solution for demanding image processing tasks. Embracing FPGA technology unlocks new possibilities and drives innovation in the field, meeting the growing demands for faster and more sophisticated image processing capabilities.

REFERENCES

[1] K. Raymenants, I. H. Huang, N. Goelen, P. Janssen, N. Van Tichelen, D. Burton, and J. Tack. "Clinical validation of the VIPUN™ gastric monitoring system versus manometry for the evaluation of gastric motility." *Neurogastroenterol Motil.*, vol.36, no. 6, e14783, 2024. doi: 10.1111/nmo.14783.

[2] B. M. Quinn, Y. Gao, U. Mahmood, et al. "Patient-adapted organ absorbed dose and effective dose estimates in pediatric 18F-FDG positron emission tomography/computed tomography studies." *BMC Med Imaging*, vol. 20, p. 9, 2020. https://doi.org/10.1186/s12880-020-0415-4

[3] V. Dakić, M. Kovač, and J. Slovinac. "Evolving high-performance computing data centers with Kubernetes, performance analysis, and dynamic workload placement based on machine learning scheduling." *Electronics*, vol. 13, no. 13, p. 2651, 2024. https://doi.org/10.3390/electronics13132651

[4] D. Merkel. "Docker: lightweight Linux containers for consistent development and deployment." *Linux J.*, vol. 2014, p. 239, 2014.

[5] H. Gantikow, S. Walter, and C. Reich. Rootless containers with Podman for HPC. In High performance computing: ISC high performance 2020 International Workshops, Frankfurt, Germany, June 21–25, 2020, Revised Selected Papers. Springer, Berlin, Heidelberg, pp. 343–354, 2020. https://doi.org/10.1007/978-3-030-59851-8_23

[6] S. Agarwal, A. Rani, V. Singh, and A. P. Mittal. FPGA Based wireless emergency medical system for developing countries, *2015 Annual Global Online Conference on Information and Computer Technology (GOCICT)*, Louisville, KY, USA, 2015, pp. 80–84. doi: 10.1109/GOCICT.2015.23

[7] H. Pfister, J. Hardenbergh, J. Knittel, H. Lauer, and L. Seiler, "The volume pro real-time ray-casting system." *Comput. Graph.*, vol. 33(Annual Conference Series), pp. 251–260, 1999.

[8] M. Levoy. "Efficient ray tracing for volume data." *ACM Trans. Graphics*, vol. 9, no. 3, pp. 245–261, 1990.

[9] M. F. Mohammed El Birek, M. F. L. Abdullah, A. A. M. Ukasha, and A. A. Elrowayati. "Digital image watermarking based on joint (DCT-DWT) and Arnold transform." *Int. J. Security Appl.*, vol. 10, no. 5, pp.107–118, 2016.

[10] R. Phade, R. Mahajan, S. Mankar, and P. Patil. "Digital image watermarking using DCT and ZIP compression technique." *Glob. J. Comput. Sci. Technol. Graphics Vis.*, vol. 13, no. 3, 2013.

[11] V. Swetha, "Design of DCT hardware accelerator using FPGA for medical image authentication." In 2023 International Conference on Bio Signals, Images, and Instrumentation (ICBSII). doi:10.1109/ICBSII58188.2023.10181061

[12] J. Xing, S. Liu, and W. Zhao. FPGA-accelerated real-time volume rendering for 3D medical image, *2010 3rd International Conference on Biomedical Engineering and Informatics*, Yantai, China, 2010, pp. 273–276. doi: 10.1109/BMEI.2010.5639475

13) R. Phani Vidyadhar et al. "FPGA implementation of medical image fusion using PCA." In 2023, 9th International Conference on Advanced Computing and Communication Systems (ICACCS).

[14] S. Sreekrishna Yadav and V. Mittal, "FPGA Implementation of segmented feature fusion in MRI images using wavelet." In 2019 International Conference on Communication and Electronic Systems (ICCES), Coimbatore, India, 2019, pp. 1946–1951. doi:10.1109/ICCES45898.2019.9002032

[15] M. A. Mohamed and B. M. El-Den. "Implementation of image fusion techniques for multi-focus images using FPGA." In 2011 28th National Radio Science Conference (NRSC), Cairo, Egypt, 2011, pp. 1–11. doi:10.1109/NRSC.2011.5873618

QUESTIONS AND ANSWERS

Q1) Describe HPC and give at least two examples of its use in biomedical applications. Using supercomputers and parallel processing techniques to solve complex computational problems beyond the capabilities of standard computers is known as high-performance computing.

Q2) What distinguishes Docker from Kubernetes and describes its use in high-performance computing. 2. What roles do Kubernetes and Docker play in the container ecosystem?

Q3) Describe the difficulties encountered when utilizing HPC containers.

Q4) How does vector offloading improve application performance?

Q5) Explain CPU, GPU, and FPGA.

Q6) Differentiate between (i) CPU and GPU, (ii) CPU and FPGA, (iii) GPU and FPGA

Chapter 10

Quantum computing in medical informatics

Unlocking revolutionary potential

10.1 QUANTUM COMPUTING AND HEALTHCARE

The convergence of quantum computing (QC) and medical informatics presents a remarkable opportunity to address key challenges in healthcare and revolutionize patient care. From the expedited discovery of life-saving drugs to the precision analysis of genomic data, QC has the potential to transform the entire healthcare ecosystem. By leveraging the power of quantum information, researchers and healthcare professionals can not only accelerate the pace of discovery but also enhance diagnostics, improve treatment outcomes, and ensure data security and privacy.

10.1.1 Fundamental concepts

Qubits: In QC, qubits are the fundamental units of information that can exist in a superposition of states. Unlike classical bits that can be in a definite state of 0 or 1, qubits are represented by vectors in a complex vector space and can be in a linear combination of the 0 and 1 states. They can be manipulated through quantum gates to perform quantum computations.

Superposition: Superposition refers to the ability of a qubit to be in a coherent combination of multiple states simultaneously. In mathematical terms, superposition is represented by a linear combination of basis states. A qubit in superposition can be in a state that is a weighted combination of both 0 and 1, denoted as 0 and 1. The superposition allows quantum algorithms to explore multiple computational paths in parallel, potentially providing exponential speedup in certain applications.

Entanglement: Entanglement is a quantum phenomenon that occurs when two or more qubits become correlated in such a way that their states cannot be described independently. Entangled qubits are in a joint state that cannot be expressed as a simple product of individual qubit states. Measuring one entangled qubit instantly

 DOI: 10.1201/9781003503033-10

determines the state of the other, regardless of their spatial separation. This nonlocal correlation enables quantum computers to perform highly interconnected operations and enables applications such as quantum teleportation and quantum cryptography.

However, harnessing the potential of QC in medical informatics is not without its challenges. The current limitations of quantum hardware, such as fragile qubits and high error rates, pose significant obstacles. Additionally, scalability remains a critical concern as quantum systems strive to process large-scale healthcare datasets efficiently. Overcoming these hurdles requires interdisciplinary collaboration, innovative algorithms, and advancements in quantum technology.

This write-up explores the revolutionary potential of QC in medical informatics, discussing specific applications and showcasing the impact that quantum information can have on healthcare. By delving into the advancements and ongoing research, we can uncover the exciting possibilities that lie at the intersection of QC and medical informatics. We can create a future where quantum technologies become an integral part of healthcare. This will lead to a new era of precise and personalized medicine, resulting in better treatments and improved outcomes for patients. Table 10.1 gives comparison between classical and quantum computing.

Table 10.1 Comparison between classical and quantum computing

	Classical computing	*Quantum computing*
Basic unit	Binary bit (1 or 0)	Qbit (vector)
State	Two possible exclusive states	Two simultaneous possible states
Computing	Logical operation	Unitary operation
Description	Truth table (true/false)	Unitary matrix
Direction	Most gates run forward	Gates are reversible
Power increases	Linearly with no. of transistors	Exponentially in proportion to the no. of qubits
Storage	n-bit storage holds 1 value. From 0 to $2^n - 1$	n-qubit storage holds 2^n value
Computation approach	Sequential processing	Parallel processing
Read	0 or 1, deterministic	0 or 1, probabilistic
Error rates	Lower	Higher
Information delivered	Can be copied without being disturbed	Cannot be copied or read without being disturbed
Security	Lower	Higher
Computation/communication cost	Higher as computing or communication volume increases	Lower as computing or communication volume increases
Computing purpose	General purpose	Optimization and factoring
Practical Implementation	Widely available and practical	Still in early stages, facing technical challenges

10.2 ROLE OF QUANTUM COMPUTING ADVANCING HEALTHCARE

QC has the potential to revolutionize healthcare by enabling faster and more accurate analysis of complex medical data. Its computational power can accelerate drug discovery, optimize treatment plans, and advance personalized medicine by processing and interpreting large-scale genomic datasets. QC can contribute to the progress of healthcare as shown in Figure 10.1.

Molecular Simulations: Quantum-based healthcare systems leverage artificial intelligence (AI), machine learning (ML), deep learning (DL), and optimization technologies to address computationally complex challenges, particularly in the domain of molecular simulations [1]. These simulations involve intricate relationships among highly coupled components, such as chemical compounds with multiple protons, and offer significant potential for efficient healthcare processing [2]. Consequently, QC provides a promising solution for overcoming traditional computing limitations, including computational power and resource requirements, enabling enhanced management of molecular simulations within healthcare systems.

Diagnosis Pricing Analysis: The application of QC improves risk analysis in diagnosis pricing by accurately forecasting a patient's current health status and predicting their likelihood of developing a specific illness. This leads to

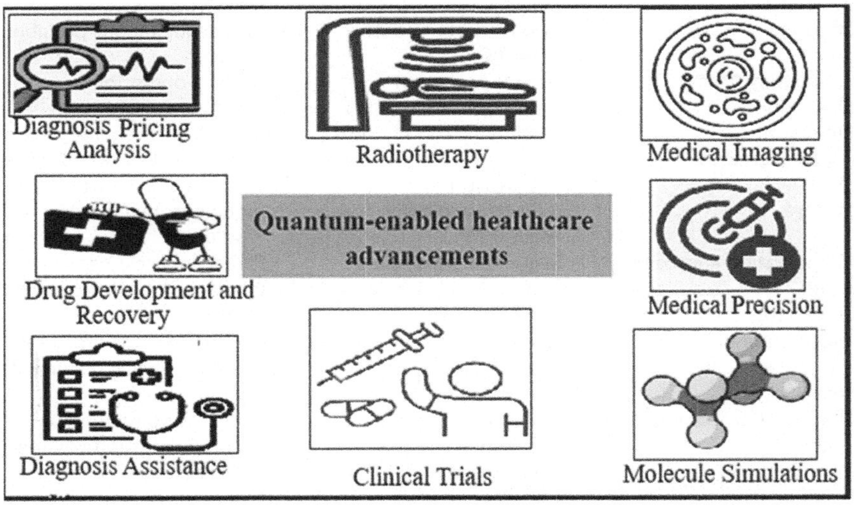

Figure 10.1 Quantum-enabled health care advancements.

optimized insurance pricing and rates. Additionally, when combined with quantum risk models, it enables a detailed examination of illness risks at a specific level, facilitating accurate computation of pricing and financial risks. Furthermore, QC enhances the accuracy of classifying and identifying malicious behavior in medical claims through advanced pattern recognition techniques, surpassing traditional approaches [3].

Clinical Trials: Clinical studies focusing on coronaviruses and their variations, as well as other diseases like AIDS and TB, play a crucial role in identifying the necessary tools and strategies to combat chronic and complex illnesses. The coronavirus, which is a component of the SARS virus, poses a significant threat to human health today [4]. While pharmaceutical companies have developed several vaccines, there is currently a lack of vaccines specifically designed for children aged 0 to 18. Clinical trials serve as an essential method for verifying and enhancing the effectiveness and reliability of medications and vaccines. Typically, these trials involve testing on animals or human subjects, but the use of in silico tests, where quantum computers can simulate human responses, could potentially eliminate the need for such carriers [5].

Medical Precision: The primary goal of medical precision is to provide personalized treatment tailored to an individual patient's specific disease. In the future, patient-centric medical care will be crucial to addressing the complexities of the human biological system. However, the cost of medication only accounts for 10-20% of healthcare expenses, while the remaining 80–90% is attributed to other factors such as socioeconomic conditions, environmental influences, and health-related behavioral challenges. Furthermore, traditional drug-based therapies may not yield effective results for certain individuals, potentially leading to adverse drug reactions and even fatalities. Therefore, early intervention and preventive measures can improve healthcare outcomes and reduce costs through the use of QC [3]. While predicting future disease risks using electronic health records can be accomplished using conventional methods, challenges such as noise, data quality, dataset size, and complexity often arise. Quantum-based ML techniques enhance the precision of early disease detection. Additionally, healthcare practitioners can leverage medical devices for continuous monitoring, allowing for the timely identification of diseases and the provision of appropriate treatments. Quantum ML facilitates patient-centric treatment by enabling continuous data streaming through medical devices, ensuring uninterrupted services for patients.

Drug Development and Recovery: QC plays a crucial role in healthcare by enabling medical professionals to conduct research at the atomic level, particularly in complex molecular interactions [2]. This technology allows for exploration in various areas, including diagnosis, drug discovery, therapy, and analysis. With advancements in QC, it is possible to simulate interactions with proteins within the human genome. However, alongside QC, AI approaches are extensively utilized to aid in patient diagnosis. ML algorithms, specifically pattern recognition, are trained on large-scale datasets and can accurately analyze current data based on the patterns learned during training. This combination of QC and AI empowers healthcare professionals to make rapid decisions based on appropriate patterns, contributing to improved patient treatment and diagnosis.

Diagnosis Assistance: QC has emerged as a valuable tool in healthcare by enabling early disease detection, leading to reduced healthcare costs and improved diagnosis and treatment outcomes [3]. For example, the early detection of diseases like cancer and COVID-19 can significantly decrease treatment expenses. Traditional diagnostic tools such as X-rays, magnetic resonance imaging (MRIs), and CT scans are computationally intensive and costly devices that are continuously advancing [6]. However, these devices face challenges related to noise, image quality, reproducibility, and safety. QC helps address these challenges by enhancing medical image analysis through techniques like edge detection, thereby improving computer-aided diagnosis. Additionally, the classification of cells based on biochemical and physical characteristics requires substantial computational resources due to the large number of predictor variables involved [7]. Quantum-enhanced ML techniques, such as quantum vector space, can effectively address these challenges and enhance single-cell diagnosis. The integration of QC allows for more efficient and accurate diagnosis, reduces the need for repetitive testing and treatment, and facilitates continuous monitoring of individual health status.

Medical Imaging: In this section, various procedures related to medical image processing are introduced, encompassing image generation, visualization, analysis, and manipulation. The term "processing biomedical images" refers to the manipulation of digital images within the realm of biomedical sciences. The key domains of digital image processing in the field of biomedical sciences are depicted in Figure 10.2.

Image construction encompasses the entire process of obtaining an image and creating a digital pattern. In the field of medicine, medical images have played a crucial role in diagnostics, treatment planning, and follow-up investigations since the advent of X-rays. These images are utilized for learning, documentation, and analysis, providing insights into the morphology, biological aspects, and physical properties of various image data dimensions [8]. A wide range of imaging techniques have been explored, involving the transmission, absorption, or refraction of light, scattering, temperature, sound, or rotation. Figure 10.3 highlights the tradeoff between contrast and image quality for different imaging modalities. It is important to note that algorithms designed for a specific imaging modality may not

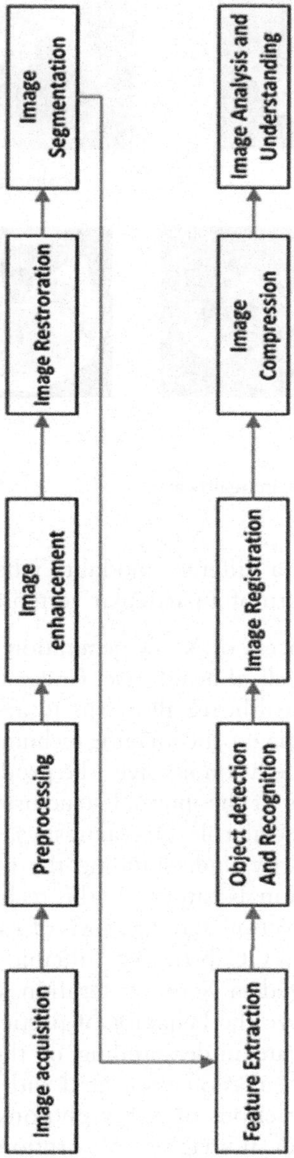

Figure 10.2 Various stages of image manipulation.

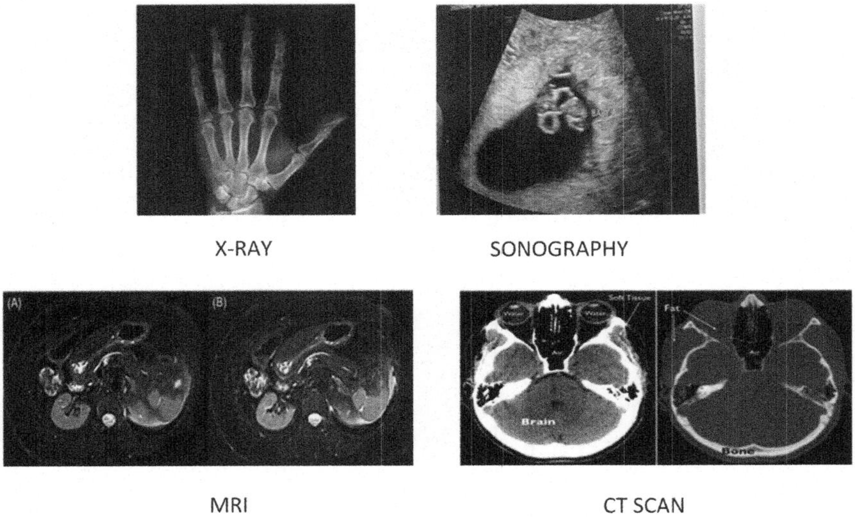

Figure 10.3 Imaging modalities in healthcare.

be directly applicable to a different modality when representing a specific pattern, such as the pattern of a particular vertebra.

X-Ray Imaging: The process of X-ray generation and interaction is of significant importance in medical healthcare. Understanding these processes in the context of medical healthcare allows us to appreciate the fundamental principles that underpin diagnostic imaging techniques and their applications in patient care. X-ray generation involves the production of photons, which are used to create images of the internal structures of the human body [8]. These images play a crucial role in diagnostics, treatment planning, and follow-up examinations. By understanding the principles of X-ray generation, healthcare professionals can utilize this technology to obtain detailed images that aid in the detection and diagnosis of various medical conditions.

In medical healthcare, QC provides valuable insights into the underlying mechanisms involved in X-ray generation and interaction. It allows us to simulate and analyze the behavior of particles at the quantum level, providing a more accurate understanding of the energy levels, electron interactions, and photon emission associated with X-rays.

Furthermore, the interactions of X-ray photons with human tissues and organs are critical in medical imaging. Absorption and scattering processes are key phenomena to consider. Absorption occurs when X-ray photons are fully absorbed by the body tissues, and this effect is utilized to generate contrasted images that highlight specific structures or abnormalities.

Scattering, on the other hand, involves the redirection of X-ray photons due to their interaction with atoms in the body. Understanding scattering phenomena helps healthcare professionals interpret X-ray images correctly and eliminate unwanted scattered radiation that may obscure diagnostic information.

By incorporating the principles of QC into the understanding of X-ray generation and interaction, medical healthcare professionals can optimize imaging techniques, improve image quality, and enhance diagnostic accuracy. This, in turn, leads to better patient outcomes, more precise treatment planning, and a deeper understanding of the human body's internal structures and functions.

Computed Technology: By leveraging QC, we can develop more efficient algorithms for image reconstruction in computed tomography (CT) scans, leading to faster and more accurate diagnoses. Quantum sensors and detectors can enhance image acquisition, resulting in higher-resolution images and improved visualization of anatomical structures [9]. Quantum ML (QML) algorithms enable automated analysis of medical images, aiding in the detection of abnormalities and the quantitative analysis of image features. Additionally, QC offers advanced encryption and secure communication protocols to protect patient data, ensuring privacy and regulatory compliance. Integrating QC into medical imaging has the potential to improve diagnostic accuracy, enhance patient outcomes, and safeguard sensitive medical information [8].

Magnetic Resonance Imaging (MRI): QC offers exciting possibilities for revolutionizing medical healthcare, specifically in the field of MRI. It can optimize data acquisition, improve image reconstruction, study relaxation processes, and enhance data analysis through QML.

By leveraging quantum principles, data acquisition during MRI scans can be made more efficient, leading to faster diagnosis and treatment decisions. Quantum-inspired algorithms enable better image reconstruction, even with incomplete or sparse data, resulting in high-quality images for accurate medical analysis.

Quantum simulators provide insights into the complex relaxation processes involved in MRI, aiding in pulse sequence design and imaging parameter optimization. Additionally, QML algorithms facilitate automated image analysis, including segmentation, classification, and disease detection, improving diagnostic capabilities.

Integrating QC into MRI holds promise for optimizing data acquisition, enhancing image quality, and advancing diagnostic abilities in medical healthcare. Although practical implementation is still under research, its potential impact on patient care is significant.

Ultrasound: Ultrasound imaging in medical healthcare relies on the principle of sound wave reflection [9]. While QC itself may not have direct applications in ultrasound imaging, it can indirectly contribute to advancements in this technology. Quantum algorithms can enhance image processing and analysis, leading to improved diagnostic accuracy and feature extraction in ultrasound images. Quantum techniques such as data compression and encryption can enhance data processing and storage capabilities, facilitating efficient sharing and analysis of ultrasound data. Quantum simulations offer insights into optimizing ultrasound imaging techniques and improving image quality by modelling sound wave interactions with tissues. Although direct integration of QC in ultrasound is still developing, ongoing research holds promise for transformative advancements in medical imaging, resulting in better patient outcomes and enhanced healthcare delivery.

Radiotherapy: Radiotherapy is a crucial cancer treatment method that utilizes electromagnetic energy to eliminate cancer cells while sparing healthy tissues [10]. However, its success relies on precise computations to accurately target tumors and optimize treatment effectiveness. QC offers potential advancements in simulating radiotherapy procedures by leveraging its parallel processing capabilities. QC enables multiple simulations to be performed simultaneously, utilizing concepts like superposition and entanglement. By harnessing QC for radiotherapy simulations, researchers and medical practitioners can explore a wider range of treatment scenarios and devise personalized approaches within compressed timeframes. This has the potential to improve treatment planning, enhance patient outcomes, and enable tailored therapeutic interventions. However, the practical implementation and validation of QC in radiotherapy simulations are still in early stages, requiring further research and development to fully realize its potential in this field [11].

10.3 QUANTUM COMPUTING REQUIREMENTS IN HEALTHCARE

The healthcare sector has shown great potential for incorporating QC technologies to address various challenges and advance medical research and patient care. QC offers unique capabilities that can revolutionize areas such as drug discovery, genomics, precision medicine, medical imaging, and healthcare optimization. However, the integration of QC into the healthcare sector requires addressing certain requirements as shown in Figure 10.4.

Computational Power: QC offers enhanced computational power by utilizing the principles of quantum physics. It surpasses the capabilities of classical computers in solving complex problems, making it valuable in the healthcare sector. Quantum computers leverage multidimensional spaces to represent and process large-scale problems. The Grover's search algorithm

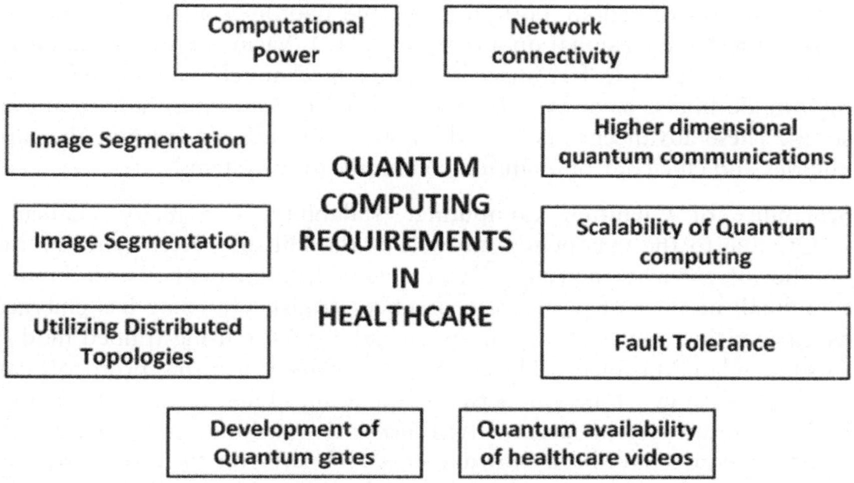

Figure 10.4 Quantum computing needs in the healthcare industry.

exemplifies the computational efficiency of QC, allowing for faster search operations compared to classical algorithms [11]. For instance, searching through a trillion items can be accomplished in just one second with a quantum computer. These advancements have the potential to revolutionize healthcare by enabling faster data analysis, precision medicine, and drug discovery. Despite their current large size, ongoing developments aim to shrink the physical footprint of quantum computers while maintaining their computational power.

High Speed Connectivity: High-speed connectivity networks like 5G and upcoming 6G are revolutionizing healthcare by providing robust connectivity for smart medical devices. QC, a rapidly advancing technology, can leverage these networks to deliver novel services and solutions in healthcare. Quantum walks, inspired by random walks, offer a universal processing model and inherent cryptographic features that can be utilized for secure data management in healthcare. By integrating quantum technologies with 5G networks, innovative cryptographic protocols and applications can be developed to enhance data security and enable secure storage and transmission of healthcare information. This research area holds great potential in addressing the evolving security challenges in healthcare and improving overall performance in data management.

Higher Dimensional Quantum Communications: High-dimensional quantum communication is a growing field in quantum information technology. It utilizes an enlarged Hilbert space to achieve higher information capacity and better noise resilience. Researchers have explored multiple photonic degrees of freedom, both in integrated photonics and bulk optics, to generate high-dimensional quantum states [12]. Various types of channels, including single-mode, free-space links, aquatic channels, and multicore and multimode fibers, have been investigated for transmitting these quantum states. These advancements have the potential to greatly improve the capabilities and efficiency of quantum communication systems.

Scalability of Quantum Computing: Scalability is a major challenge in QC due to the exponential growth of the Hilbert vector space as the number of particles increases. Exact diagonalization methods are limited to a small number of particles in practice. Transfer learning has emerged as a promising approach to improve scalability by reusing trained models to solve related problems. Physics-inspired transfer learning protocols can leverage features of neural network quantum states to describe many-body quantum systems accurately. Boltzmann machines and other simple neural networks have been shown to effectively describe the ground state of quantum systems [13]. Transfer learning enables the transfer of neural network quantum state parameters from an initial system to a larger system of similar characteristics, enhancing scalability. Physics-inspired protocols can be employed for transfer learning, but achieving efficiency and effectiveness as system size grows remains a challenge.

Fault Tolerance: Fault tolerance is of utmost importance in quantum computers due to the fragile and entangled nature of their components. It ensures the robustness of quantum computers and enables the reliable solving of quantum problems, ensuring the fidelity of quantum computations. This capability allows quantum computers to tackle computational challenges that are difficult for traditional computing systems.

However, errors in qubits or in the measurement mechanisms can have devastating consequences during computations. The error correction system itself faces significant challenges. One approach to monitor these systems is by using ancillary qubits, which continuously analyze logical errors for detection and correction. While ancillary qubits have shown promise, errors in the ancillary qubits can propagate to the qubits, introducing additional errors in the operations.

Embedding error correction codes among the qubits is a viable solution to address this issue. This approach allows the system to correct the code when errors occur in certain bits. It mitigates the propagation of faulty errors by ensuring that a single faulty gate or time stamp results in a single faulty gate. By reducing the likelihood of catastrophic failures, this method contributes to the robustness and reliability of quantum computers.

Quantum Availability of Healthcare System: The availability of quantum computers in the healthcare system poses unique challenges compared to traditional computing systems. Unlike traditional systems where computing is performed near the location of devices, quantum computers are typically located at remote facilities. This presents difficulties in accessing virtual machines hosted on quantum computers.

To ensure the availability of quantum computers in the healthcare system, careful consideration is needed. It is necessary to establish robust and reliable mechanisms for accessing and utilizing virtual machines on quantum computers. This may involve the development of secure and efficient remote access protocols, network infrastructure optimization, and implementation of redundancy measures to mitigate potential downtime.

Addressing the availability requirements of quantum computers in the healthcare system is crucial to ensure seamless access and utilization of QC resources. It requires careful planning, technological advancements, and collaboration between QC providers and healthcare organizations to overcome the unique challenges associated with the remote nature of QC facilities.

Deployment of Quantum Gates: The deployment of quantum gates is a critical requirement in layered QC, where each gate performs specific operations on quantum systems. However, hardware limitations, such as the no-cloning theorem, pose challenges in coordinating multiple gates simultaneously within a quantum system. To address these challenges, researchers have proposed various techniques and algorithms [14, 15].

Furthermore, innovative approaches have been introduced to program gate-model quantum computers without considering error correction and compilation requirements. These methods utilize parameterized unitaries to generate quantum states, enabling efficient quantum computations.

In the realm of multicomputer architectures, a quantum multicomputer optimized for Shor's factoring algorithm has been developed. This architecture employs numerous interconnected nodes linked through a quantum bus, with a focus on optimizing the factorization process. Various optimization techniques are utilized to reduce latency and improve circuit paths, enhancing overall performance. These advancements in quantum gate deployment and optimization techniques contribute to enhancing the efficiency and efficacy of QC systems [16]. They enable the resolution of complex problems and the attainment of desired outcomes in diverse applications.

Utilizing Distributed Topologies: Distributed topologies present a promising solution for realizing large-scale quantum computers, addressing the physical challenges associated with the distribution of quantum states. The deployment of a quantum bus for communication, coupled with distributed execution of quantum algorithms and error-correction techniques, is essential for achieving efficient distributed computation, communication, and quantum error correction in quantum applications.

To facilitate the management of arbitrary quantum hardware and ensure effective communication, the establishment of system area networks becomes crucial, supported by appropriate communication protocols. Furthermore, the development of quantum metropolitan area networks and quantum wide area networks emerges as viable options for scaling up QC capabilities.

Researchers have conducted experimental evaluations of diverse quantum error correction models to evaluate their scalability in the context of QC [17]. Additionally, the pursuit of a million-qubit quantum computer has highlighted the need for extensive component integration and reliable hardware technologies, substantiated through comprehensive simulation and modelling tools [18].

Overall, these research efforts contribute significantly to the advancement of distributed QC systems, facilitating efficient communication, robust error correction, and the realization of large-scale quantum architectures.

Physical Implementation Requirements: The physical implementation of quantum computers can be classified into four generations based on their characteristics and technologies used [17].

First-generation quantum computers are implemented using ion traps, with physical speeds in the kilohertz (kHz) range and logical speeds in the hertz (Hz) range [18–24]. These systems have a footprint size in the range of millimeters to centimeters.

Second-generation quantum computers employ distributed diamonds, superconducting quantum circuits, and linear optical strategies. They operate at physical speeds in the megahertz (MHz) range, while their logical speeds are in the kilohertz (kHz) range. The footprint size of these computers is typically in the millimeter range.

Third-generation quantum computers utilize monolithic diamonds, donor-based systems, and quantum dot technologies. They achieve logical speeds in the megahertz (MHz) range and physical speeds in the gigahertz (GHz) range and have a footprint size in the micrometer (um) range.

Fourth-generation quantum computers are based on topological QC, an evolutionary stage where quantum error correction is not required due to natural protection against decoherence. One open problem in this generation is the realization of distributed QC using anionic particles across distant points.

In terms of practical realizations, Monz et al. propose a scalable implementation of the Shor algorithm on quantum computers, focusing on the factorization algorithm. While various implementations of this algorithm have been demonstrated using different quantum computer architectures, the general scalability of the algorithm remains a topic of discussion.

In another study, the authors propose an improved operation of exchange-coupled semiconductor quantum dots, contributing to advancements in quantum dot-based QC.

These advancements in physical implementation offer insights into the scalability, efficiency, and performance of quantum computers across different generations and technologies.

Quantum Machine Learning: QML and quantum AI (QAI) are rapidly developing fields that leverage experimental quantum information processing. Superconducting quantum circuits have been used for implementing basic QML protocols [25]. A quantum recommendation system has been proposed, which efficiently samples from an approximation of a preference matrix without the need for complete reconstruction [26]. Furthermore, a hybrid quantum-classical DL framework has been introduced for handling high-dimensional real-world ML datasets on continuous variables [27].

In the context of healthcare systems, integrating QC requires upgrading existing infrastructure to support the high computational power provided by quantum technologies. These advancements in QML highlight the need to address specific requirements for quantum-enabled healthcare systems to ensure their effective implementation.

10.4 DESIGNING AN EFFECTIVE QUANTUM COMPUTING ARCHITECTURE FOR HEALTHCARE APPLICATIONS

This can be done by creating a well-structured and efficient framework that harnesses the power of QC to address healthcare-related challenges. It involves identifying the specific requirements and constraints of healthcare applications and developing a tailored architecture that leverages QC capabilities to provide advanced computational solutions [28, 29]. This entails designing the configuration of quantum hardware, optimizing algorithms and protocols, and integrating the architecture with existing healthcare systems. The goal is to ensure that the QC infrastructure effectively supports various healthcare tasks such as medical imaging analysis, drug discovery, genomics, personalized medicine, and optimization of healthcare processes. The design process involves careful consideration of QC principles, the unique characteristics of healthcare datasets, and the specific needs of healthcare providers and patients [30, 31]. The ultimate aim is to create a robust and scalable architecture that maximizes the benefits of QC for healthcare applications, leading to improved diagnosis, treatment, and overall healthcare outcomes.

10.5 QUANTUM COMPUTING SECURITY CONSIDERATIONS IN HEALTHCARE

Ensuring the security of healthcare applications is crucial due to their critical impact on human lives. The siloed nature of healthcare systems poses a significant challenge for innovation, data sharing, and systematic progress. To address this, effective security implementation should foster collaboration among academia, industry, researchers, and governments. Chuck Brooks, an expert in cyber security and chair in the Quantum Security Alliance, emphasizes the need for such collaboration.

Security is equally important for QC systems, as they have the potential to exponentially enhance computing capacities, thereby posing risks to current cryptographic mechanisms. However, QC also presents an opportunity for improved security by leveraging the unique properties of subatomic particles and the principles of quantum mechanics. Cryptography has long served as the theoretical foundation for healthcare information security. QC in cryptography combines classical cryptography with quantum mechanics to provide unconditional security for healthcare communication between objects and service consumers. Quantum cryptography, being the first commercially available use case of QC, is grounded in the fundamental laws of mechanics rather than unproven complex computational assumptions.

The literature highlights various approaches to address security and privacy challenges in quantum-based healthcare applications. Researchers have proposed cloud-based quantum computers, encryption mechanisms, and blockchain integration to protect patient data and ensure data integrity. These solutions aim to resist quantum attacks, optimize data encryption, and provide secure access to medical records. However, some approaches require further evaluation for real-time medical data and potential overhead considerations. Overall, these efforts aim to enhance the security and privacy of healthcare data in the QC paradigm.

10.6 OUTSTANDING CHALLENGES AND FUTURE RESEARCH AVENUES

The critical research issues/problems, challenges, and possible futuristic directions are briefly discussed [32, 33–36].

Classical Healthcare Data Loading: The integration of classical healthcare data with quantum circuits for loading onto blockchain systems is an important aspect that has not received significant attention thus far. Cost-effective approaches for loading classical healthcare data onto quantum circuits are yet to be explored. However, it is recommended to consider this area for future initiatives, as it holds potential for advancing the field of quantum-based healthcare data management.

Quantum Blockchain Healthcare Data Structure Presentation: The presentation and standardization of healthcare data structure within a quantum blockchain framework is currently lacking. The absence of a standardized approach for formulating a healthcare data structure using QC poses a significant challenge for efficient implementation. Addressing this challenge and establishing standardization in the presentation of data within quantum blockchain systems will be crucial for the future development and adoption of quantum-based healthcare applications.

AI/ML for Drug and Other Healthcare Analysis: QC offers researchers greater opportunities to leverage AI, ML, and DL techniques in healthcare analysis. By harnessing the power of QC, AI/ML operations can be performed at an accelerated pace, leading to enhanced performance of decision support systems in various healthcare applications. These include but are not limited to diagnosis pricing analysis, molecular simulation, drug development and discovery, medical imaging analysis, and recommendation systems. QC opens up new avenues for advanced data analysis and optimization, enabling more efficient and effective healthcare analysis and decision-making processes.

Quantum-Based Attack Analysis for Electronic Medical Records/Data: The security of electronic medical records (EMRs) and healthcare data is of paramount importance, and the emergence of QC poses new challenges in this regard. As QC advances, traditional encryption algorithms that currently protect sensitive medical data may become vulnerable to attacks by quantum computers.

To ensure the robustness of medical data protection using blockchain functionalities, it is crucial to analyze the potential threats posed by QC. This involves assessing the vulnerabilities of existing encryption mechanisms and cryptographic protocols that underpin blockchain-based healthcare systems.

By conducting a QC-based attack analysis, researchers can identify potential weaknesses and develop countermeasures to safeguard EMRs and healthcare data from quantum threats. This analysis helps in evaluating the resilience of blockchain-based healthcare systems against quantum attacks and enables the development of quantum-resistant encryption algorithms and protocols to enhance the security of medical data stored on the blockchain.

Quantum threat analysis for EMRs/data is essential to stay ahead of potential risks and ensure the long-term security and privacy of healthcare information in the face of advancing quantum technologies.

Developing Quantum Marketplace: Developing a quantum marketplace presents a significant challenge in implementing QC solutions, particularly in terms of pricing and resource allocation for quantum services. Similar to existing web services marketplaces, the development of a QC marketplace aims to provide a platform where service subscribers can access quantum services on a pay-per-use basis.

To establish a successful quantum marketplace, a coordinated quantum strategy is essential. This strategy should encompass the distribution of quantum services, the development of pricing models, and the allocation of resources. It requires collaboration among experts from various domains, including quantum systems, finance, service distribution mechanisms, and control strategies for quantum resource management.

The development of a distributed quantum marketplace requires careful consideration of factors such as service availability, service quality, security, and scalability. The marketplace should enable users to select and subscribe to specific quantum services based on their requirements. The pricing of these services should be determined based on the resources consumed by the users.

Overall, the development of a quantum marketplace necessitates a multidisciplinary approach, bringing together experts from QC, finance, and related fields. By establishing such a marketplace, users can access quantum services efficiently while providers can offer their services in a structured and economically viable manner.

Quantum Web and Cloud Services: Enabling QC services on commodity hardware is a crucial challenge to unlock the full potential of QC capabilities. Given the significant resource requirements of QC implementations, accessing QC for general-purpose problem-solving becomes increasingly difficult. However, there are efforts being made to bring QC services to web and cloud platforms.

One example of implementing quantum web services is Amazon Braket. Amazon Braket serves as a platform that allows researchers and experts to analyze and evaluate QC models in a real-time testing environment. It offers an experimental setting where users can design, test, and assess QC algorithms using simulated quantum environments, as well as run them on actual QC hardware. Amazon Braket provides access to various QC technologies, including quantum annealing hardware from D-Wave, ion-trap devices from IonQ, and systems based on superconducting qubits from Rigetti.

In addition to the Amazon web services ecosystem, other QC solutions are needed to offer quantum web services to users. Software development kits (SDKs) can be developed and implemented to simulate QC algorithms. These SDKs provide a way for developers to test and validate their QC algorithms without the need for physical quantum hardware.

Overall, the development of quantum web services on platforms like Amazon Braket, along with the availability of SDKs for quantum simulation, is a step towards democratizing access to QC. It allows users to explore and harness the power of QC even without dedicated quantum hardware, opening up possibilities for broader adoption and innovation in this exciting field.

Large-Scale Optimization: Optimization problems are common across various fields, but many of them become intractable and face combinatorial explosion challenges when dealing with large instances. The traveling salesman problem (TSP) is a well-known example of such a problem, where finding the shortest route that visits each city exactly once and returns to the starting point becomes increasingly difficult as the number of cities increases. TSP is classified as NP-hard, and finding an optimal solution becomes impractical for large numbers of cities using traditional computing systems.

In such cases, heuristics are often employed as approximate solutions because solving these problems on classical computers would take an impractically long time. QC offers potential solutions to address these challenges, utilizing two approaches: quantum annealing and universal quantum computers.

Quantum annealing is an optimization heuristic that can overcome the limitations of traditional computing systems in solving optimization problems. It can be implemented on specialized quantum annealers, which are relatively easier to develop compared to universal quantum computers. However, the effectiveness of quantum annealing compared to classical computers is still an area of exploration. Lightweight digital annealers offer a simulation of quantum annealers using classical computing, providing cost-effective solutions.

On the other hand, universal quantum computers have the capability to solve a wide range of QC problems, including optimization problems. However, commercial implementations of universal annealers are currently rare, making them more costly for solving optimization problems.

10.7 CONCLUSION

In conclusion, the convergence of QC and medical informatics presents a remarkable opportunity to revolutionize healthcare. Quantum information can revolutionize drug discovery by rapidly simulating molecular interactions and optimizing therapeutic compounds. In genomics, quantum algorithms can expedite the analysis of vast genomic datasets, unraveling complex genetic relationships and enhancing personalized medicine. QC can also enhance medical imaging, enabling more accurate diagnoses and treatment plans. Furthermore, quantum cryptography can bolster data security and privacy, safeguarding sensitive patient information. While challenges such as hardware limitations and scalability need to be overcome, the potential of QC in medical informatics is vast. As quantum technology advances and more researchers explore this intersection, we can anticipate unprecedented breakthroughs that will reshape the healthcare landscape, improve patient outcomes, and propel medical informatics into an era of boundless possibilities. The time is ripe for researchers, practitioners, and policymakers to embrace the potential of QC and chart a course towards a brighter, more efficient, and data-driven healthcare future.

REFERENCES

[1] S. W. Hwang et al. "Symbiosis of semiconductors, AI and quantum computing." In 2020 IEEE International Electron Devices Meeting (IEDM), 2020, doi:10.1109/IEDM13553.2020.9372061

[2] C. Choudhury, N. Arul Murugan, and U. D. Priyakumar. "Structure-based drug repurposing: Traditional and advanced AI/ML-aided methods." *Drug Discov. Today*, vol. 27, no. 7, pp. 1847–1861, 2022. doi:10.1016/j.drudis.2022.03.006

[3] H. Doga, et al. How can quantum computing be applied in clinical trial design and optimization?, *Trends Pharmacol Sci*, vol. 45, no. 10, pp. 880–891, 2024. https://doi.org/10.1016/j.tips.2024.08.005.

[4] J. M. Abduljalil and B. M. Abduljalil. "Epidemiology, genome, and clinical features of the pandemic SARS-CoV-2: a recent view." *New Microb. New Infect.*, vol. 35, p. 100672, May 2020. doi:10.1016/j.nmni.2020.100672

[5] F. Pappalardo, G. Russo, F. M. Tshinanu, and M. Viceconti. "In silico clinical trials: Concepts and early adoptions." *Brief. Bioinform.*, vol. 20, no. 5, pp. 1699–1708, Sep. 2019. doi:10.1093/bib/bby043

[6] X. Yuan et al. "Current and perspective diagnostic techniques for COVID-19." *ACS Infect. Dis.*, vol. 6, no. 8, pp. 1998–2016, Aug. 2020. doi:10.1021/acsinfecdis.0c00365

[7] A. Ruffino, T.-Y. Yang, J. Michniewicz, Y. Peng, E. Charbon, and M. F. Gonzalez-Zalba. "A cryo-CMOS chip that integrates silicon quantum dots and multiplexed dispersive readout electronics." *Nat. Electron.*, vol. 5, no. 1, pp. 53–59, 2022. doi:10.1038/s41928-021-00687-6

[8] T. M.Deserno. Fundamentals of biomedical image processing. In: Deserno, T. (Eds), *Biomedical Image Processing. Biological and Medical Physics, Biomedical Engineering*. Berlin, Heidelberg: Springer. https://doi.org/10.1007/978-3-642-15816-2_1]

[9] G. Dougherty. Medical image processing techniques and applications. Springer, New York, 2011.

[10] Strategy and pwc. "The future of healthcare has arrived | Strategy& Middle East." 2020. Available at https://www.strategyand.pwc.com/m1/en/reports/2021/the-future-of-healthcare-has-arrived.html. Accessed 14 October 2022.

[11] P. Kwiat, J. Mitchell, P. Schwindt, and A. White. "Grover's search algorithm: an optical approach." *J. Modern Optics*, vol. 47,no. 2-3, pp. 257–266, 2000.

[12] N. Young. An introduction to Hilbert space. Cambridge University Press, 1988.

[13] R. Salakhutdinov and G. Hinton. "Deep Boltzmann machines." in Artificial intelligence and statistics. PMLR, 2009, pp. 448–455.

[14] H. Neven, V. S. Denchev, G. Rose, and W. G. Macready. "Training a large scale classifier with the quantum adiabatic algorithm." arXiv preprint arXiv:0912.0779, 2009.

[15] H. Neven, V. S. Denchev, G. Rose, and W. G. Macready. "Training a binary classifier with the quantum adiabatic algorithm." arXiv preprint arXiv:0811.0416, 2008.

[16] A. Paler, I. Polian, K. Nemoto, and S. J. Devitt. "Fault-tolerant, high level quantum circuits: form, compilation and description." *Quantum Sci. Technol.*, vol. 2, no. 2, p. 025003, 2017.

[17] R. Van Meter and S. J. Devitt. "Local and distributed quantum computation." arXiv preprint arXiv:1605.06951, 2016.

[18] M. Ahsan, R. V. Meter, and J. Kim. "Designing a million-qubit quantum computer using a resource performance simulator." *ACM J. Emerg. Technol. Comput. Syst. (JETC)*, vol. 12, no. 4, pp. 1–25, 2015.

[19] R. Blakestad, C. Ospelkaus, A. VanDevender, J. Amini, J. Britton, D. Leibfried, and D. J. Wineland. "High-fidelity transport of trapped ion qubits through an X-junction trap array." *Phys. Rev. Lett.*, vol. 102, no. 15, p. 153002, 2009.

[20] K. R. Brown, J. Kim, and C. Monroe. "Co-designing a scalable quantum computer with trapped atomic ions." *NPJ Quantum Inform.*, vol. 2, no. 1, pp. 1–10, 2016.

[21] J. I. Cirac and P. Zoller. "Quantum computations with cold trapped ions." *Phys. Rev. Lett.*, vol. 74, no. 20, p. 4091, 1995.

[22] L.-M. Duan, M. Madsen, D. Moehring, P. Maunz, R. Kohn Jr, and C. Monroe. "Probabilistic quantum gates between remote atoms through interference of optical frequency qubits." *Phys. Rev. A*, vol. 73, no. 6, p. 062324, 2006.

[23] W. Hensinger, S. Olmschenk, D. Stick, D. Hucul, M. Yeo, M. Acton, L. Deslauriers, C. Monroe, and J. Rabchuk. "T-junction ion trap array for two-dimensional ion shuttling, storage, and manipulation." *Appl. Phys. Lett.*, vol. 88, no. 3, p. 034101, 2006.

[24] D. Hucul, I. V. Inlek, G. Vittorini, C. Crocker, S. Debnath, S. M. Clark, and C. Monroe. "Modular entanglement of atomic qubits using photons and phonons." *Nat. Phys.*, vol. 11, no. 1, pp. 37–42, 2015.

[25] L. Lamata. "Basic protocols in quantum reinforcement learning with superconducting circuits." *Scientif. Rep.*, vol. 7, no. 1, pp. 1–10, 2017.

[26] I. Kerenidis and A. Prakash. "Quantum recommendation systems." arXiv preprint arXiv:1603.08675, 2016.

[27] M. Benedetti, J. Realpe-G´omez, and A. Perdomo-Ortiz. "Quantum assisted Helmholtz machines: A quantum–classical deep learning framework for industrial datasets in near-term devices." *Quantum Sci. Technol.*, vol. 3, no. 3, p. 034007, 2018.

[28] N. C. Jones, R. Van Meter, A. G. Fowler, P. L. McMahon, J. Kim, T. D. Ladd, and Y. Yamamoto. "Layered architecture for quantum computing." *Phys. Rev. X*, vol. 2, no. 3, p. 031007, 2012.

[29] K. M. Svore, A. V. Aho, A. W. Cross, I. Chuang, and I. L. Markov. "A layered software architecture for quantum computing design tools." *Computer*, vol. 39, no. 1, pp. 74–83, 2006.

[30] A. M. Steane. "Quantum computer architecture for fast entropy extraction." arXiv preprint quant-ph/0203047, 2002.

[31] "How to build a 300 bit, 1 giga-operation quantum computer." arXiv preprint quant-ph/0412165, 2004.

[32] S. S. Gill et al. "Quantum computing: A taxonomy, systematic review, and future directions." *Softw. Pract. Exp.*, vol. 52, no. 1, pp. 66–114, 2022. doi:10.1002/spe.3039
[33] A. Kumar et al. "Survey of promising technologies for quantum drones and networks." *IEEE Access*, vol. 9, pp. 125868–125911, 2021. doi:10.1109/ACCESS.2021.3109816
[34] A. Kumar, C. Ottaviani, S. S. Gill, and R. Buyya. "Securing the future internet of things with post-quantum cryptography." *Secur. Priv.*, vol. 5, no. 2, Mar. 2022. doi:10.1002/spy2.200
[35] A. Kumar, D. Augusto de Jesus Pacheco, K. Kaushik, and J. J. P. C. Rodrigues. "Futuristic view of the Internet of Quantum Drones: Review, challenges and research agenda." *Veh. Commun.*, vol. 36, p. 100487, Aug. 2022. doi:10.1016/j.vehcom.2022.100487
[36] K. Kaushik and A. Kumar. "Demystifying quantum blockchain for healthcare." *Secur. Priv.*, vol. 6, no.3, e284, Oct. 2022. doi:10.1002/spy2.284

Objective-Type Questions:

1. **True/False**: Quantum computing uses qubits, which can exist in both 0 and 1 states simultaneously.
2. **Multiple Choice**: Which of the following phenomena allows qubits to influence each other regardless of distance?
   a) Superposition
   b) Entanglement
   c) Classical bits
   d) Encryption
3. **Multiple Choice**: What is the primary computational advantage of quantum computing in molecular simulations?
   a) Sequential processing
   b) Parallel processing
   c) Low energy consumption
   d) Deterministic algorithms
4. **One-word answer**: Which quantum algorithm is known for faster search operations in databases?
5. **True/False**: Classical bits can be in superposition states like qubits.
6. **Multiple Choice**: Quantum computing can significantly reduce healthcare costs in diagnosing diseases such as:
   a) Cancer
   b) COVID-19
   c) Tuberculosis
   d) All of the above
7. **Multiple Choice**: What percentage of healthcare costs are attributed to socioeconomic conditions, environmental influences, and behavioral challenges?

a) 10–20%
b) 30–50%
c) 80–90%
d) 100%

8. **One-word answer:** Which quantum phenomenon makes it difficult to copy or read quantum information without disturbance?
9. **True/False:** Quantum-enhanced machine learning can help classify cells in single-cell diagnosis.
10. **True/False:** Quantum entanglement allows qubits to be correlated in such a way that their states are dependent on each other, no matter the distance.
11. **Multiple Choice:** Which of the following is a significant challenge in using quantum computing for healthcare?
    a) Quantum entanglement
    b) High error rates in qubits
    c) Faster computation
    d) Increased data storage
12. **One-word answer:** What quantum algorithm can be used for factoring large numbers, potentially breaking classical encryption systems?
13. **Multiple Choice:** In quantum computing, which of the following contributes to faster data analysis in drug discovery?
    a) Classical parallel computing
    b) Quantum superposition
    c) AI pattern recognition
    d) Molecular modeling
14. **True/False:** Quantum computers are particularly effective at performing tasks that involve large, sequential data processing.
15. **Multiple Choice:** Which aspect of quantum computing is crucial for improving secure communication in healthcare?
    a) Quantum superposition
    b) Quantum entanglement
    c) Quantum cryptography
    d) Quantum gates
16. **Multiple Choice:** Which medical application of quantum computing involves using simulations to predict drug interactions at the molecular level?
    a) Genomics
    b) Radiotherapy
    c) Molecular simulations
    d) Diagnosis assistance
17. **One-word answer:** What term is used to describe the ability of quantum computers to perform multiple calculations simultaneously, making them ideal for large-scale optimization problems?

18. **True/False:** Quantum computing helps optimize radiotherapy by simulating multiple treatment scenarios at the same time.
19. **Multiple Choice:** What is the primary purpose of quantum-enhanced machine learning in healthcare?
    a) To improve drug manufacturing
    b) To enhance data storage
    c) To improve diagnostic accuracy and disease detection
    d) To simplify healthcare administration
20. **Multiple Choice:** Which of the following medical imaging technologies is enhanced by quantum computing through improved image reconstruction and data acquisition?
    a) MRI
    b) Ultrasound
    c) X-rays
    d) PET scans
21. **Multiple Choice:** What challenge does quantum computing face when trying to handle large-scale healthcare datasets?
    a) High computational power
    b) Low error rates
    c) Fragile qubits and high error rates
    d) Limited memory
22. **Multiple Choice:** Which of the following areas is NOT directly mentioned as a quantum computing application in healthcare?
    a) Genomics
    b) Medical imaging
    c) Vaccination programs
    d) Diagnosis assistance
23. **Multiple Choice:** What role does quantum computing play in improving the accuracy of classifying and identifying malicious behavior in medical claims?
    a) Enhanced memory storage
    b) Advanced pattern recognition techniques
    c) Higher computational power
    d) Quantum cryptography
24. **Multiple Choice:** In the context of quantum computing in healthcare, which of the following is essential to optimize data privacy and regulatory compliance?
    a) Quantum sensors
    b) Quantum machine learning
    c) Quantum cryptography and secure communication protocols
    d) Medical imaging algorithms
25. **True/False:** Quantum-enhanced algorithms in medical imaging, such as edge detection, can improve the classification of cells based on biochemical and physical characteristics.

Short Answer Questions:

1. What is the significance of superposition in quantum computing for healthcare applications?
2. How does quantum computing improve medical imaging techniques?
3. Explain the role of quantum computing in drug discovery.
4. What are the primary challenges of integrating quantum computing into healthcare?
5. Why is quantum computing important in optimizing diagnosis pricing in healthcare?
6. What are the advantages of using quantum computing in genomic analysis?
7. Explain how quantum computing enhances data security in healthcare.
8. What makes quantum computing suitable for solving optimization problems in healthcare?
9. How does quantum computing support medical imaging advancements?

Long Answer Questions:

1. Discuss the key differences between classical and quantum computing, and how these differences affect healthcare applications.
2. Analyze the impact of quantum computing on personalized medicine and how it can revolutionize patient treatment.
3. Explain the ethical concerns surrounding the use of quantum computing in healthcare, particularly regarding data privacy and security.
4. What are the future challenges and research directions necessary for the widespread adoption of quantum computing in healthcare?
5. Discuss a real-world case study where quantum computing has shown promise in healthcare, such as in drug development or disease diagnosis. What were the results, and what challenges remain?
6. Discuss the potential of quantum computing in revolutionizing drug discovery and development. How does it overcome current limitations in the pharmaceutical industry?
7. Analyze the ethical implications of using quantum computing in healthcare, especially regarding data privacy and accessibility.
8. Explain how quantum computing can transform personalized medicine and how it enhances patient-specific treatment approaches.
9. Describe the technological challenges of integrating quantum computing into healthcare. How can these challenges be addressed?
10. Evaluate the role of quantum-enhanced AI in healthcare, focusing on how it can assist in early disease detection and improve diagnostic accuracy.

Index

Abstraction, 45
Accuracy, 26 118
Acids (lncRNAs), 75
Activation functions, 21
Acute myeloid leukemia (AML), 74
AdaBoost, 84
Adam optimization, 108
Adaptability, 21
Adaptive Haar wavelet-based, 105
AI applications, 7
AI-powered technologies, 98
Alzheimer disease, 112
Alzheimer's Disease Neuroimaging Initiative (ADNI), 117
Ambient-assisted living (AAL), 194
Amyotrophic lateral sclerosis (ALS), 51
Analysis, 33
Area under ROC curve (AUC), 73
Area under the receiver operating characteristic curve (AUC-ROC), 118
Arrhythmias, 127
Artificial intelligence (AI), 2, 20
ASIC, 219
The Australian Imaging Biomarkers and Lifestyle (AIBL), 117
Autoencoders, 24
Autonomous vehicles, 25

Backpropagation, 21
Binary grasshopper optimization algorithm (AHW-BGOA), 105
Bioinformatics, 50
Biomarker discovery, 100
Biomedical image analysis, 42
Biomedical image fusion, 52
Biomedical signals, 43
Bradykinesia, 135
Brain network analysis, 134
Breast cancer, 79

Cancer, 55; recurrence, 78; research, 55; survival, 80; susceptibility, 73
Capsule networks, 24
Cardiovascular Disease Risk Assessment, 49
Classification, 68
Clinical challenges, 83
Clinical decision support systems (CDSS), 7
Clinical integration, 101
Cloud segment, 104
Cluster computing, 1
Clustering, 69
Colorectal cancer, 75
Computational biology, 50
Computed tomography, 97
Computer vision, 23
Congenital heart disease, 127
Convolutional layer, 135
Convolutional neural networks (CNNs), 24
Coronary Artery Disease (CAD), 127
CPLD, 222
Cross-modal, 132
Cross-validation, 118

Data augmentation, 28
Data collection, 16
Data preprocessing, 16
Data storage, 45
Deep belief networks (DBNs), 136
Deep CNN (DCNN), 71
Deep learning, 20
Deep reinforcement learning, 24
Dental imaging, 45
Diffusion tensor imaging (DTI), 116
Digital patient records, 125
Dimensionality reduction, 69
Discrete wavelet transform, 105
Disease diagnosis, 49
Disease prediction, 33
Disease progression monitoring, 100
DL techniques, 120
Dragonfly algorithm, 109

Drug development, 100
Drug discovery, 9, 19
Drug response prediction, 50

ECG signal processing, 47
EEG (electroencephalogram) interpretation, 45, 52
Effective data management, 116
Electrocardiograms (ECGs), 45
Electromyography (EMGs), 45, 47
Electronic health record (EHR), 55
Electronic medical record (EMR), 55, 249
EMD method, 107
Emergency medical service (EMS), 218
Empirical mode decomposition (EMD), 106
Endoscopy, 45
End-to-end learning, 21
Ensemble learning, 81
Entanglement, 234
Epidemic protection, 19
Epidemiological modelling, 8
Epilepsy, 101
Evaluation, 46

False negative (FN), 26
False positive (FP), 26
Fault tolerance, 245
Feature extraction, 39
Feedforward neural networks (FNNs), 24
Fluoroscopy, 45
Fourier-domain optical coherence tomography (FDOCT), 201
FPGA, 219
Functional connectivity, 134
Functional MRI (fMRI), 132

Gait analysis, 50
Generalization, 46
Generative adversarial networks (GAN), 24, 149, 160
Glioblastoma, 80
Gradient-weighted class activation, 106
Graphics processing units (GPUs), 1

Healthcare, 6
Healthcare operations, 8
Heart attack (myocardial infar3ction), 127
Heart failure, 127
Heart valve disease, 127
Hemorrhagic stroke, 121
Herlev dataset, 182
Higher dimensional quantum communications, 244
High-performance computing (HPC), 1, 213
Hybrid models, 120
Hypertension, 121

Image analysis, 124
Image fusion, 39
Imagenet, 118
Image processing, 39
Image recognition, 17
Image registration, 39
Image segmentation, 30, 39, 170
Independent component analysis (ICA), 135
Indicators, 125
Internet of Things (IoT), 31
Ischemic stroke, 121
Iterative refinement, 101

k-fold cross-validation, 118
Kubernetes, 215

Liver cancer, 79
Logistic regression, 68
Long noncoding ribonucleic, 75
Long short-term memory, 24

Machine learning, 14, 20
Magnetic resonance imaging (MRI), 44, 116, 125
Mammography, 45
Mapping (Grad-CAM), 106
Mechanical thrombectomy, 121
Medical image modalities, 43
Medication response prediction, 103
Medications, 122
Mendeley data, 181
Metastasis, 78
Minimum redundancy maximum relevance (MRMR), 76
Model architecture design, 101
Model complexity, 17
Model evaluation, 101
Model interpretability, 16
Model learning, 16
Model selection, 16
Model training, 101
Morphological features, 134
Motor neuron diseases (MNDs), 98
Multidomain multiview discriminant correlation analysis (mmDCA), 54
Multimodal fusion, 120
Multivariate adaptive regression splines (MARS), 80
Myocardial Infarction, 127

The Naive Bayes (NB), 68
National Cancer Institute (NCI), 56
Natural language processing (NLP), 17, 18, 125
Networks (RBFNs), 24
Neural networks, 67, 68
Neuroimaging, 116
Neurological disorders diagnosis, 49

Oncology, 83
the Open Access Series of Imaging Studies (OASIS), 117
Oral squamous cell carcinoma (OSCC), 78

Parkinson's disease, 135
Performance superiority, 120
Personalized risk assessment, 125
Personalized seizure prediction models, 103
Personalized treatment planning, 50, 128
Pharmacogenomics, 52
Physiological, 29, 38, 42, 45, 50–55, 63, 75, 97, 98, 103–104, 124, 125, 128–30, 134, 167
Physiological signal fusion, 52
Population health management, 57
Positron emission tomography (PET), 116
Postischemic stroke, 121
Postural instability, 136
Precision, 26
Precision medicine, 31
Principal component analysis (PCA), 135
Professional challenges, 86
Psychiatry, 132
Python, 229

Quantum blockchain, 248
Quantum machine learning, 247
Qubits, 234

Radial basis function, 24
Radiographic Bone Levels (RBL), 156, 161
Recurrent neural networks (RNNs), 24
Reduction, 41
Region of converge curve, 73
Regression, 68
Regularization techniques, 120
Regulatory compliance, 57
Rehabilitation technologies, 52
Reinforcement learning, 15, 69
Remote patient monitoring, 7, 19, 49
Representation learning, 21
Residue number system (RNS), 202
Riemannian geometry, 54
Rigidity, 136
Risk prediction, 124, 128

Scalability, 21
Seizure detection, 103
Semisupervised learning (SSL), 69
Sensitivity, 26
Siamese networks, 24
SIPaKMeD database, 178
skrGAN, 151
Specificity, 26
Speech recognition, 17
Stationary wavelet, 109
Structural health monitoring (SHM), 31
Structural MRI (sMRI), 132
Superposition, 234
Supervised learning, 15
Support vector machine (SVM), 68
Swarm intelligence based optimization, 109
System Verilog, 229

Technical challenges, 87
Telemedicine, 104
Tensor processing units (TPUs), 1
3D reconstruction, 39
Thrombolytic therapy, 121
Tool challenges, 87
Training set expansion, 28
Transcriptomic study, 72
Transfer learning, 120
Transformer networks, 24
Transform (SWT), 109
Treatment response prediction, 100
Tremors, 135
True negative, 26
True positive (TP), 26

UCI risk factors, 180
Ultrasound imaging, 45
Unsupervised DL techniques, 120
Unsupervised learning, 15
User segment, 104

Vaccine development, 10, 19
Verilog, 228
VHDL, 229
Virtual machines (VMs), 216
Voice signal analysis, 136

Xilinx Vivado, 228
X-ray imaging, 44

For Product Safety Concerns and Information please contact our EU representative GPSR@taylorandfrancis.com Taylor & Francis Verlag GmbH, Kaufingerstraße 24, 80331 München, Germany

Printed and bound by CPI Group (UK) Ltd, Croydon, CR0 4YY
14/09/2026
02216256-0012